Aortic Valve Preservation

Takashi Kunihara • Shuichiro Takanashi
Editors

Aortic Valve Preservation

Concepts and Approaches

Springer

Editors
Takashi Kunihara
Department of Cardiac Surgery
The Jikei University School of Medicine
Tokyo
Japan

Shuichiro Takanashi
Cardiovascular Surgery
Sakakibara Heart Institute
Fuchu
Tokyo
Japan

The Work was first published in 2015 by Bunkodo Co., Ltd. with the following title: DAIDOUMYAKUBEN KEISEIJUTSU NO SUBETE.

ISBN 978-981-13-2067-5 ISBN 978-981-13-2068-2 (eBook)
https://doi.org/10.1007/978-981-13-2068-2

Library of Congress Control Number: 2018964763

This Springer imprint is published by the registered company Springer Nature Singapore Pte Ltd.
The registered company address is: 152 Beach Road, #21-01/04 Gateway East, Singapore 189721, Singapore

Foreword (Japanese Version)

The first attempts at aortic valve repair were undertaken in the 1950s. At that time understanding of the normal and pathologic anatomy and function of the aortic valve was still limited; consequently the results of repair were unpredictable and replacement became the standard of care. Later better imaging techniques and more detailed understanding of aortic valve form and function provided the basis for further development.

In the past 30 years reconstructive procedures for aortic regurgitation have evolved into an increasingly practiced alternative to valve replacement. Initially this was an approach primarily for patients with aortic dilatation and preserved cusps. In the past 15 years the evolution has progressed, and repair is now increasingly performed also in patients with isolated cusp disease or the combination of aortic dilatation and cusp prolapse. Thus, aortic valve repair is currently where mitral valve repair was 30 years ago.

Many colleagues have participated in this evolutionary process, and a number of these dedicated surgeons have come together to generate this book. It covers all important facets dealing with aortic valve repair, and the authors have made an excellent effort to cover the topic thoroughly. The result is an excellent overview and current description of the state of the art. It will help those who want to refresh their memory or focus on specific details of this changing area. Even more it will help those surgeons who plan to start or expand their repair activities on the aortic valve. They must thus be congratulated for this excellent accumulation and description of current knowledge.

Homburg, Germany H.-J. Schäfers

Foreword (English Version)

Aortic valve-sparing and repair procedures have emerged in the last 25 years as alternative options to root and valve replacement with prostheses for patients with root dilatation with or without aortic regurgitation and those with isolated aortic insufficiency. Nowadays there is a wealth of data on the results of root and valve replacement with prostheses whether in the context of the Bentall procedure or isolated valve replacement. It is well established that with the currently available prostheses and protocols, mechanical valves bring the risk of the complications associated with life-long oral anticoagulation (mainly bleeding and thromboembolic events) whereas the bioprostheses mainly have the risks of valve deterioration and reoperation over time. Nonetheless, recent large studies show that survival is similar regardless of the type of prosthesis used and is suboptimal compared to the expected survival of a matched general population. There is also an increasing amount of data on the results of aortic valve-sparing and repair procedures, and we now have the results at 20 years. Available studies show that valve-sparing and repair procedures are associated with much lower rates of thromboembolism, bleeding events, and infective endocarditis but carry a certain risk of reoperation on the valve over time that seems nonetheless very reasonable and acceptable. Further and more importantly, long-term survival of these patients is significantly improved, most likely due to the lower incidence of valve-related complications.

Since its first description, valve-sparing root replacement procedures (the remodeling technique—the Yacoub operation—and the reimplantation technique—the David operation) have very much evolved and improved so much so that on the one hand, an external annuloplasty is now routinely added to the remodeling, and on the other, we are at the fifth modification of the original David operation (David-V) along with having the Stanford modification and our specific Brussels technique. Also, the techniques of cusp repair and annuloplasty, particularly for patients with isolated aortic regurgitation, have greatly evolved.

Extensive research works have allowed a better understanding of the aortic valve anatomy and function, particularly the role of the functional aortic annulus and the mechanism of leaflet coaptation. Currently, we have reference measures for the size of the aortic annulus, the geometric and effective height of the leaflet, and the length of coaptation. We also have new tools in the operating room, such as the caliper, to quantitatively assess the impact of the repair.

However, the acceptance of these techniques by both the surgical community and the referring physicians has progressed quite slowly compared to that for the mitral valve repair techniques and even now, these procedures are performed only in highly specialized centers by a handful of surgeons. Consequently, the number of patients that indeed benefit from these procedures remains very low. Therefore, every initiative aimed to promote advancement in the field of aortic valve repair and the diffusion of these techniques is to be praised and supported.

Kunihara, Takanashi, and colleagues are within this handful of surgeons who routinely perform aortic valve repair procedures and have largely contributed to the advancement of this field. In this book, they have done great work in presenting and discussing the indications for valve sparing and repair, the techniques in a large variety of clinical settings and valve phenotypes, current annuloplasty techniques, and finally, a full section on specific situations. We believe that this book shows that aortic valve repair techniques are nowadays well described and are currently standardized and reproducible. We are sure that cardiologists, cardiac surgeons, and anesthesiologists will enjoy reading this text and benefit from it. Cardiologists will learn how to improve echo assessment to precisely define the mechanism of regurgitation and help the surgeon plan the repair. Cardiac surgeons will learn the principles behind the techniques of repair and the goals to pursue during the procedure. Anesthesiologists will learn what to expect after repair and how to reveal potential pitfalls predictive of late failure. We hope that this book will have the large diffusion that it deserves.

Brussels, Belgium Gebrine El Khoury

Preface (Translation of the Japanese Version)

According to statistics published by the Japanese Association for Thoracic Surgery in 2012, mitral valvuloplasty accounted for 66% of the total number of isolated mitral valve surgeries during that year in Japan, whereas aortic valvuloplasty accounted for only 4%. Aortic valvuloplasty was also only performed in 23% of patients who underwent isolated aortic root surgery for non-dissecting aneurysm. Our special survey also indicated that both groups only comprised 8% and 30%, respectively. It is presumed that the majority of lesions in patients who require aortic root replacement are ectatic, and when accompanied by aortic regurgitation, this is still presumed to represent a good indication for valvuloplasty. Among the surgeons who are active at the forefront of clinical practice, we believe that at least some of these individuals must be disappointed with the fact that valves in some patients could have been preserved instead of replaced. Many wonder why these differences exist between the mitral and aortic valves.

First, aortic valvuloplasty is by no means a novel technique. Concerted efforts were already being made by some surgeons in the 1970s, although the long-term outcomes were abysmal. So for quite some time thereafter, it was not possible to appreciate the fact that this form of surgery would eventually achieve superior outcomes to valve replacement. However, in the early 1990s, the outcomes of aortic valvuloplasty that included the aortic root were reexamined, and at the start of the 2000s, an objective method was proposed to evaluate the morphology of the aortic valve. Since then, aortic valvuloplasty has become standardized and recognized as a reproducible surgical technique, and in recent years it has rapidly increased in popularity.

However, aortic valvuloplasty has not been well disseminated in Japan, and it is no exaggeration to say that this is because Japanese surgeons lack experience in and knowledge of aortic valvuloplasty. If we can increase the degree of comprehension of this type of surgery among cardiologists, then going forward, the surgical indications will gradually increase. If patients are also referred to surgeons at an early stage before valve leaflet degeneration or annuloaortic ectasia has occurred, then valvuloplasty can be performed with greater precision, and this should result in a virtuous cycle. The main point of publishing this book is that by popularizing and developing aortic valvuloplasty in Japan, patients who would have been treated with valve replacement to date can undergo valvuloplasty instead, and if this occurs, we believe this will be a great boon to patients.

For this book, we mainly worked with coauthors who are members of the Aortic Valve Academy established in December 2013. However, to improve surgical outcomes, it is essential to have a good understanding of aortic valve anatomy and pathophysiology and its diagnosis, so we also added authors who are expert cardiologists. The main target readers are cardiovascular surgeons and cardiologists; however, to make the book accessible to other readers, such as cardiac anesthesiologists, medical interns, clinical engineering technicians, and scrub nurses, we aimed to make the contents as easy as possible to understand by including numerous illustrations. It would be a great delight to everyone involved in the planning of this book if it would become the standard reference text for cardiovascular surgery teams who are starting to perform aortic valvuloplasty.

On a fine day in November 2015

Tokyo, Japan Takashi Kunihara
Tokyo, Japan Shuichiro Takanashi

Preface (English Version)

This book was originally published in Japanese in November 2015 with the aim of popularizing aortic valvuloplasty in Japan. This field of practice has subsequently increased in visibility, although actual dissemination of the techniques is progressing slowly. As we see abroad, successive leaders in the field are continuing to publish new findings while the gap between them and surgeons in the general community level continues to widen. For this reason, we received numerous, fervent requests for an English translation of this book from top foreign surgeons who knew of its existence, and we are now pleased to finally release the English edition of the book. These requests arrived just as we were considering the incorporation of new knowledge into the book, so it was very convenient for us, and we started the project immediately.

Although this new knowledge has been incorporated throughout the English edition, we specifically expanded the general considerations and added new chapters. This also includes attempts to clarify our current positions and address global trends in the field. It will be extremely interesting to see how this data will change in the near future. Originally, all of our authors were Japanese nationals, but we wanted to include the latest knowledge on computational models in this edition, so for the first time, we have invited a foreign author to contribute. In addition, the limited number of references present in the Japanese edition has been expanded in the English edition so that we can better support the readers in their research.

We are deeply grateful to all of the authors who contributed to the current revision.

This book will be available not only to foreign surgeons but also to staff members on multidisciplinary cardiac treatment teams. If we are hereby able to deepen the common understanding of this type of surgery, improve surgical outcomes, and popularize aortic valvuloplasty, we believe that achieving these goals will be of enormous benefit to patients around the world suffering from aortic regurgitation as well as to editors and authors working in the field.

Tokyo, Japan — Shuichiro Takanashi
Tokyo, Japan — Takashi Kunihara

The original version of the book was revised: Previous publication details has been updated in copyright page. The erratum to the book is available at https://doi.org/10.1007/978-981-13-2068-2_41.

Acknowledgments

As stated in the Preface, this book was originally published in Japanese in November 2015. We would like to offer our deepest gratitude to Prof. Tina Tajima of St. Marianna University School of Medicine for her assistance with the translation of the book and English editing of all the chapters.

Tokyo, Japan — Takashi Kunihara
Tokyo, Japan — Shuichiro Takanashi

Contents

Part I

Introduction

Anatomy of the Aortic Valve and its Morphological Characteristics

1

Osamu Igawa

Abbreviations

AAo	Ascending aorta
AMFC	Aorto-mitral fibrous continuity
AML	Anterior mitral leaflet
AoV	Aortic valve
APC	Anterior pulmonary cusp
APM	Anterior papillary muscle
ATL	Anterior tricuspid leaflet
AVJ	Aorto-ventricular junction, artero-ventricular junction
BR	Basal ring
CS	Coronary sinus
HB	His bundle
HBb	Branching portion of His bundle
HBp	Penetrating portion of His bundle
IAS	Interatrial septum
ILT	Interleaflet triangle
IVFT	Intervalvular fibrous trigone
IVS	Interventricular septum
LA	Left atrium
LAA	Left atrial appendage
LAD	Left anterior descending coronary artery
LAFT	Left anterior fibrous trigone
LAS	Left aortic sinus of Valsalva
LCAos	Left coronary artery ostium
LCC	Left coronary cusp of aortic valve
LCX	Left circumflex coronary artery
LFT	Left fibrous trigone
LIPV	Left inferior pulmonary vein
LMT	Left main trunk
LV	Left ventricle
LVAW	Anterior wall of left ventricle
LVM	Left ventricular muscle
LVOT	Left ventricular outflow tract
MS	Membranous septum
MV	Mitral valve
NAS	Non-coronary aortic sinus of Valsalva
NCC	Non-coronary cusp of aortic valve
PML	Posterior mitral leaflet
PPC	Posterior pulmonary cusp
PPM	Posterior papillary muscle
PS	Pulmonary sinus
PT	Pulmonary trunk
PTL	Posterior tricuspid leaflet
PTS	Pericardial transverse sinus
PV	Pulmonary valve
RA	Right atrium
RAA	Right atrial appendage
RAFT	Right anterior fibrous trigone
RAS	Right aortic sinus of Valsalva
RCA	Right coronary artery of aortic valve
RCAos	Right coronary artery ostium
RCC	Right coronary cusp
RFT	Right fibrous trigone
RV	Right ventricle
RVM	Right ventricular muscle
RVOT	Right ventricular outflow tract

O. Igawa (✉)
Department of Internal Medicine / Cardiology, Nippon Medical School, Tama Nagayama Hospital, Tokyo, Japan
e-mail: oigawa@nms.ac.jp

T. Kunihara, S. Takanashi (eds.), *Aortic Valve Preservation*,
https://doi.org/10.1007/978-981-13-2068-2_1

SMT	Septomarginal trabecula
SPC	Septal pulmonary cusp
STJ	Sinotubular junction
STL	Septal tricuspid leaflet
SVC	Superior vena cava
TV	Tricuspid valve

1.1 Introduction

The aortic root is a structure consisting of the lower part of the ascending aorta, sinotubular junction (STJ), annulus, cusps, aortic sinus of Valsalva, and coronary artery ostia. When considering the structure of the aortic root and its surroundings, confirming the structure of (1) the junction of the root of the pulmonary trunk (PT) with the right ventricular outflow tract (RVOT) as a basic concept makes it simpler to understand the precise structure of (2) the junction of the aortic root with the left ventricular outflow tract (LVOT).

In this chapter, human cardiac preparations are used to provide accurate images of the aortic root and the structure of (1) and (2), and (3) to verify the surrounding structures. This chapter also intends to confirm the relation between these structures and logically build an image of the aortic root. Furthermore, it aims to consider the potential issues that may occur when operative procedures are performed on the aortic root from the perspective of its anatomical structure [1].

1.2 Positional Relationship of the Root of the Pulmonary Trunk and the Aortic Root

Figure 1.1 illustrates the sampled human cardiac preparation observed from the superior-dextral angle after sectioning through the superior portion of the roots of the two great vessels (aorta and PT). The aortic valve (AoV) and pulmonary valve (PV) can be seen in the sample. From this figure, it can be observed that the left main trunk (LMT) originates from the left aortic sinus of Valsalva (LAS) and descends to encircle the root of the PT from the posterior side. On the opposite side, the right coronary artery (RCA) originates from the right aortic sinus of Valsalva (RAS) and runs along the right atrioventricular groove posteriorly to the right atrial appendage (RAA).

Observing the aorta from the superior side, the right ventricular free wall is situated anteriorly to RAS, the left ventricular free wall is situated laterally to the anterior half of the LAS, and the left atrial wall is situated posteriorly to the posterior half of the LAS. Also, each of the left and right atrial walls is located on the posterior-sinistral and posterior-dextral parts of the non-coronary aortic sinus of Valsalva (NAS), respectively.

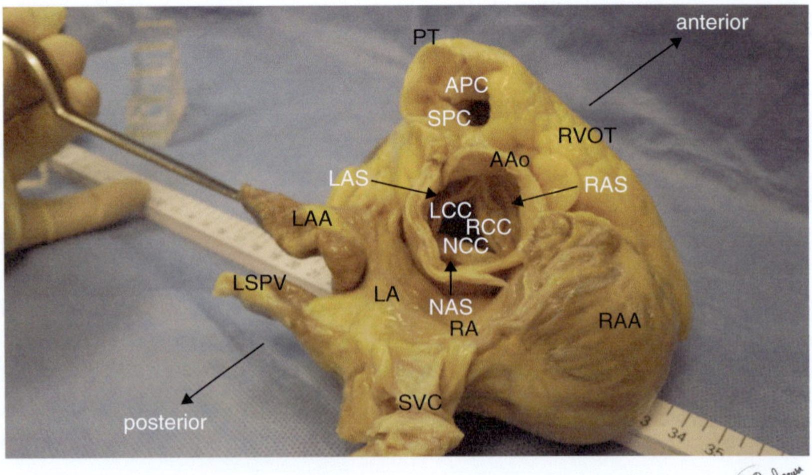

Fig. 1.1 Observation of the cardiac preparation from the superior-dextral angle after transverse dissection superior to the STJ. This position allows a clear view of the aortic valve and pulmonary valve and their surrounding structures

The view of the AoV from the superior aspect shows that the PV is located in the left anterior position, the tricuspid valve (TV) is in the right posterior position, and the mitral valve (MV) is in the left posterior position. The AoV annulus, TV annulus, and MV annulus are connected by firm fibrous tissues that comprise the fibrous cardiac skeleton, which is discussed later in this chapter. The aortic root and PT are connected by ligaments.

The next section of this chapter looks at the aortic root from the lumen and intends to establish the connection between the aortic root and its surrounding structures.

1.3 Anatomy of the Junction Between the Root of the Pulmonary Trunk and the Right Ventricle Outflow Tract

Figure 1.2 is a schematic diagram that clarifies the structure of the junction between the right ventricular outflow tract (RVOT) and the root of the PT. The myocardium of the RVOT is firmly connected to the root of the PT. The boundary of this connection is called the artero-ventricular junction (AVJ). The PV cusps are not attached along the AVJ; rather, they are attached to the lumen of the root of the PT cranially to the AVJ and not in a ring shape but in a crown-like shape. This crown-like attachment line of the PV cusps creates a strong PV annulus and is also a part of the fibrous skeleton, which is further described later in this chapter. The ring connecting the tops of the crown of the pulmonary attachment line (annulus) along the wall of the PT is called the sinotubular junction (STJ). The crown-like attachment line (annulus) passes through the AVJ and then continues to the myocardium of the RVOT. The ring (black line) linking the nadir of the caudal part of the attachment line (annulus) on the myocardial side running along the wall of the RVOT is called the basal ring (BR).

Figure 1.3 is a schematic diagram of the lumen observed when the junction of the PT-RVOT is dissected at the commissure of the anterior and posterior PV and is then exposed vertically after extending the incision line towards the RVOT. The attachment line (annulus) passes through the AVJ and continues into the myocardial region, and the

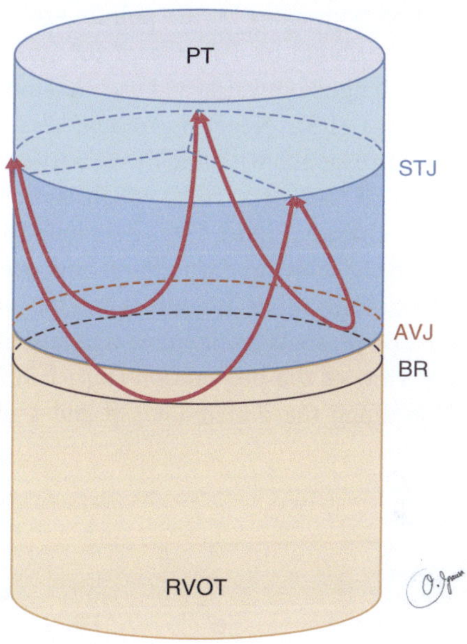

Fig. 1.2 Schematic diagram of the conjunction of the pulmonary trunk with the right ventricular outflow tract. The borderline between the PT and RVOT musculature is clear and is called the artero-ventricular junction (AVJ). The borderline connecting the three tops of the crown-shaped pulmonary valve annulus is called the sinotubular junction (STJ). Also, the circular boundary connecting the three nadirs of this crown is called the basal ring (BR)

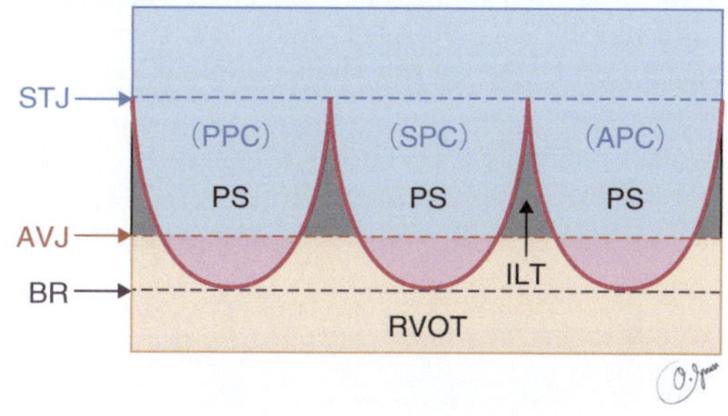

Fig. 1.3 Schematic diagram of the junction of the pulmonary trunk-right ventricular outflow tract. This view can be seen by opening the junction after incising the commissure of the APC and PPC and then extending the incision line along a vertical axis from the pulmonary trunk to the right ventricular outflow tract. (The APC, PPC, and SPC are incised at the annulus, and the annulus is exposed in this image.) The region surrounded by the STJ superiorly, by the AVJ inferiorly, and by the pulmonary valve annuluses on both sides bulges outside and is called the pulmonary sinus

BR, the line which connects the caudal part of the attachment line (annulus) on the myocardial region, can be seen. This region, which is surrounded superiorly by the STJ, inferiorly by the AVJ, and on both sides by the pulmonary annuluses, can be found on PT side of the junction. This part is bulged outwards and is called the pulmonary sinus (PS). Needless to say, this construction corresponds with that of the aortic sinus of Valsalva of the aortic root, which is covered later in this chapter. Figure 1.4 is a schematic diagram precisely showing the relation between the attachment of the valves (annulus) and the sinus.

Figure 1.5 presents a schematic diagram of the sectional view of the preparation (Fig. 1.3) after dissection along the dotted lines p and s along with the actual sectional histological images. It can be seen in the sectional view "p" (Fig. 1.5b) that this region lacks ventricular muscle although it is functionally in the right ventricle (RV). In contrast, the sectional view "s" (Fig. 1.5c) shows that although this region contains ventricular muscle, it is functionally in the PT. At first glance, it seems as if ventricular muscle has strayed into the PT, but it has not. This is a quite natural organization occurring due to the attachment points of the valves extending over to both the pulmonary root and the RVOT myocardium. It can be said that the RVOT myocardium exists within the functional PT. In many of our experiments, we have not found myocardial tissue straying into the PT by passing through the STJ.

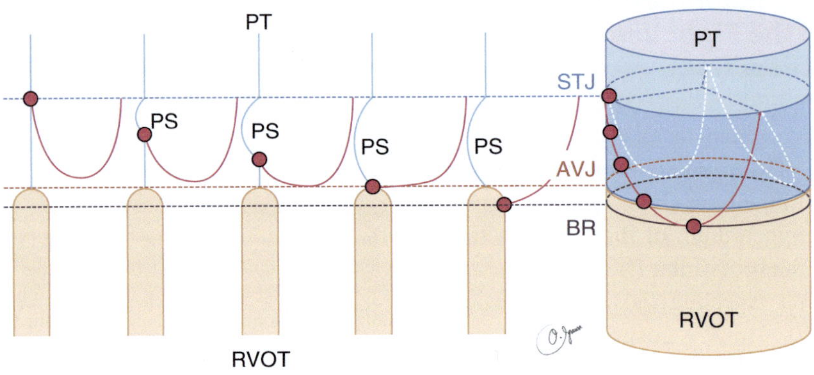

Fig. 1.4 Perceived form of the pulmonary annulus and the structure of the pulmonary sinus. This serial cross-sectional view on the left side shows the pulmonary sinus (PS) (which is the wall of the vessel bulged outward) represented as light blue lines, the annulus as a red closed circle, and the cusps as red lines

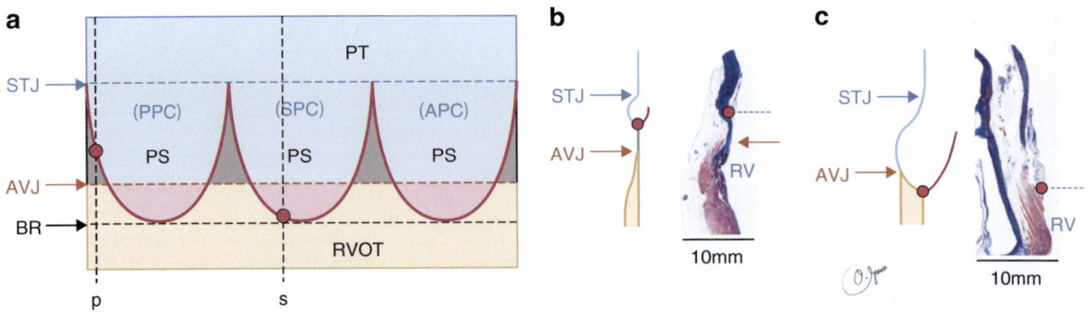

Fig. 1.5 Schematic diagram and histological image of a sagittal section view of the junction of the pulmonary trunk with the right ventricular outflow tract (**a**). Creating a cross-section by incising the preparation along the dotted lines p (**b**) and s (**c**) allows us to observe in (**b**) that this region in the right ventricle does not contain myocardial tissue whereas that in (**c**), although it is a region in the pulmonary trunk, does contain myocardial tissue

1.4 Comparison of the Junction Between the Root of the Pulmonary Trunk and Right Ventricular Outflow Tract and that Between the Aortic Root and Left Ventricular Outflow Tract

The structure of the junction of the root of the PT with the RVOT and that of the aortic root with the LVOT can be compared in the schematic diagrams shown in Fig. 1.6a, b. Figure 1.6b shows the relation of the aortic root and the left ventricular muscle (LVM) in the LVOT. Figure 1.6c shows a schematic diagram representing the addition of the structure of the RV to the connection of the aortic root-LVOT. From these illustrations it can be concluded that the interventricular septum (IVS) is a joint structure consisting of LVM and right ventricular muscle (RVM).

As represented in Fig. 1.6a, at the junction with the RVOT, the root of the PT has an annulus that has an equal relation with the myocardium of the RVOT throughout its whole circumference. However, as viewed in Fig. 1.6b, at the junction with the LVOT, only some parts of the aortic annulus (parts of the right and left coronary cusps) connect with the myocardium of the LVOT (discussed later).

1.5 Fibrous Cardiac Skeleton

The fibrous cardiac skeleton is a structure that controls the basic construction and configuration of the heart. When comparing the heart to a building, the fibrous cardiac skeleton functions as girders. This skeleton consists of "4 annuluses (2 fibrous rings and 2 fibrous crowns) and supporting fibrous tissues located between them" (Fig. 1.7). To improve viewing of the fibrous cardiac skeleton in the physical heart, the right/left fibrous rings, right/left fibrous trigones, and aortic root are exposed after removing the atria by incising at the atrioventricular groove. Both the image of the dissected preparation and its schematic diagram are provided in Fig. 1.7. As shown in the schematic diagram of the heart in Fig. 1.8, two fibrous rings, the right/left fibrous rings, respectively support the TV and MV. The two fibrous coronets respectively consist of those of the PV and AoV, and they provide support to these structures. These four structures are linked and supported by firm fibrous tissues.

Looking at the connection of these structures, the link between the AoV annulus, MV annulus, and TV annulus is connected by three fibrous trigones (right/left anterior fibrous trigone [R/LAFT] and intervalvular fibrous trigone [IVFT]) under the commissure of the aortic annulus and two fibrous trigones (right/left fibrous trigone) situated in the center of the aortic annulus.

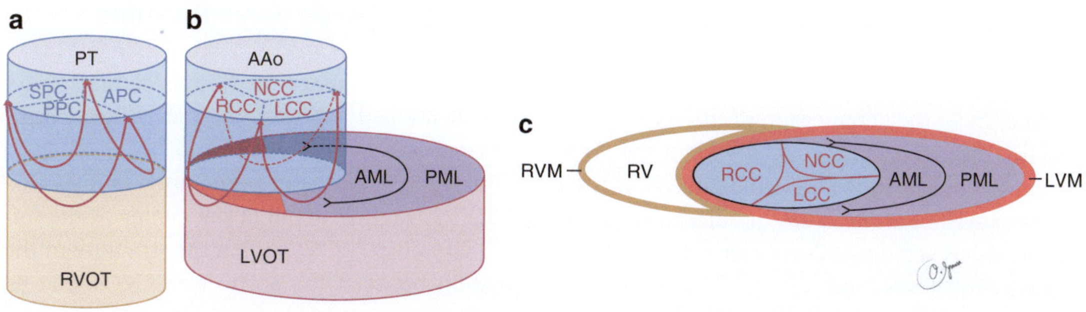

Fig. 1.6 Schematic diagram comparing the structure of the junction of the root of the pulmonary trunk-right ventricular outflow tract (**a**), the junction of the aortic root-left ventricular outflow tract (**b**), and the junction of the aortic root-left ventricular outflow tract after the addition of the structure of the right ventricle (**c**)

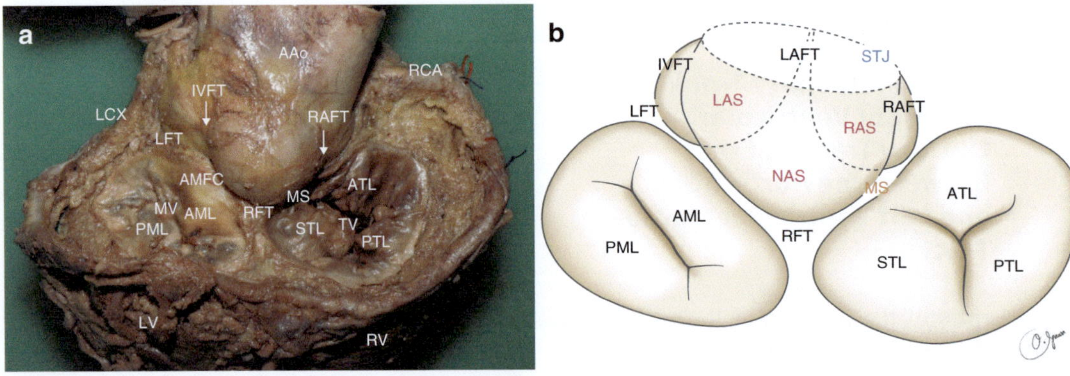

Fig. 1.7 (**a**) Aortic root and the atrioventricular fibrous ring. The right/left fibrous ring, right/left fibrous trigone, and aortic root are exposed after dissecting the heart at the atrioventricular groove and removing the atria to gain a clear view of fibrous cardiac skeleton. (**b**) Aortic root and the atrioventricular fibrous ventricular ring (schematic diagram of **a**)

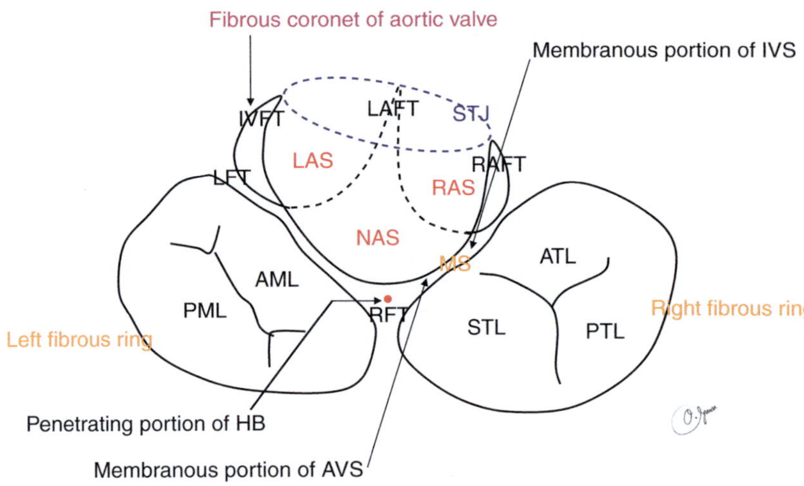

Fig. 1.8 Schematic diagram of the fibrous cardiac skeleton. The His bundle (HB) of the cardiac conduction system enters the right fibrous trigone at the red dot and passes through (penetrating portion of the HB). *AVS* atrioventricular septum, *IVS* interventricular septum

Additionally, the TV annulus is linked to the MV annulus by the fibrous membrane (the extension of the membranous portion of atrioventricular septum). Three interleaflet triangles are located under the commissure of the PV, and the junction between the PV annulus and the AoV annulus is linked by the conoid ligament situated on the LAFT. Furthermore, the aforementioned membranous septum (MS) is consistent with the fibrous cardiac skeleton.

1.6 The Structure just Beneath the Aortic Valve Annulus

This section discusses the fibrous cardiac skeleton mentioned above on the actual heart preparation.

In Fig. 1.9, the heart preparation is dissected along the sagittal plane at the center of the left coronary cusp (LCC) so that the structure of the junction between the aortic root-LVOT can be

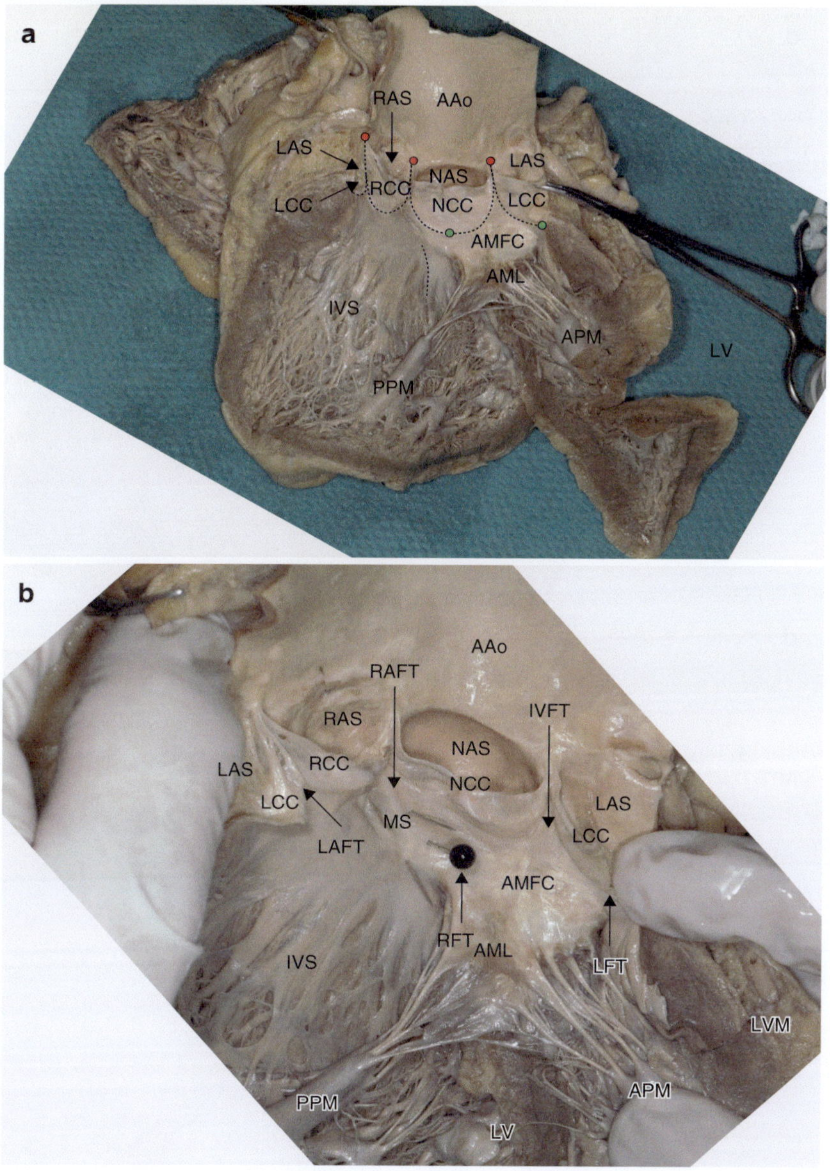

Fig. 1.9 (**a**) View of the junction of the aortic root-left ventricular outflow tract. Regarding the junction of the aortic root-left ventricular outflow tract, the ascending aorta and interventricular septum can be observed simultaneously in the sideways preparation after dissection at the center of the left coronary cusp of the aortic valve in the sagittal plane. Tendinous cords extend from the anterior and posterior papillary muscles of the left ventricle to the anterior mitral leaflet (AML). In addition, the AML connects with the left coronary and non-coronary cusps of the aortic valve by the aorto-mitral fibrous continuity. (**b**) Internal view of the aortic root. (**c**) View directly under the aortic valve. Light from the right side of the heart allows a clear view of the membranous septum (MS) region. The black dotted line in the MS indicates a part of annulus of the septal tricuspid leaflet (STL). (**d**) Schematic diagram of the internal view under the aortic annulus at the junction of the aortic root-left ventricular outflow tract

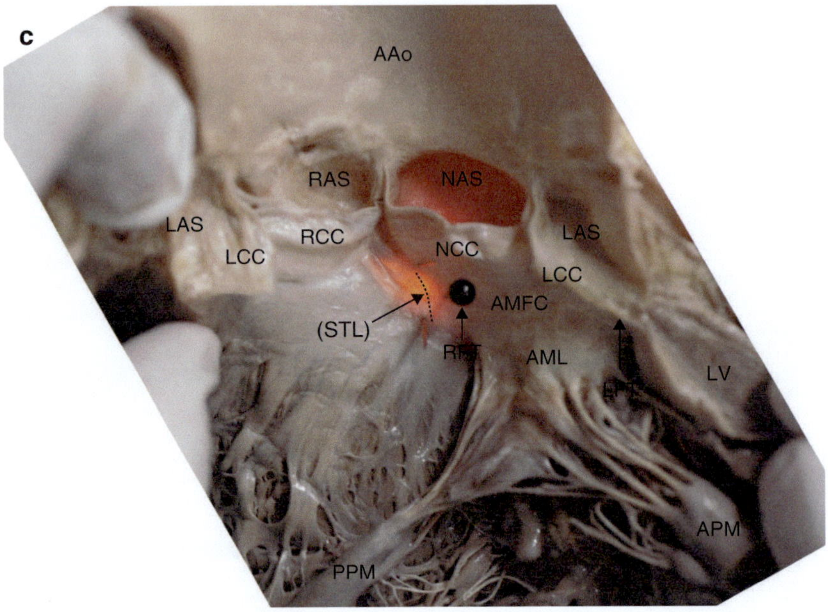

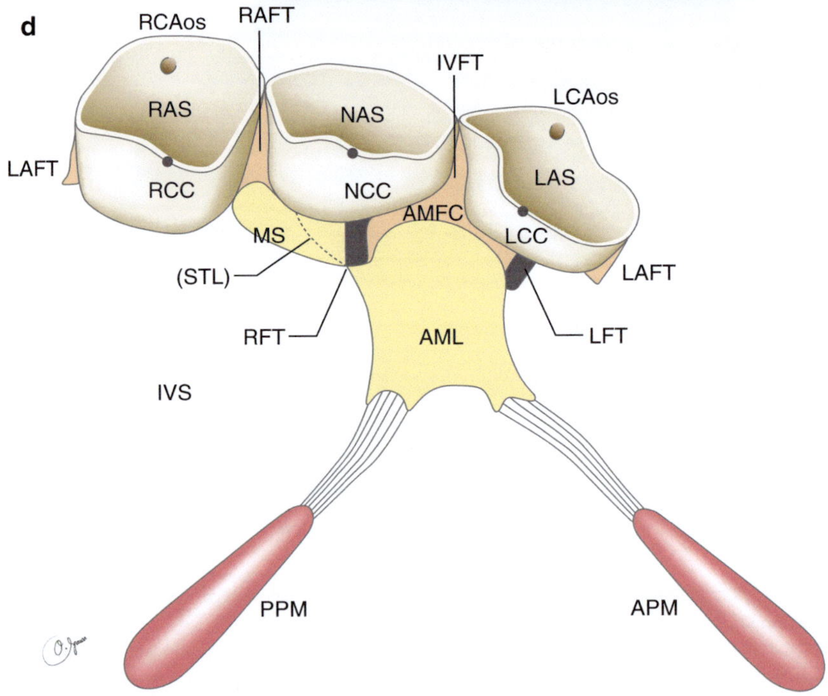

Fig. 1.9 (continued)

observed; the photo of the preparation lying sideways after dissection (Fig. 1.9a), magnified images (Fig. 1.9b, c), and a schematic diagram of the area (Fig. 1.9d) are shown. Structures confirmed above, including the STJ, BR, L/R/NAS, and left/right coronary artery ostia can be seen. Triangular-shaped fibrous tissue can be found to the side of the area just beneath each commissure between the AoV cusps. The RAFT and LAFT can be seen caudal to the commissure of the right coronary cusp-non-coronary cusp (RCC-NCC) of the aortic valve (CRCC-NCC) and the commissure of the RCC-LCC (CRCC-LCC), and the IVFT is located under the commissure of the NCC-LCC (CNCC-LCC). The aortic root remodeling procedure spares these ILTs and maintains the distensibility of the aortic root; therefore, the procedure can be considered to be quite more physiological than the aortic valve reimplantation procedure [2]. The caudal portion of CRCC-NCC, the RAFT, has a membranous structure called the MS attached to it. The annulus of the posterior part of the RCC and the anterior part of the NCC are directly attached to the MS.

As can be seen in Fig. 1.9, the IVFT, which is located on the caudal portion of CNCC-LCC, is connected to the anterior mitral leaflet by firm fibrous tissue called the aorto-mitral fibrous continuity (AMFC).

The LAFT, which is positioned directly under the CRCC-LCC, connects to left ventricular myocardial tissue. On the right side of the LAFT, the IVS consisting of overlapping LVM and RVM is present, whereas the left ventricular free-wall consisting of LVM is observed on the left side.

1.7 Muscular Portion and Fibrous Portion

The abovementioned contents should be comprehended to realize that the AoV annulus is connected to two distinct kinds of tissues: muscular tissue (IVS and LVM) and fibrous tissue (MS, R/LFT, RAFT, and LAFT). Therefore, the AoV annulus is divided into a muscular portion connected to muscular tissues and a fibrous portion connected to fibrous tissue. The former comprises (1) the anterior part of the RCC (the overlapping structure of the RVM and LVM of the IVS) and (2) the anterior part of the LCC (LVM); the latter comprises (1) the posterior part of the RCC (anterior to the MS), (2) the anterior part of the NCC (posterior to the MS), (3) the posterior part of the NCC (RFT and the right side of the IVFT), and (4) the posterior part of the LCC (LFT and the left side of the IVFT). The IVFT connects to the anterior mitral leaflet through the AMFC. This is summarized in Fig. 1.10. Thus, during the aortic root remodeling procedure, David's team previously applied annuloplasty to the fibrous portion alone, but this would appear to be insufficient because the procedure lacks any recruitment of the muscular portion [3].

Figure 1.11 shows a sectional image of the junction of the aortic root-LVOT with regards to the posterior region of the NCC. The relation of the structures connected to the anterior mitral leaflet (AML) from the NCC (this also applies to the LCC) can be seen. In the same area, the firm structure of the AMFC, which does not contain any myocardial tissue, can also be found.

Figure 1.12 presents a sectional image of the junction of aortic root-LVOT with regards to the anterior region of the NCC. The relation of the structures connected to the IVS via the MS from the NCC (this also applies to the RCC) can be seen. The branching portion of the HB (HBb) is running along the point where it transitions from the MS to the IVS.

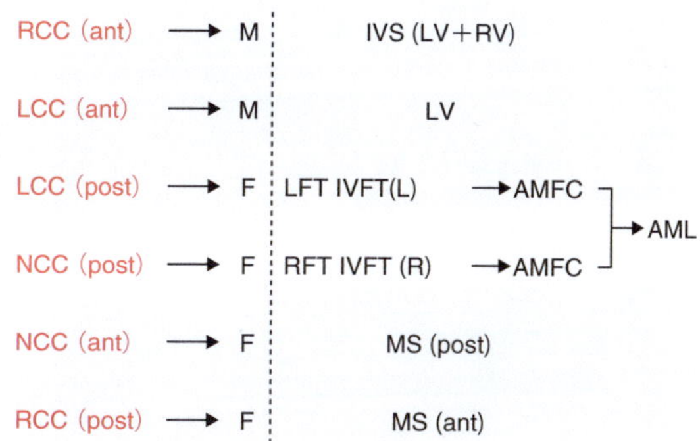

Fig. 1.10 Structures connecting to the aortic root. The aortic root is divided into two portions depending on their points of connection: the muscular portion is connected to muscular tissue, and the fibrous portion is connected to fibrous tissue

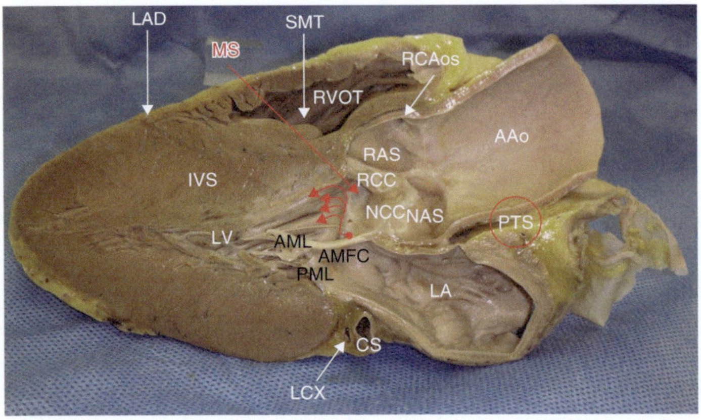

Fig. 1.11 Relation of the aortic root to the left ventricular outflow tract. The transitional portion from the aortic non-coronary cusp (also from the left coronary cusp) to the anterior mitral leaflet (AML) consists of fibrous tissue that contains no myocardium called the aorto-mitral fibrous continuity (AMFC). The pericardial transverse sinus (PTS), septomarginal trabecula (SMT), coronary sinus (CS), left anterior descending coronary artery (LAD), and left circumflex coronary artery (LCX) are also shown

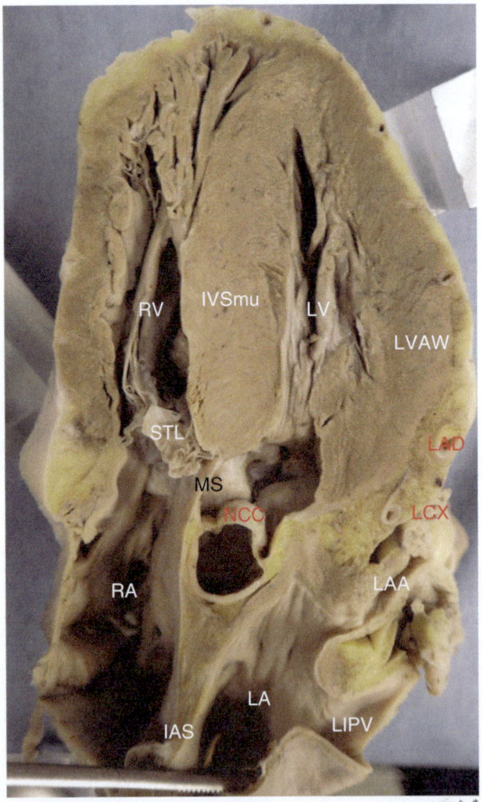

Fig. 1.12 Sectional image of the junction of the aortic root-left ventricular outflow tract focusing on the anterior half of the non-coronary cusp of the aorta. There is structural continuity from the non-coronary cusp of aorta (also from the right coronary cusp) to the muscular portion of the interventricular septum through the membranous septum

1.8 Relation with the Electrical Conduction System

As mentioned above, the MS lies under the CRCC-NCC. From the left ventricular view, the MS appears to be only one fibrous membrane but when viewed from the right ventricular side, it is separated into the MS of the right atrial (RA) region and that of the right ventricular region by the septal tricuspid leaflet. In other words, it is separated into two portions: the membranous portion of the atrioventricular septum, i.e., the boundary of the left ventricle (LV)-RA (AVSme), and the membranous portion of the IVS, i.e., the boundary of the LV-RV (IVSme). The important point is that the HB portion of the electrical conduction system of the heart runs along the lower edge of the MS (i.e., the superior edge of the muscular portion of the IVS [IVSmu]) (Fig. 1.13). The HB consists of the penetrating portion of the HB (HBp), located on the RA side and which penetrates through the RFT (central fibrous body), and the subsequent HBb, located on the ventricular side and which runs along the lower edge of the MS. The HBb is so named because it branches after entering the ventricular side. Therefore, surgery in the region under the CRCC-NCC carries the risk of damaging the conduction system of the heart.

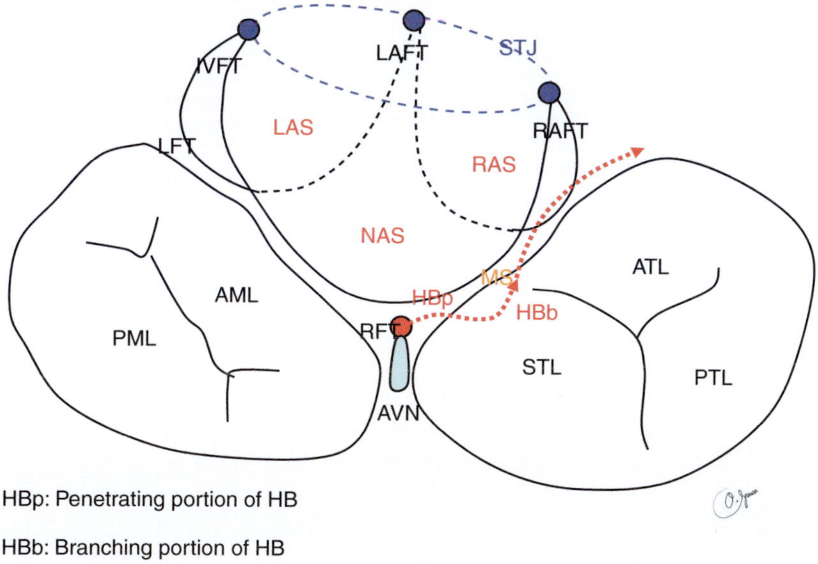

Fig. 1.13 Relation between the fibrous cardiac skeleton and the electrical conduction system. The A-V node (AVN) located on atrioventricular septum connects to the His bundle (HB), which penetrates the right fibrous trigone (central fibrous body) (penetrating portion of the HB [HBp]). The HB runs along the lower edge of the membranous septum (i.e., the superior edge of the muscular portion of interventricular septum [IVSmu]) and then branches (branching portion of the HB [HBb]).

1.9 Conclusion

The structure of the aortic root is quite complicated. A complete explanation is beyond the scope of this chapter, and thus only a limited part was explained. However, this chapter intends for the reader to consider the structure of the AoV from the aspect of the "logic of structure" of the heart. It would be appreciated if this explanation could contribute to future clinical practice.

References

1. Igawa O. Clinical cardiac structurology. Tokyo: Igaku-Shoin; 2011.
2. Wuliya M, Sleilaty G, Di Centa I, Khelil N, Berrebi A, Czitrom D, et al. An expansible aortic ring to preserve aortic root dynamics after aortic valve repair. Eur J Cardiothorac Surg. 2015;47:482–90.
3. David TE. Aortic root aneurysms: remodeling or composite replacement? Ann Thorac Surg. 1997;64:1564–8.

2 Pathophysiology and Natural History of Aortic Regurgitation

Masao Daimon

2.1 Introduction

Aortic regurgitation (AR) causes left ventricular (LV) volume overload through the regurgitant flow from the aorta into the left ventricle (LV) due to incomplete aortic valve closure in diastole. There are a wide variety of causes of AR including not only changes to the leaflets themselves but also geometric changes to the perivalvular tissues, such as aortic root enlargement. Furthermore, AR causes progressive myocardial injury by means of complex mechanisms, such as both LV volume overload and increased afterload, myocardial ischemia, and energy loss due to turbulence. In addition, when compensatory mechanisms for these myocardial injury factors become inadequate, heart failure ensues for which the prognosis is poor. For this reason, when significant LV enlargement and/or systolic dysfunction is observed in severe AR, then surgery is required before patients develop symptomatic heart failure. It is essential to comprehend the pathophysiology and natural history of AR to make an appropriate diagnosis of AR and determine the optimal therapeutic strategy.

2.2 Etiology

The causes of AR are extremely diverse and can be divided into primary causes, such as degeneration of the leaflets themselves, or secondary causes, such as abnormalities of the perivalvular tissues, including aortic root dilatation (Table 2.1). The prevalence of AR due particularly to degenerative changes associated with aging is increasing with the growth of the aging society in the current era. Secondary AR occurs when there is inadequate coaptation of the leaflets due to dilatation or geometric changes of the aortic root, despite an absence of leaflet degeneration. The etiology of AR includes aortitis and systemic disorders such as Behçet's disease, syphilis, or ankylosing spondylitis, and sometimes these systemic disorders are overlooked until AR occurs. Thus, careful assessments of not only valve but also systemic disorders are required in patients with AR. Because the risk of anastomotic leakage in the early postoperative period has been reported to be high in patients with Behçet's disease [1], the indications for surgery must be considered carefully particularly in this subgroup. In addition, AR may sometimes be caused by ergot alkaloids, such as pergolide, which is used to treat Parkinson disease. Thus it is essential to perform a thorough investigation of the cause of AR when determining the therapeutic strategy.

The original version of this chapter was revised. A correction to this chapter can be found at https://doi.org/10.1007/978-981-13-2068-2_41

M. Daimon (✉)
Department of Clinical Laboratory, The University of Tokyo Hospital, Tokyo, Japan
e-mail: daimon@muf.biglobe.ne.jp

T. Kunihara, S. Takanashi (eds.), *Aortic Valve Preservation*,
https://doi.org/10.1007/978-981-13-2068-2_2

Table 2.1 Etiology of AR

Primary valve disease	Secondary disease
• Rheumatic • Degenerative (sclerotic) • Prolapse • Congenital – Bicuspid (or unicuspid) aortic valve – Quadricuspid aortic valve – Others • Infective endocarditis • Other inflammatory disorders (SLE, etc.) • Drug induced	• Aortic root dilatation (including Marfan syndrome) • Aortic inflammatory disorders – Aortitis – Syphilis – Behçet's disease – Others (ankylosing spondylitis, etc.) • Aortic dissection • VSD

SLE systemic lupus erythematosus; *VSD* ventricular septal defect

2.3 Pathophysiology and Hemodynamics

AR is not merely a disorder enhancing LV volume overload; there are several other factors involved in this pathological condition, and myocardial injury progresses due to a number of interrelated factors (Fig. 2.1). First, the blood ejected from the LV returns to the LV again due to regurgitation, which results in LV volume overload. In addition, the regurgitant blood volume is added to the output required for the peripheral circulation, resulting in a high LV stroke volume, which in turn causes compensatory LV enlargement and hypertrophy, which may increase as the severity of the AR increases. Furthermore, the pulse pressure widens as the stroke volume increases, which increases the systolic blood pressure. Thus, AR is a complex pathological condition that involves both LV pressure overload and increased afterload. According to the American Heart Association (AHA)/American College of Cardiology (ACC) guidelines [2], reducing the systolic blood pressure to 140 mmHg by anti-hypertensive medication is a class I recommendation. This indicates the importance of controlling afterload in AR. Angina pectoris is also a well-known symptom of AR, although the coronary flow reserve decreases as the diastolic blood pressure decreases in patients with AR; thus, myocardial ischemia may also cause the progression of myocardial injury [3]. Recent technological advancements of echocardiography such as that of vector flow mapping provide us with a more detailed analysis of the hemodynamics in AR. The AR jet flowing from the high-pressure aorta into the LV causes turbulence within the LV, and this turbulence causes energy loss in the LV and increases the LV myocardial work load consecutively [4]. Furthermore, the number of elderly patients with AR has increased in recent years, and aging itself can be one of the causes of LV diastolic dysfunction with increased myocardial stiffness. Accordingly, complex mechanisms, such as the increased LV pressure load or energy loss by turbulence, are involved in the pathophysiology of AR in addition to LV volume overload. Compared to mitral regurgitation, which is also a disorder of LV volume overload, the mechanism of progressive LV myocardial injury in AR appears to be more complex. During the early stages of chronic AR, LV enlargement and hypertrophy compensate for this overload and maintain the LV contractility. However, progressive myocardial injury, such as myocardial hypertrophy or myocyte fibrosis, results in failure of these compensatory mechanisms and heart failure ensues. If AR is treated surgically by valve replacement or valvuloplasty at the early stage when myocardial damage is reversible, the LV function can be recovered and preserved. However, at the late stage when myocardial damage is severe and irreversible, LV dysfunction would persist, resulting in a poor prognosis, even after surgical intervention for AR. Therefore, it is advisable to perform surgical treatment before irreversible myocardial injury occurs, even in patients with asymptomatic chronic AR.

Meanwhile, in acute AR, the compensatory mechanisms of LV enlargement and hypertrophy are not yet active, so the patient experiences rapid hemodynamic deterioration and develops heart failure. Specifically, acute heart failure may occur in cases of acute and severe AR, even in the absence of LV enlargement or a decreased left ventricular ejection fraction (LVEF). Thus, emergency surgical treatment is mandatory for hemodynamic improvement in this setting.

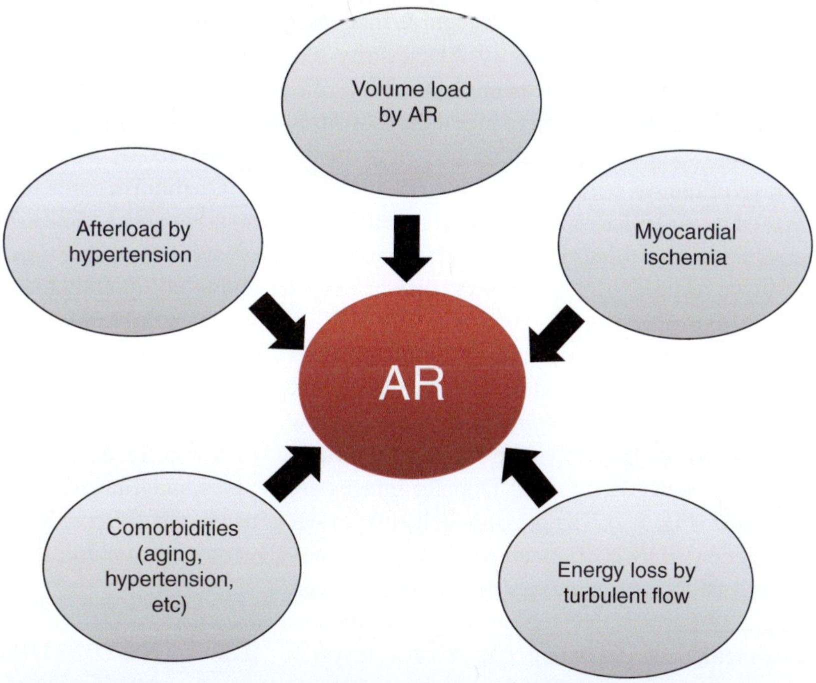

Fig. 2.1 Pathophysiology of aortic regurgitation. Aortic regurgitation is not merely a disorder affecting left ventricular volume overload; there are several other factors related to the progression of this pathological condition

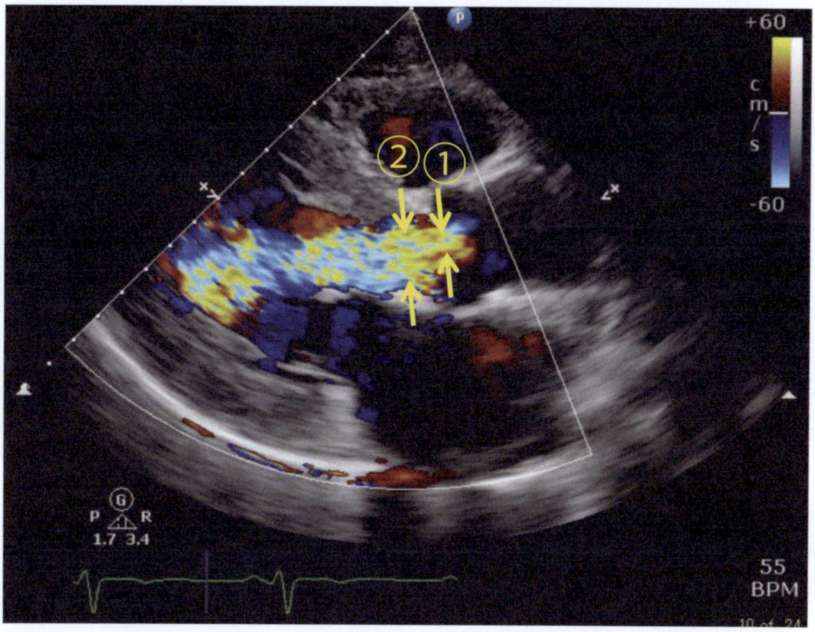

Fig. 2.2 Echocardiographic evaluation of aortic regurgitation (AR) severity by color Doppler imaging. Vena contracta width is measured as the narrowest site of the AR color Doppler signal (①), and AR color Doppler jet width is measured at the left ventricular outflow tract (②)

2.4 Grading of AR

Echocardiography is the most widely used noninvasive modality for evaluating the severity of AR [2]. Details are provided in the American Society of Echocardiography (ASE) guidelines. There are some well-known echocardiographic parameters for assessing AR severity. Among these, the simplest parameters for routine use are the vena contracta width at the regurgitant orifice and the jet width at the left ventricular outflow tract (Fig. 2.2). The AR jet distance, which was used previously, is no longer used because it may be frequently incorrect due to mixture of the AR jet with the mitral inflow. However, we need to recognize that each echocardiographic parameter of AR severity has its intrinsic limitations. For example, the vena contracta may not form a perfect circle on short-axis sections in some cases, which may result in misdiagnosis of the AR severity, or it could be underestimated based on jet width due to an eccentric AR jet. Other echocardiographic parameters also have their own respective advantages and disadvantages [2, 5]. For this reason, wherever possible, a comprehensive evaluation using multiple parameters should be performed when evaluating AR severity by echocardiography. Holo-diastolic flow reversal can be observed in the abdominal aorta in cases of severe AR if pulsed Doppler images are examined (Fig. 2.3). The pressure half-time of AR flow, recorded by continuous-wave Doppler measurements, shortens as the severity of AR increases (Fig. 2.3). Furthermore, the most precise and reliable method of evaluating AR severity involves quantitative estimation of the regurgitant volume using Doppler images. The regurgitant volume can be calculated from the difference between the stroke volume in the left ventricular outflow tract and inflow at the mitral valve using pulsed-wave Doppler images. Otherwise, the proximal isovelocity surface area (PISA) of the regurgitant color flow jet can be used to estimate the regurgitant volume [2, 5]. Routine quantitative evaluation of AR severity is recommended in patients with suspected moderate or greater AR to avoid overlooking severe AR.

Qualitative catheter-based aortography is an invasive and non-physiological investigation that involves the rapid injection of a contrast agent and is not quantitative. Despite these limitations it is a useful test when an adequate evaluation of AR severity cannot be achieved by echocardiography. Recently, heart magnetic resonance imaging (MRI) has also emerged as a novel technique to assess AR severity [5]. Cardiac MRI also provides quantitative assessment of the AR volume using the difference between the left and right ventricular volumes. (Table 2.2).

2.5 Natural History and Follow-Up

As previously mentioned, LV myocardial injury would progress as long as severe AR persists, even if the patient is asymptomatic, and ultimately, the patient would develop symptoms of heart failure. The prognosis for heart failure

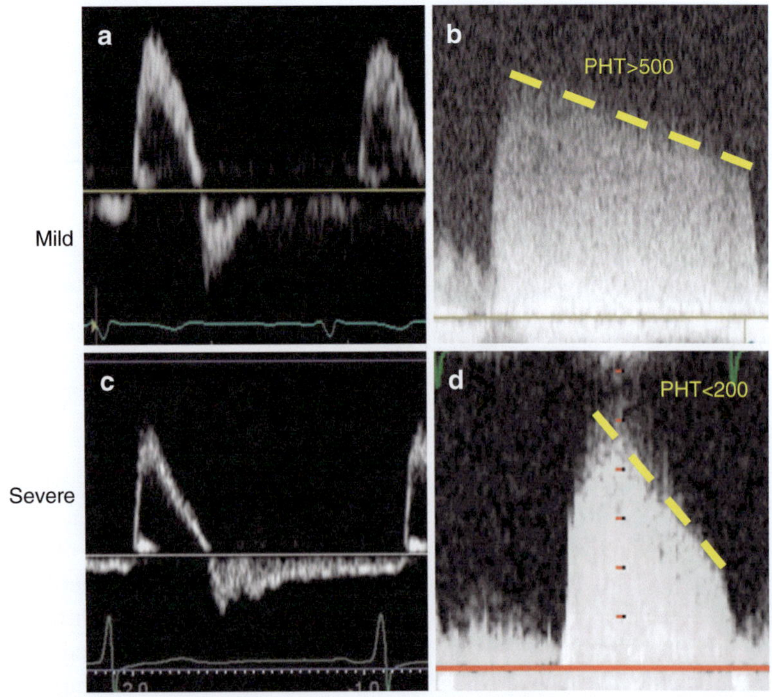

Fig. 2.3 Supportive signs of aortic regurgitation (AR) grading by echocardiography. Pulsed-wave Doppler imaging of blood flow from the abdominal aorta in mild AR (**a**) and severe AR (**c**). Continuous-wave Doppler imaging of the AR jet in mild AR (**b**) and severe AR (**d**). *PHT* pressure half time

caused by AR is poor [6] (Fig. 2.4). The annual mortality rate for patients with NYHA class III and IV symptoms is high at 24.6% if surgery is not performed after the onset of symptomatic heart failure. An annual mortality rate of 6.3% was reported even in patients with NYHA class II symptoms [2]. Accordingly, the indication for surgery is a class I recommendation for patients with severe AR who suffer from symptoms of heart failure [2], and surgical indications must be investigated on an urgent basis.

It was reported that the risk of sudden death in asymptomatic AR patients with normal LV ejection fraction is not so high, but approximately 25% of asymptomatic AR patients will develop symptoms of heart failure within a year if they have LV dysfunction [2, 7]. For this reason, it is important to search for patients with a poor prognosis and who are at elevated risk for the onset of heart failure and to advise surgical treatment, even if they are asymptomatic. Detaint et al., who investigated mortality in asymptomatic AR, divided patients on the basis of a quantitative evaluation of their AR severity according to ASE guidelines and reported on their results [8] (Fig. 2.5). This graph shows that certainly severe AR has a poor prognosis, but also moderate AR cannot unequivocally be said to have a favorable prognosis. As mentioned previously, the pathological condition of AR is complex, and it is not merely a disorder affecting LV volume overload. Thus, there are patients who may develop progressive LV dysfunction and the onset of heart failure, even when quantitative evaluation by echocardiography indicates that their

Table 2.2 Grading of aortic regurgitation severity (cited in modified form from references 2 and 5)

	Mild	Moderate	Severe
Qualitative			
Angiographic grade	1+	2+	3–4+
Color Doppler jet width	Central jet, <25% of LVOTd	25–64% of LVOTd	Central jet, ≥65% LVOTd
Vena contracta width (cm)	<0.3	0.3–0.6	>0.6
Quantitative			
Regurgitant volume (mL)	<30	30–59	≥60
Regurgitant fraction (%)	<30	30–49	≥50
Regurgitant orifice area (cm²)	0.10	0.10–0.29	≥0.30
Additional			
LV size			Usually dilated
Flow in the abdominal aorta			Prominent holodiastolic reversal
Aortic regurgitation PHT	Incomplete or faint Slow, >500		Steep, <200

LVOTd left ventricular outflow tract diameter, *PHT* pressure half time

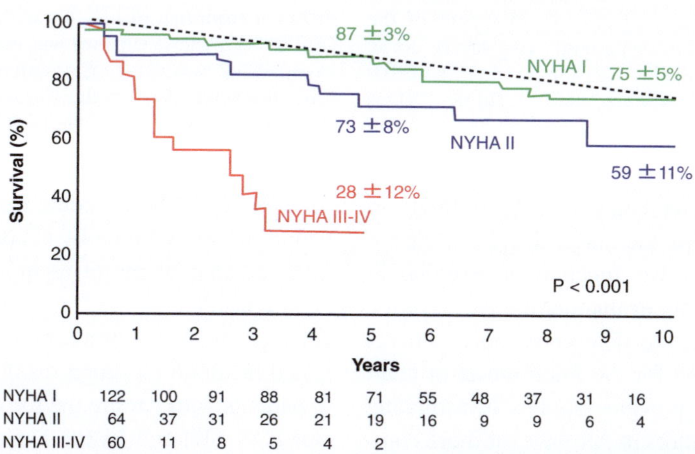

Fig. 2.4 Survival with conservative treatment of the entire study population of patients with severe aortic regurgitation stratified according to NYHA class at baseline. When symptoms ≥ NYHA grade II appear, conservative treatment has a poor prognosis (cited from Reference 6). The dotted line indicates the natural prognosis of healthy individuals of the same age

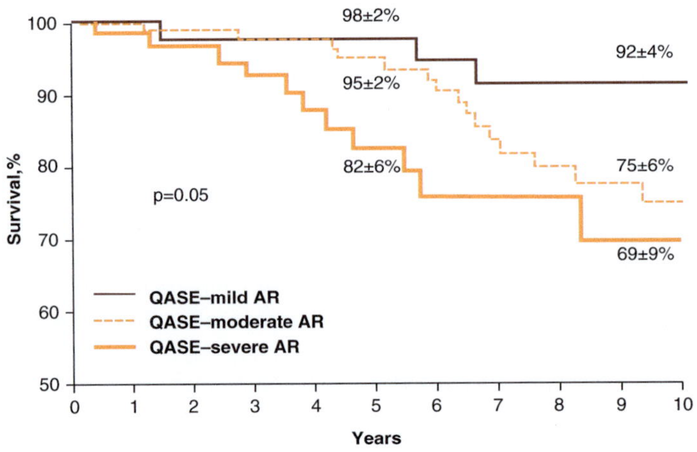

Fig. 2.5 Survival under conservative management after the diagnosis of asymptomatic aortic regurgitation (AR). Patients are stratified according to quantitative American Society of Echocardiography AR grading [5]. The prognosis of AR worsens as the severity increases, even in asymptomatic patients. However, we also know that the prognosis for moderate AR is not necessarily favorable (cited from Reference 8)

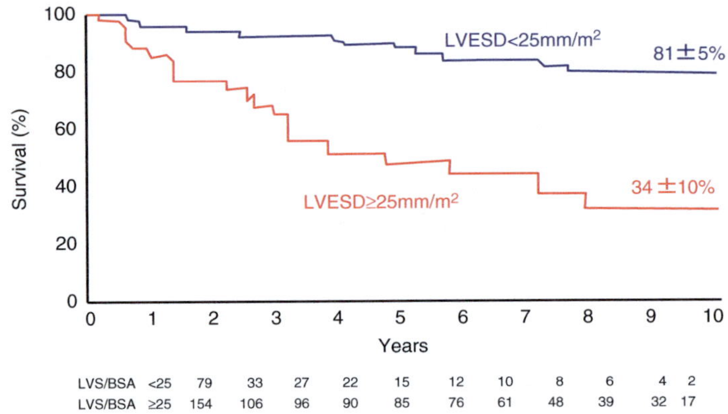

Fig. 2.6 Survival with conservative treatment of the entire study population of patients with severe aortic regurgitation stratified according to LVESD/BSA. Survival of patients with baseline values ≥25 mm/m² was lower than expected ($P < 0.001$) and different from that of patients with values <25 mm/m² ($P < 0.001$), whose survival was not different from that expected ($P = 0.52$). *LVESD* left ventricular end systolic diameter, *BSA* body surface area (cited from Reference 6)

AR is moderate rather than severe. Accordingly, to accurately determine the surgical indications for AR, assessment of LV function is essential in addition to accurately evaluating the AR severity. It is also imperative to determine those patients who are at high risk for the future onset of heart failure. In reality, previous studies investigating poor prognostic factors in AR have far more commonly reported on LV function rather than AR severity [2]. In these studies, the quantitative evaluation of regurgitation by echocardiography contradicted that of mitral regurgitation, which has been considered as an incremental and accurate value predictive of prognosis [2]. The two established factors for a prognosis of poor LV function in patients with AR are the LV end-systolic diameter (LVESD) and LVEF. Dujardin et al. studied patients with advanced LV dilatation, as indicated

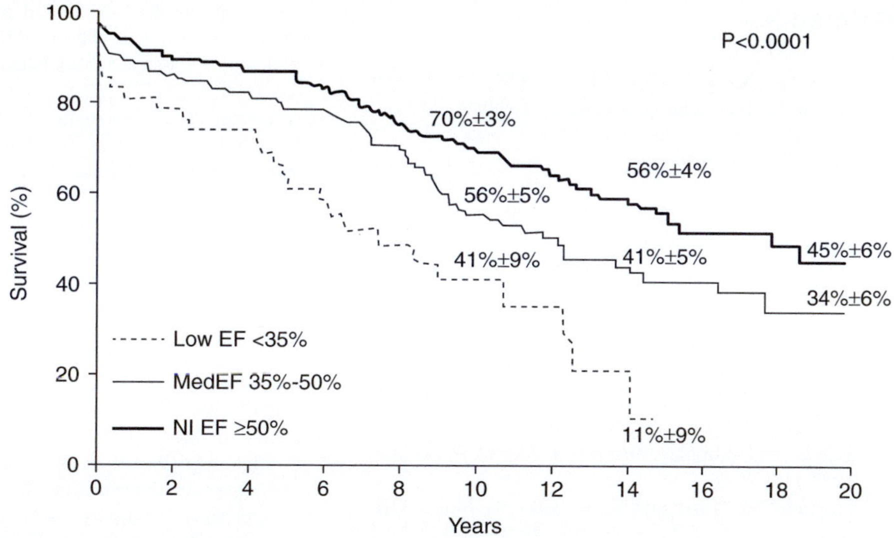

LoEF (EF <35%)	43	35	31	21	15	8	6	3			
MedEF (EF 35%-50%)	134	115	108	95	78	50	34	30	19	9	2
Nl EF (EF ≥50%)	273	245	231	184	141	112	83	60	32	17	1

Fig. 2.7 Survival after aortic valve replacement (AVR) for the entire study population with significant aortic regurgitation stratified according to ejection fraction (EF). Patients with a markedly low EF had significantly lower survival rates than those with a normal or moderately reduced EF before AVR (cited from Reference 9)

by an LVESD/body surface area (BSA) ratio ≥25 mm/m^2, and reported a poor prognosis of approximately 34% for 10-year survival if these patients were only treated conservatively [6] (Fig. 2.6). This was one of the reasons for establishing an LVESD/BSA ratio ≥25 mm/m^2 as one criterion for determining the indications for surgery in the AHA/ACC guidelines [2]. The LVEF is also an important prognosticator in AR, and the postoperative long-term prognosis is poorer for patients with lower LVEF values, even if they undergo surgery. Reports indicate that 50% is the LVEF cut-off value at which the prognosis is the same as that of healthy individuals of the same age [9] (Fig. 2.7). This was the basis for establishing an LVEF of 50% as a criterion for surgical indications in the AHA/ACC guidelines [2]. Plasma brain natriuretic peptide (BNP), which is used to assess heart failure, has also been thought to be a useful prognosticator for AR. Pizarro et al. reported that groups with a plasma BNP ≥ 130 pg/mL had a significantly higher incidence of subsequent heart failure and mortality due to heart events [10]. This was also the case even among patients with an LVEF ≥55%. Naturally, periodic history taking and examination and echocardiography should be performed during AR follow-up, although we must ensure that we do not omit plasma BNP tests to achieve accurate timing of surgery.

2.6 Conclusion

This chapter has reviewed the pathophysiology and natural history of AR. As clinicians, we must have a good understanding of the pathological condition and natural history of AR and strive to perform accurate determination of both disease severity and the therapeutic strategy.

References

1. Ma WG, Zheng J, Zhu JM, Liu YM, Li M, Sun LZ. Aortic regurgitation caused by Behçet's disease: surgical experience during an 11-year period. J Card Surg. 2012;27:39–44.
2. Nishimura RA, Otto CM, Bonow RO, Carabello BA, Erwin JP 3rd, Guyton RA, et al. 2014 AHA/ACC guidelines for the management of patients with valvular heart disease: a report of the American College of Cardiology/American Heart Association Task Force on Practice Guidelines. J Am Coll Cardiol. 2014;63:e57–e185.
3. Nitenberg A, Foult JM, Antony I, Blanchet F, Rahali M. Coronary flow and resistance reserve in patients with chronic aortic regurgitation, angina pectoris and normal coronary arteries. J Am Coll Cardiol. 1988;11:478–86.
4. Stugaard M, Koriyama H, Katsuki K, Masuda K, Asanuma T, Takeda Y, et al. Energy loss in the left ventricle obtained by vector flow mapping as a new quantitative measure of severity of aortic regurgitation: a combined experimental and clinical study. Eur Heart J Cardiovasc Imaging. 2015;16:723–30.
5. Zoghbi WA, Adams D, Bonow RO, Enriquez-Sarano M, Foster E, Grayburn PA, et al. Recommendations for noninvasive evaluation of native valvular regurgitation: a report from the American Society of Echocardiography developed in collaboration with the Society for Cardiovascular Magnetic Resonance. J Am Soc Echocardiogr. 2017;30:303–71..
6. Dujardin KS, Enriquez-Sarano M, Schaff HV, Bailey KR, Seward JB, Tajik AJ. Mortality and morbidity of aortic regurgitation in clinical practice. A long-term follow-up study. Circulation. 1999;99:1851–7.
7. Bonow RO, Carabello BA, Chatterjee K, de Leon AC Jr, Faxon DP, Freed MD, American College of Cardiology/American Heart Association Task Force on Practice Guidelines, et al. 2008 Focused update incorporated into the ACC/AHA 2006 guidelines for the management of patients with valvular heart disease: a report of the American College of Cardiology/American Heart Association Task Force on Practice Guidelines (Writing Committee to revise the 1998 guidelines for the management of patients with valvular heart disease). Endorsed by the Society of Cardiovascular Anesthesiologists, Society for Cardiovascular Angiography and Interventions, and Society of Thoracic Surgeons. J Am Coll Cardiol. 2008;52:e1–142.
8. Detaint D, Messika-Zeitoun D, Maalouf J, Tribouilloy C, Mahoney DW, Tajik AJ, et al. Quantitative echocardiographic determinants of clinical outcome in asymptomatic patients with aortic regurgitation: a prospective study. JACC Cardiovasc Imaging. 2008;1:1–11.
9. Chaliki HP, Mohty D, Avierinos JF, Scott CG, Schaff HV, Tajik AJ, et al. Outcomes after aortic valve replacement in patients with severe aortic regurgitation and markedly reduced left ventricular function. Circulation. 2002;106:2687–93.
10. Pizarro R, Bazzino OO, Oberti PF, Falconi ML, Arias AM, Krauss JG, et al. Prospective validation of the prognostic usefulness of B-type natriuretic peptide in asymptomatic patients with chronic severe aortic regurgitation. J Am Coll Cardiol. 2011;58:1705–14.

3 Ultrasound Measurement of Aortic Valves

Keitaro Mahara

3.1 Introduction

The standard surgical treatment for aortic regurgitation (AR) is aortic valve replacement. In the latest guidelines on valvular heart disease published in 2014 by the American Heart Association (AHA) and the American College of Cardiology (ACC) [1]. However, in cases of AR caused by enlargement of the aortic root, it is stated that valve-sparing aortic root replacement can be one of the choices when the cusp configuration is maintained. In the guidelines released in 2017 by the European Society of Cardiology (ESC) and the European Association for Cardio-Thoracic Surgery (EACTS) [2], positive results were announced for aortic valvuloplasty performed at facilities with high experience [3–6]. Although the number of aortic valvuloplasties has increased compared to that of aortic valve replacements, the guidelines state that aortic valve replacement is still the standard surgical treatment.

The effectiveness of aortic valve replacement using mechanical valves in young and biological valves in elderly patients is widely accepted, and thus, the indication for aortic valvuloplasty must carefully be considered. However, it makes logical sense to preserve the cusps and to replace the aortic root alone in case of AR associated with aortic root enlargement and in the absence of cusp pathology. On the other hand, advanced surgical technique is necessary when performing aortic valvuloplasty for AR with cusp pathology. Nevertheless, it is vital to observe the underlying mechanisms of AR in detail by echocardiography and to differentiate the normal and abnormal parts that are causing the AR.

3.2 The Mechanism of AR

AR is brought about by structural changes in the aortic complex that result in the loss of cusp coaptation. Namely, AR is caused by either cusp degeneration or enlargement of the root, which supports the aortic cusps, and the two interact with one another. Advanced AR may enlarge the aortic root structure, and the subsequent root enlargement causes alteration of the three-dimensional structure of the cusps. Boodhwani and his colleagues proposed to classify the etiology of AR according to the surgical technique required [7] (Fig. 3.1). In clinical practice, a bicuspid aortic valve and root enlargement comprise the majority of etiologies for aortic valvuloplasty; however, vasculitis should also be differentiated. Furthermore, cusp bending or fenestration can also cause AR. Aortic valvuloplasty is generally not indicated for AR caused by cusp restriction.

K. Mahara (✉)
Director of Echocardiography Laboratory, Sakakibara Heart Institute, Tokyo, Japan
e-mail: kmahara@shi.heart.or.jp

T. Kunihara, S. Takanashi (eds.), *Aortic Valve Preservation*,
https://doi.org/10.1007/978-981-13-2068-2_3

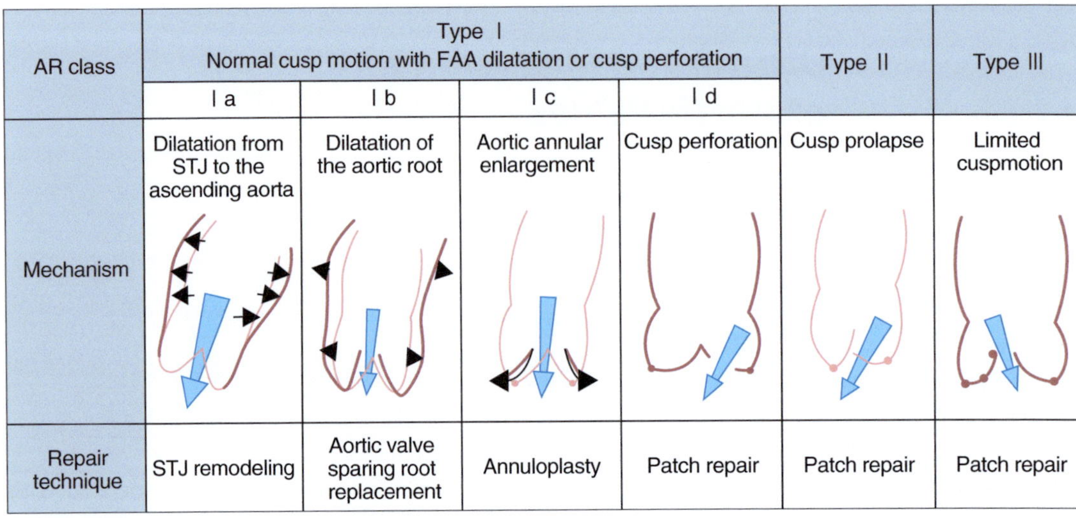

Fig. 3.1 Functional classification of AR. *FAA* functional aortic annulus (from Boodhwani M, et al. Repair-oriented classification of aortic insufficiency: impact on surgical techniques and clinical outcomes. J Thorac Cardiovasc Surg. 2013;146:264–74)

Bicuspid Aortic Valve

Prolapse of an elongated fused cusp causes AR in the majority of patients with a bicuspid aortic valve (Fig. 3.2). Care must be taken in patients with AR caused by degenerative thickening and shortening of the raphe, which will necessitate pericardial patch repair (Fig. 3.3). It is also important whether the Valsalva sinuses are nearly bisected or trisected (Fig. 3.4). Aortic valvuloplasty creating an asymmetric bicuspid valve in patients with a trisected Valsalva sinus may not secure a sufficient area of valve opening and is more likely to be associated with aortic stenosis. Additionally, because AR is often accompanied by root enlargement, 3-dimensional observation is essential. Postoperative aortic stenosis is the major concern associated with aortic valvuloplasty for the bicuspid aortic valve. Therefore, it is crucial to assess the preoperative valve area, the structure of the Valsalva sinus, and the degree of cusp degeneration, and to predict the postoperative valve area. When the ideal effective valve area cannot be determined by intraoperative transesophageal echocardiography, conversion to aortic valve replacement should be considered.

Aortic Root Enlargement

Aortic root enlargement is recognized in the majority of patients with AR. The pattern of aortic root enlargement varies depending on the patient, but overall, in the majority of instances it encompasses the aortic annulus to the Valsalva sinus, sinotubular junction (STJ), and the proximal ascending aorta. Because the morphology of aortic root enlargement affects the configuration of cusp coaptation, both should be examined. For example, the cusp coaptation area deviates to the left ventricular side in patients with annular enlargement (Fig. 3.5a) and to the aortic side in those with STJ enlargement (Fig. 3.5b). Also, asymmetric enlargement may cause asymmetric deviation of cusp height and induce an eccentric jet. Furthermore, cusp bending, which is described later, frequently occurs in the cusp within the enlarged sinus.

Cusp Prolapse

Cusp prolapse has not yet been clearly defined for the aortic valve. Here, it is defined as the presence of an eccentric jet due to asymmetric

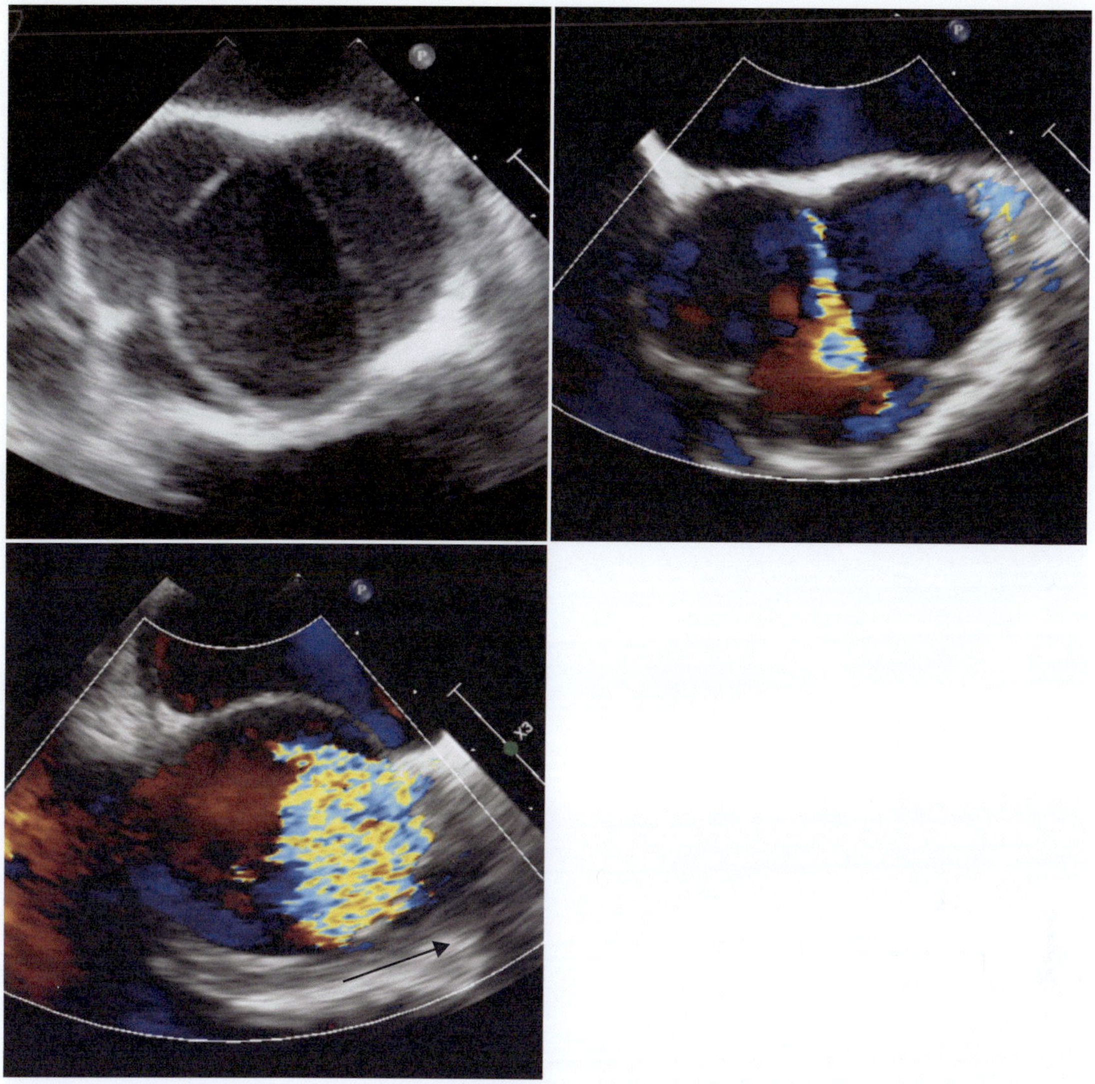

Fig. 3.2 Bicuspid aortic valve and the direction of the regurgitant jet. The regurgitant jet is directed toward the opposite side of prolapsing fused cusp

deviation of cusp height. The causes of cusp prolapse in tricuspid valves are elongation of the free margin associated with myxomatous degeneration, a large fenestration, bending, and rupture of the free edge. Elongation of the free margin and fenestration are frequently associated with cusp bending and prolapse. Pericardial patch repair is required in cases of a large fenestration (Fig. 3.6). It is essential to evaluate the location of the bending cusp (Fig. 3.7). Whether it is centrally located or localized on the commissure side and whether it causes deviation of cusp height that results in regurgitation should be carefully examined.

Cusp prolapse is assessed by 3-dimensional transesophageal echocardiography. Because the aortic valve consists of three cusps, it is difficult to evaluate left- or non-coronary cusp prolapse by conventional 2-dimensional echocardiography. The data set of 3-dimensional transesophageal echocardiography enables free cross-sectional observation; therefore, the deviation of each cusp height and the direction of the regurgitant jet can be assessed (Fig. 3.8).

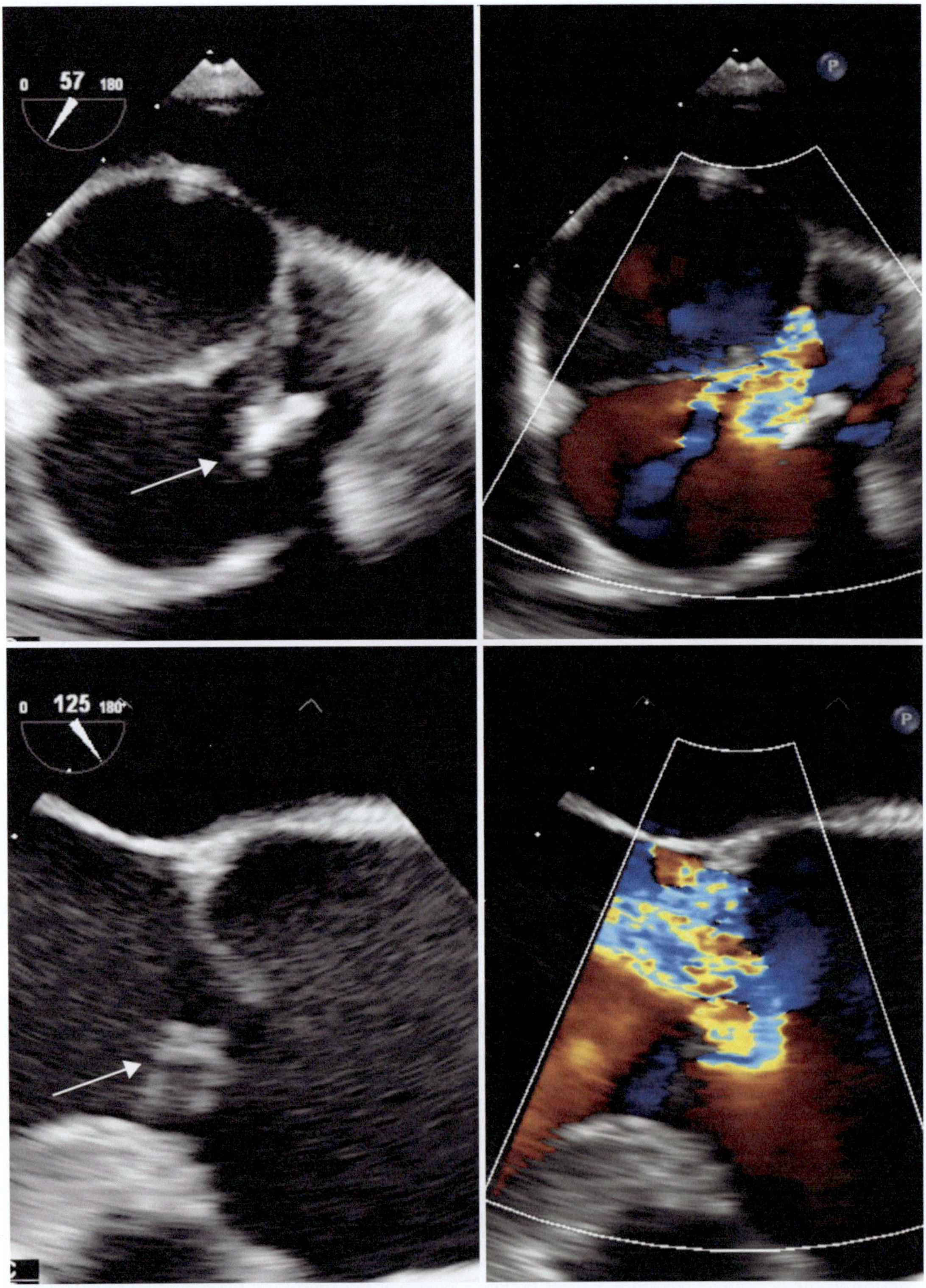

Fig. 3.3 Advanced AR associated with advanced calcification at the raphe. Calcification is seen at the raphe (arrow). A gap at the center of the raphe creates regurgitation

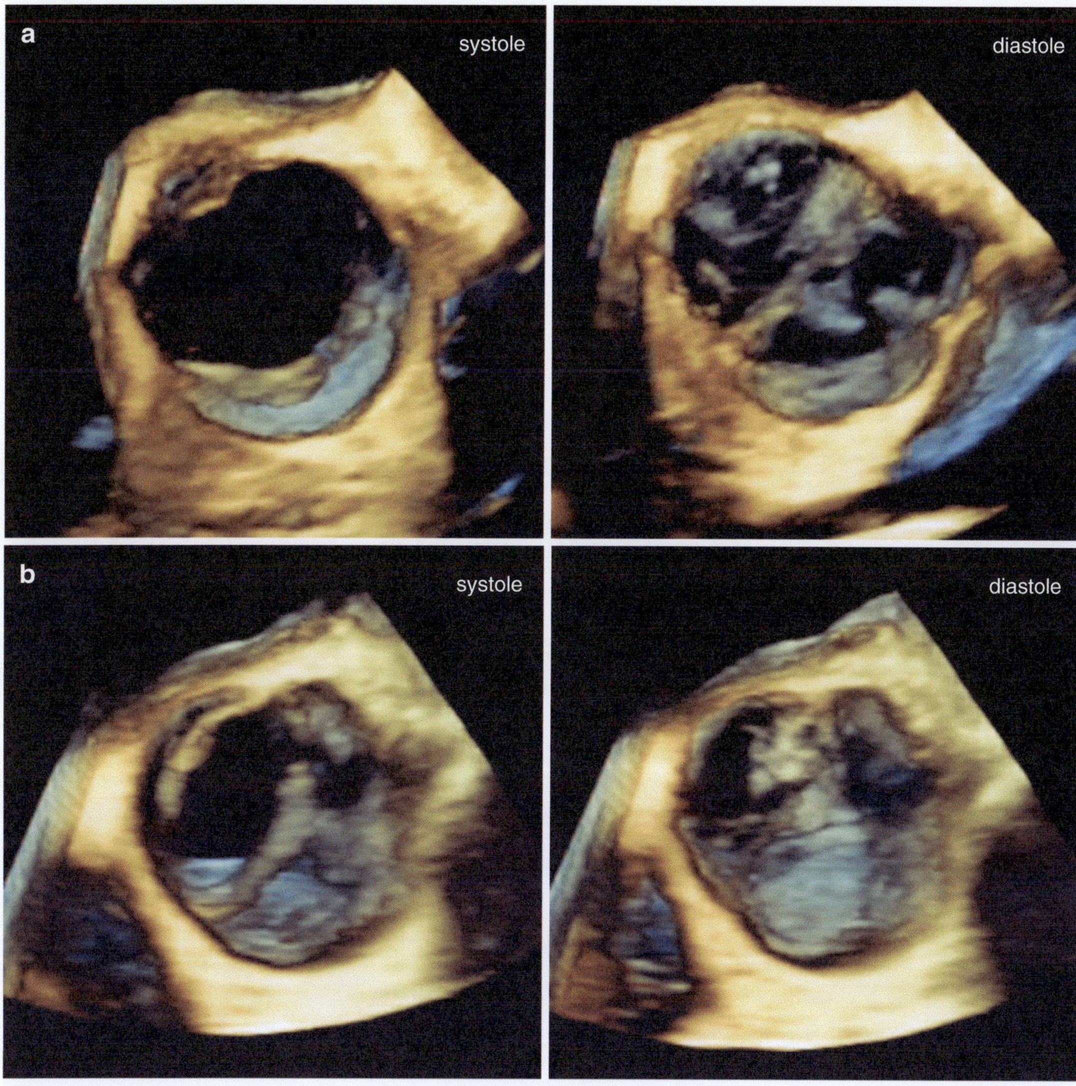

Fig. 3.4 Configuration of the Valsalva sinus in the bicuspid aortic valve. The Valsalva sinus shown in panel (**a**) is relatively bisected. However, that shown in panel (**b**) corresponds to a 2:1 ratio

Degenerative Thickening and Shortening of Cusps

In the case of rheumatic valvular heart disease, adhesion of the commissures and thickening and shortening of the cusps can be seen due to rheumatic degeneration, which causes a loss of cusp coaptation that induces the regurgitation (Fig. 3.9). Thickening and shortening can also occur due to senile degenerative changes that induce aortic regurgitation due to the insufficient coaptation depth (Fig. 3.10). In these etiologies, aortic valvuloplasty is always challenging. The cases with AR caused by a bicuspid valve or aortic root enlargement, or by cusp prolapse, are also associated with degenerative changes of the cusps that are linked to aging. Considerable attention is necessary in the case of a bicuspid valve with increased transvalvular blood flow velocity or especially in the elderly with root enlargement or cusp prolapse. It is essential to evaluate the cusp size numerically by measuring the geometric height of the aortic valve as described later.

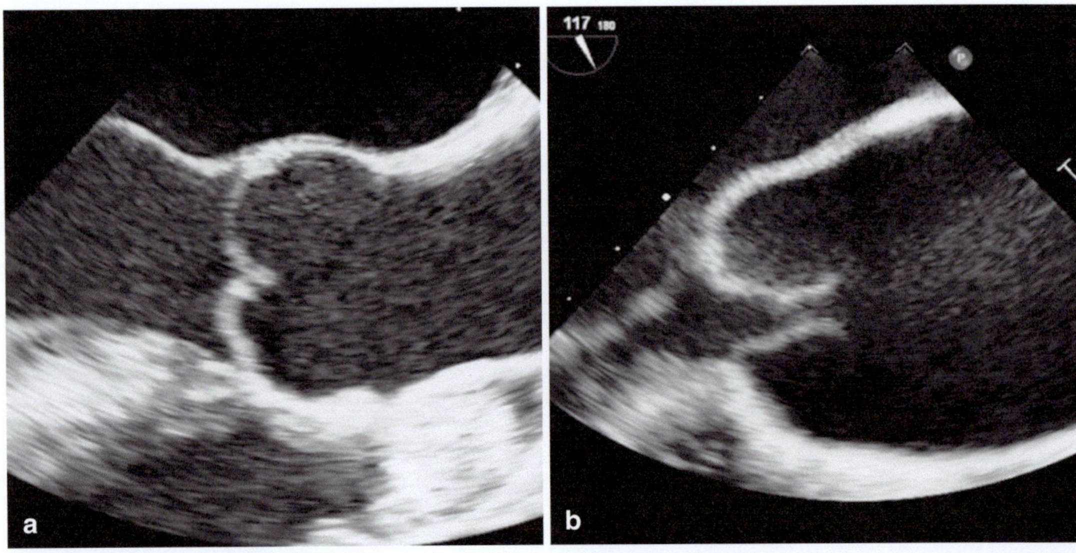

Fig. 3.5 Pattern of aortic root enlargement and cusp deviation. In panel (**a**), although the aortic annulus is enlarged, enlargement of the Valsalva sinus and STJ is not remarkable. The cusps deviate to the left ventricular side. In panel (**b**), although annular enlargement is not present, the Valsalva sinus and STJ are enlarged. The cusps deviate to the ascending aorta

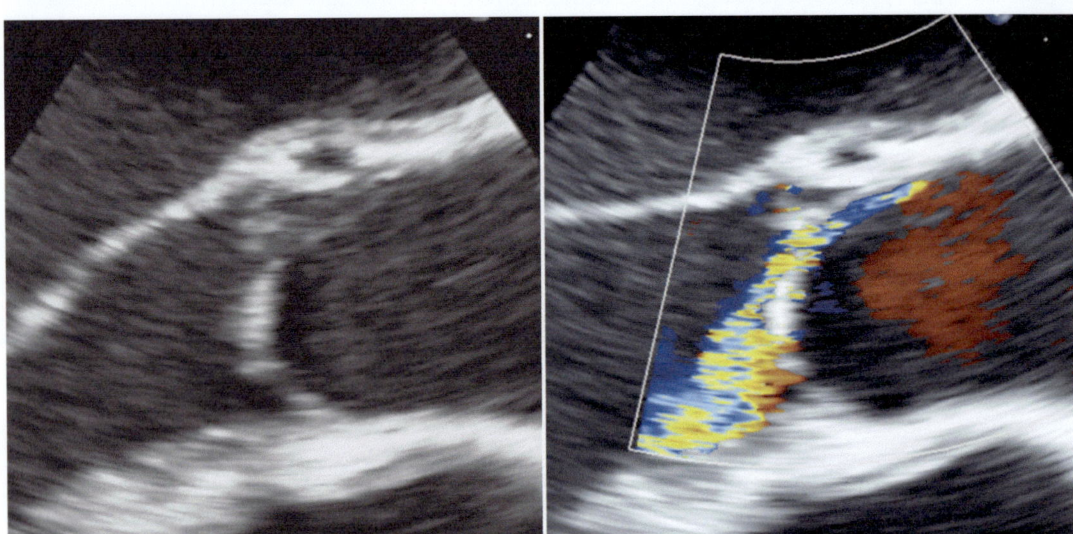

Fig. 3.6 Advanced AR due to fenestration. Regurgitation is seen from proximal to the commissure between the left- and non-coronary cusps in the direction toward the opposite side of the prolapsing non-coronary cusp. Intraoperative findings revealed fenestration at the same location, which was repaired by autologous pericardium

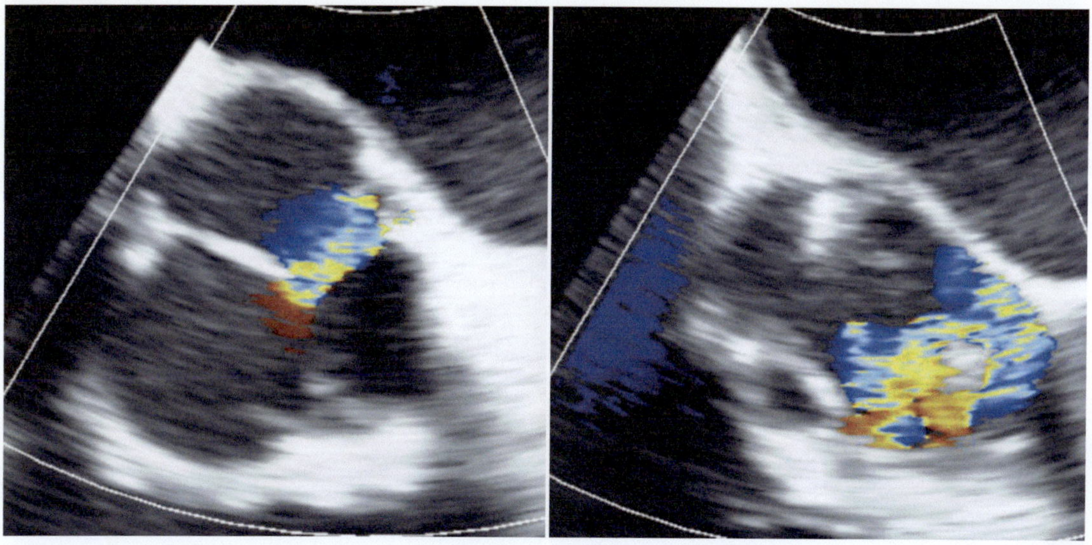

Fig. 3.6 (continued)

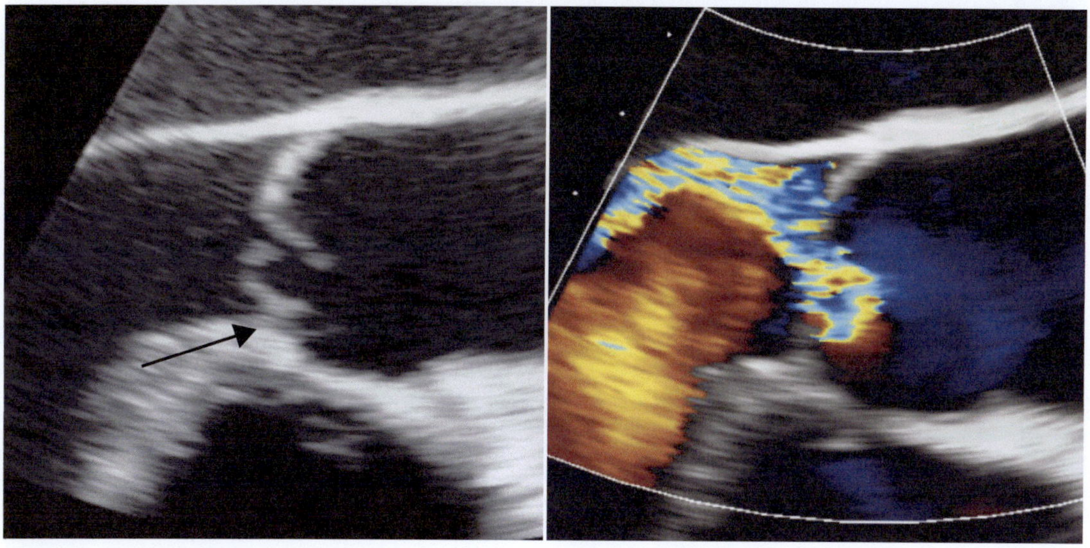

Fig. 3.7 Advanced AR due to bending. Bending can be observed in the prolapsing right coronary cusp (arrow). Regurgitation is directed toward the opposite side of the prolapsing right coronary cusp

3.3 Preoperative Assessment Before Aortic Valvuloplasty

As mentioned previously, it is important to identify the etiology of regurgitation in the assessment for aortic valvuloplasty. The geometric height is measured using 3-dimensional transesophageal echocardiography. The cross-section cutting each cusp orthogonally is extracted and measured from the hinge point to the cusp tip (Fig. 3.11). Long-term durable repair cannot be expected in patients with a geometric height below 16 mm in a tricuspid valve and below 19 mm in a non-fused cusp of a bicuspid valve [8]. Postoperative aortic stenosis will become concern in aortic valvuloplasty for a bicuspid valve, and therefore, the aortic valve area should be measured preoperatively. In the assessment of the aortic root, the diameters of the

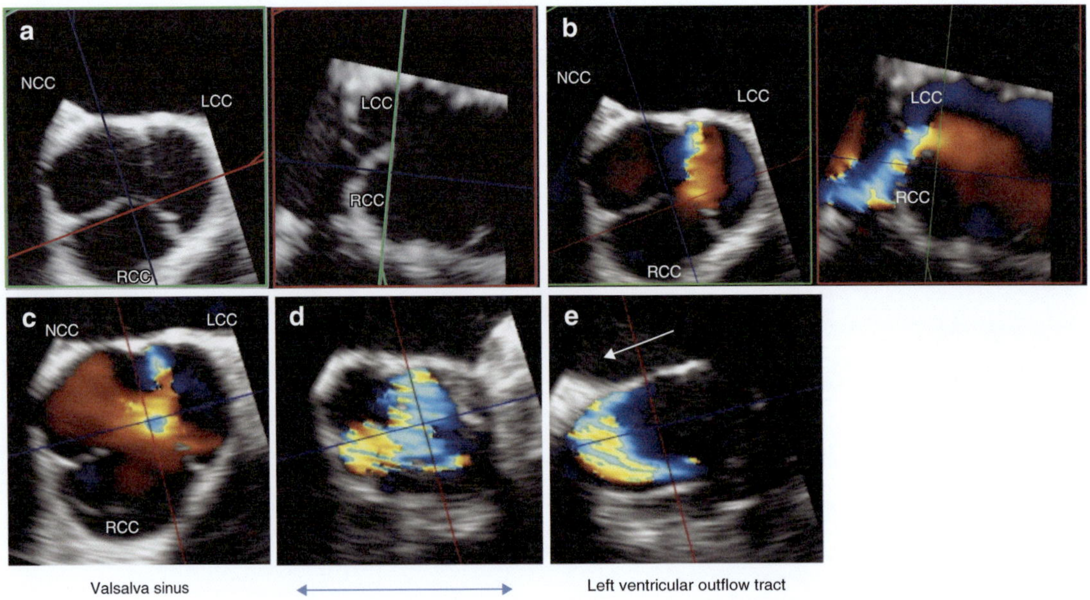

Fig. 3.8 Advanced AR due to left coronary cusp prolapse. (**a**, **b**) The long-axis view in the right image is derived from the reconstruction by cutting at the red line shown in the short-axis view on the left image. Deviation of the LCC height can be identified from the cross-sectional image across the LCC and RCC. (**c**–**e**) A short-axis view showing accelerated flow of the regurgitant jet in the direction of the left ventricular outflow tract is obtained by 3-dimensional imaging. The jet can be seen flowing toward the opposite side of the prolapsing LCC. *LCC* left coronary cusp, *NCC* non-coronary cusp, *RCC* right coronary cusp

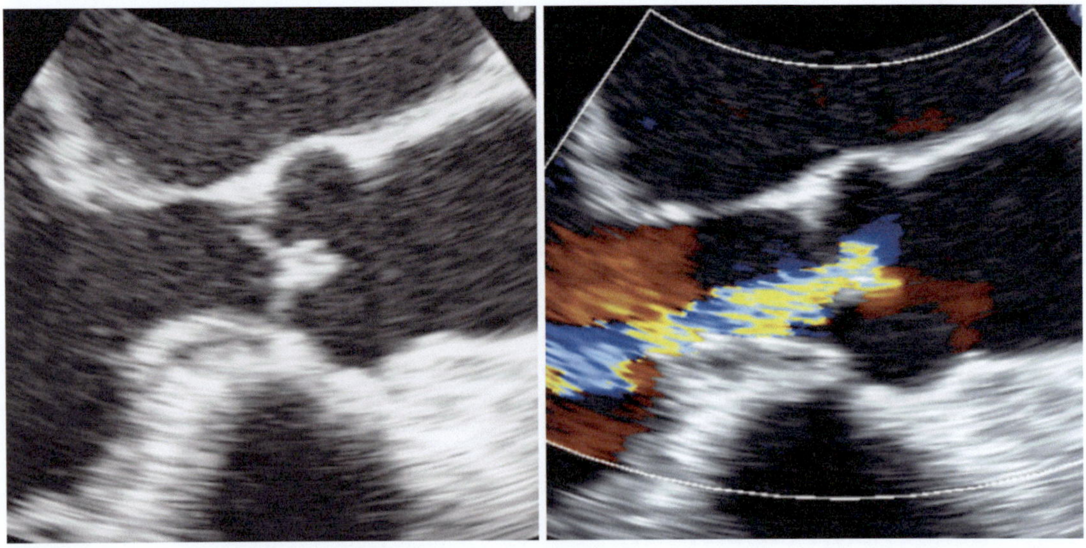

Fig. 3.9 Advanced AR due to rheumatic degeneration. Thickening and shortening of the cusps with rheumatic degeneration can be seen. Commissural fusions can also be seen in the short-axis view

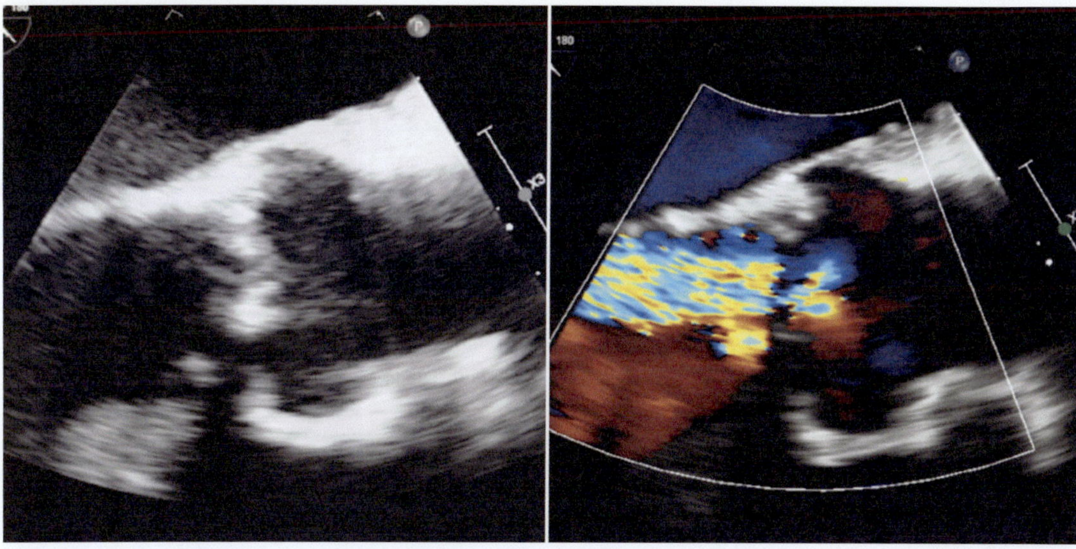

Fig. 3.10 Advanced AR due to senile degeneration. Thickening and shortening of the cusps with calcification can be seen, and aortic stenosis is also present

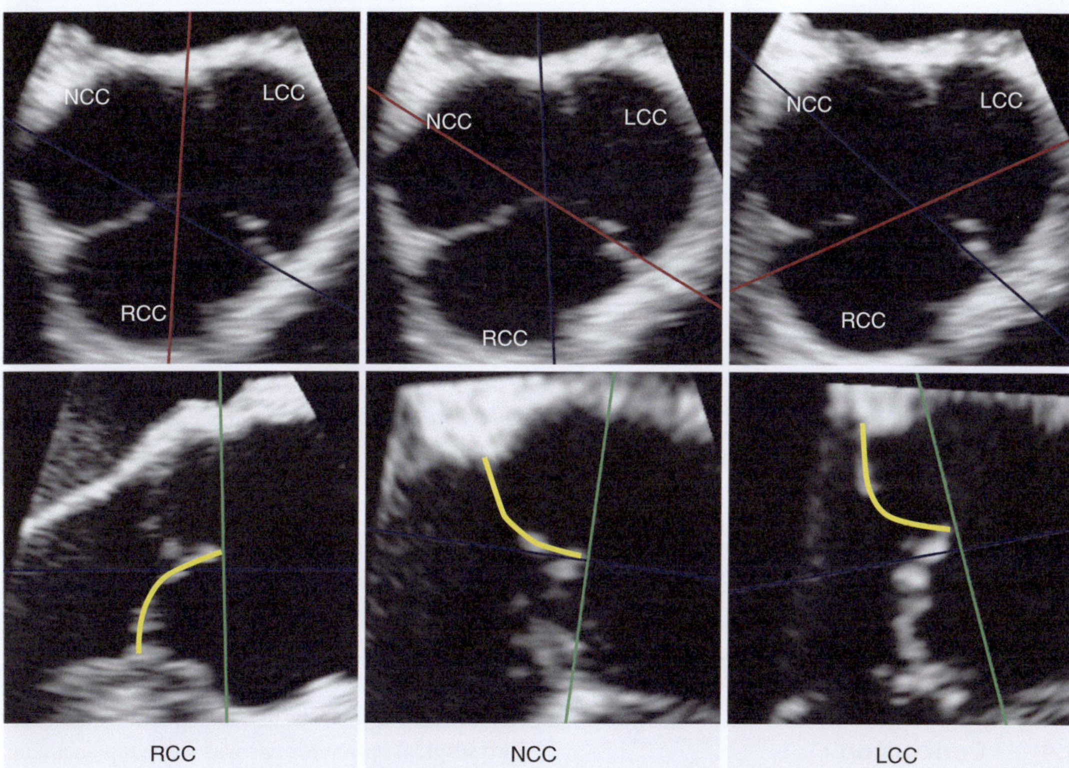

Fig. 3.11 Measurement of geometric height. The geometric height is measured by extracting the cross-section cutting of each cusp orthogonally (red lines). *LCC* left coronary cusp, *NCC* non-coronary cusp, *RCC* right coronary cusp

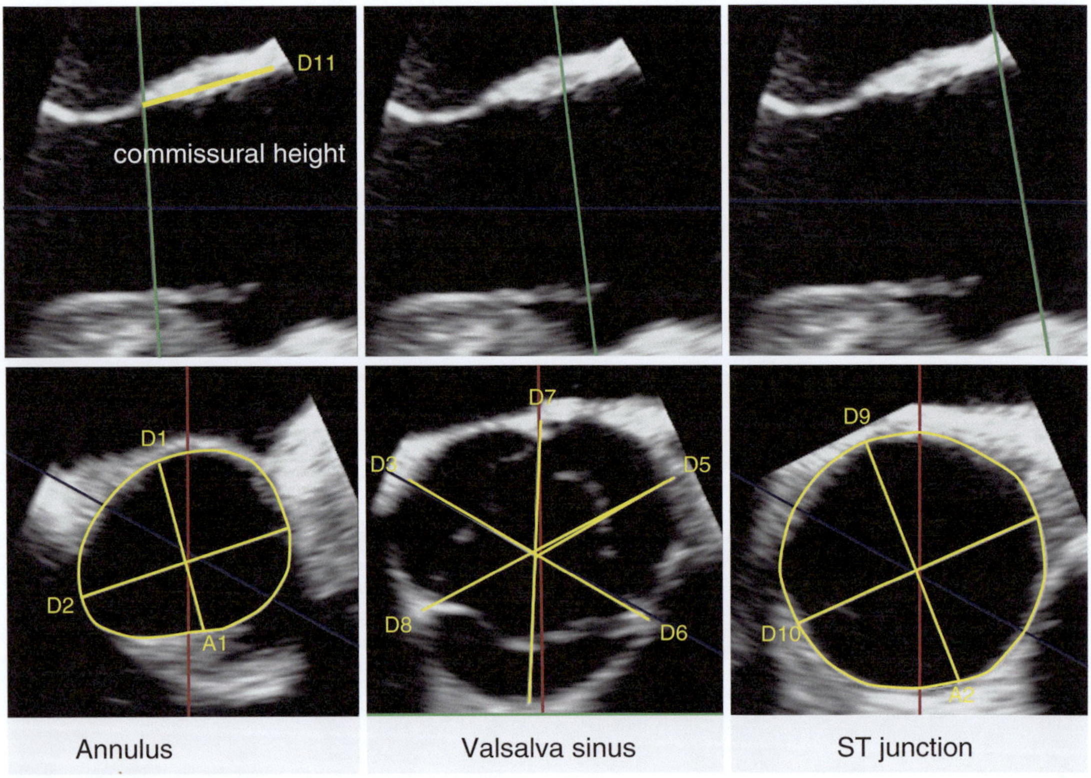

Fig. 3.12 Three-dimensional imaging measurement of the aortic root. Measurement is performed in the short-axis view by extracting the appropriate cross-section from a long-axis view

annulus, Valsalva sinus, and STJ should be measured by 3-dimensional transesophageal echocardiography (Fig. 3.12). In patients with associated aortic root enlargement, the natural curvature of the STJ can be lost and can be difficult to measure. In such cases, the STJ can be measured by finding the circular area where the bulge of the Valsalva sinus is lost in the short-axis view or by other landmarks such as the commissures or coronary artery ostia. Also, the commissural height, the length from the basal ring to the commissure between the left- and non-coronary cusp, should be measured. This data will be helpful in choosing the graft size for the aortic root reconstruction.

3.4 Conclusion

To plan aortic valvuloplasty, preoperative assessment using 3-dimensional transesophageal echocardiography is vital. First, the deviation of each cusp height is identified based on the direction of the regurgitant jet by 3-dimensional color Doppler imaging. When such deviation is documented, the cause is examined by carefully observing the cusp pathology and the commissural area. The presence of root enlargement is evaluated by investigating the degree and location of the enlargement at the annulus, Valsalva sinus, STJ, and ascending aorta. Basically, aortic valvuloplasty is feasible by reducing the size of the enlarged root, which results in enhancement of the cusp coaptation zone, followed by cusp plication to achieve an identical height for each cusp. Therefore, this operation can become difficult in patients without root enlargement or with insufficient cusp height. Previously, the etiology of AR was not discussed in detail as the standard surgical option for AR was valve replacement. However, identification of the pathological lesions that induce AR will play a key role in the success of aortic valvuloplasty similarly to the preoperative assessment for mitral valve repair.

References

1. Nishimura RA, Otto CM, Bonow RO, Carabello BA, Erwin JP 3rd, Guyton RA, ACC/AHA Task Force Members, et al. 2014 AHA/ACC Guideline for the Management of Patients with Valvular Heart Disease: executive summary: a report of the American College of Cardiology/American Heart Association Task Force on Practice Guidelines. Circulation. 2014;129:2440–92.
2. Baumgartner H, Falk V, Bax JJ, De Bonis M, Hamm C, Holm PJ, ESC Scientific Document Group, et al. 2017 ESC/EACTS Guidelines for the management of valvular heart disease. Eur Heart J. 2017;38:2739–91.
3. Aicher D, Fries R, Rodionycheva S, Schmidt K, Langer F, Schäfers HJ. Aortic valve repair leads to a low incidence of valve-related complications. Eur J Cardiothorac Surg. 2010;37:127–32.
4. Vohra HA, Whistance RN, De Kerchove L, Punjabi P, El Khoury G. Valve-preserving surgery on the bicuspid aortic valve. Eur J Cardiothorac Surg. 2013;43:888–98.
5. Arabkhani B, Mookhoek A, Di Centa I, Lansac E, Bekkers JA, De Lind Van Wijngaarden R, et al. Reported outcome after valve-sparing aortic root replacement for aortic root aneurysm: a systematic review and metaanalysis. Ann Thorac Surg. 2015;100:1126–31.
6. Lansac E, Di Centa I, Sleilaty G, Lejeune S, Khelil N, Berrebi A, et al. Long-term results of external aortic ring annuloplasty for aortic valve repair. Eur J Cardiothorac Surg. 2016;50:350–60.
7. Boodhwani M, de Kerchove L, Glineur D, Poncelet A, Rubay J, Astarci P, et al. Repair-oriented classification of aortic insufficiency: impact on surgical techniques and clinical outcomes. J Thorac Cardiovasc Surg. 2009;137:286–94.
8. Schäfers HJ, Schmied W, Marom G, Aicher D. Cusp height in aortic valves. J Thorac Cardiovasc Surg. 2013;146:269–74.

4 Computed Tomographic Measurements of Aortic Valves

Nobuo Iguchi

4.1 Introduction

Thus far, most aortic diagnostic imaging has relied on echocardiography; however, computed tomography (CT) has increasingly emerged as an efficient and essential modality, thanks to recent technological advances in CT systems and in workstation software. This chapter attempts to provide an overall comprehensive view of CT diagnosis and the framework of its effective application.

4.2 General Knowledge for CT Diagnosis

The CT Diagnostic Process

CT scanned images can be acquired in patients in whom the absence of contraindications such as renal failure or allergy to contrast media has been confirmed. Because the amount of contrast medium injected is relatively high, this author's facility uses the right median cubital vein to secure the injection route. Currently used machines can scan at high speeds, and thus, the scan time is short and, depending on the procedure, can be completed within 0.3 s, although the duration and amount of radiation exposure can vary depending on the scanning procedure (Fig. 4.1). Of note, procedures performed after determining the appropriate cardiac phase are the most time-consuming part of the procedure; they include the transfer of reconstructed images to a workstation and the display of multiple images.

Factors Associated with the Quality of CT Images

Not all diagnostic CT images are of high quality and comprehensible. Several critical factors, including heart rate, calcification, arrhythmias, and the amount of injected contrast medium, must be considered to obtain high-quality images, and "efficient" CT images can only be obtained when all of these critical factors are fulfilled.

Understanding Artifacts

Banding Artifact (Stair-Step Artifact)

Sometimes, the image appears to be stair-step like, and such an image is obtained when the patient's R-R interval is not constant. Precise observation is not possible with this type of image, and thus proper attention must be paid to avoid such images.

Blooming Artifact (Partial Volume Effect)

This refers to the enlargement of a scanned object with high Hounsfield unit (HU) values [1]. This

N. Iguchi (✉)
Department of Cardiology, Sakakibara Heart Institute, Tokyo, Japan
e-mail: niguchi@shi.heart.or.jp

T. Kunihara, S. Takanashi (eds.), *Aortic Valve Preservation*,
https://doi.org/10.1007/978-981-13-2068-2_4

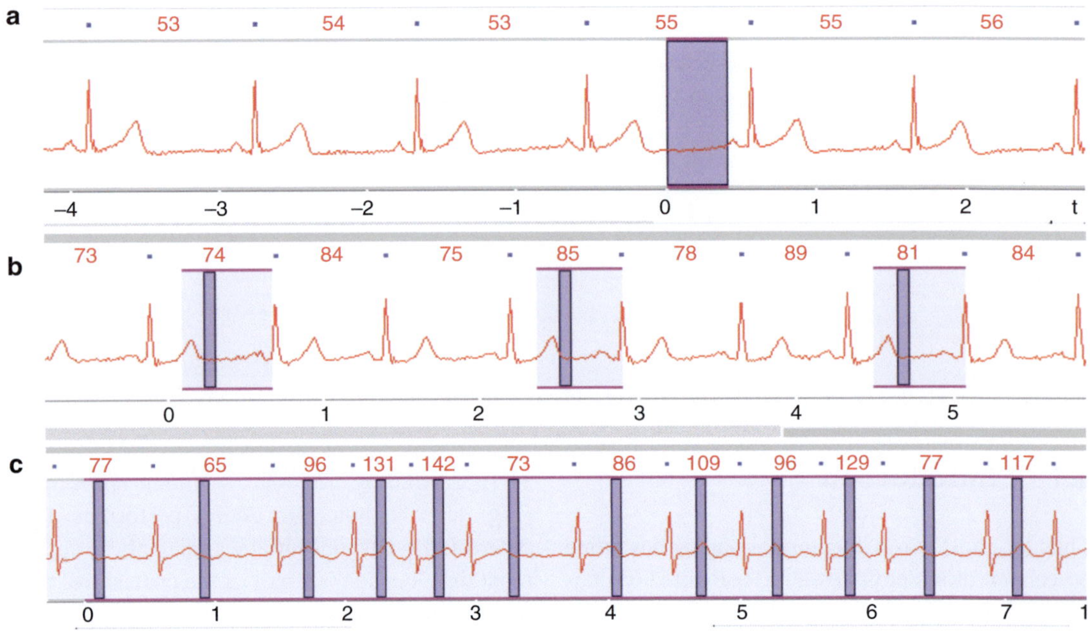

Fig. 4.1 CT scanning procedure and cardiac phase. Two types of prospective ECG gating are used during which (**a**) radiation exposure is delivered for only one cardiac phase per heartbeat and (**b**) repetitive radiation exposure is delivered over several heartbeats to obtain data for one cardiac phase. Also, retrospective ECG gating involves (**c**) obtaining total phases or relatively long scans of cardiac phases by delivering exposure over several heartbeats and then reconstructing the entire cardiac phase; however, the amount of exposure will be the highest

can be seen mostly in patients with high amounts of calcification and is conspicuous in CT systems with low spatial resolution.

Beam-Hardening Effect

This phenomenon occurs when the area surrounding an object with a high CT value is cast in a shadow. This effect may lead to underestimation during the diagnosis, and thus, careful diagnosis is required when such images are used [2].

CT Image Display Procedures

Volume Rendering

This technique can provide comprehensive, highly realistic images. However, such images cannot be used for measurement because, depending on the settings used, the image may be different than the actual morphology (Fig. 4.2).

Multi-Planar Reconstruction (MPR)

This technique is applied to the assessment of the degree of severity of stenoses in the coronary arteries, and it is the most appropriate technique for quantitative assessment. A MPR image of an aortic valve is shown in Fig. 4.3.

Maximum Intensity Projection

This technique is used to display the object with the highest CT value from a certain direction, and it can imitate invasive coronary angiography (Fig. 4.4).

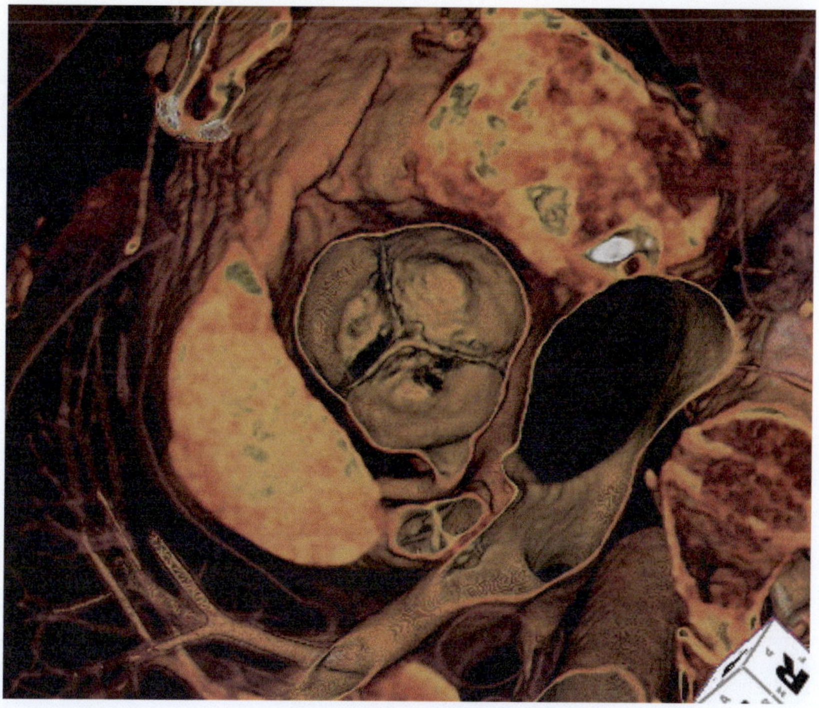

Fig. 4.2 Volume rendering display procedure. Postoperative aortic valves after an aortic root remodeling procedure by volume rendering imaging show that the anatomical relationship with surrounding tissues can be clearly observed

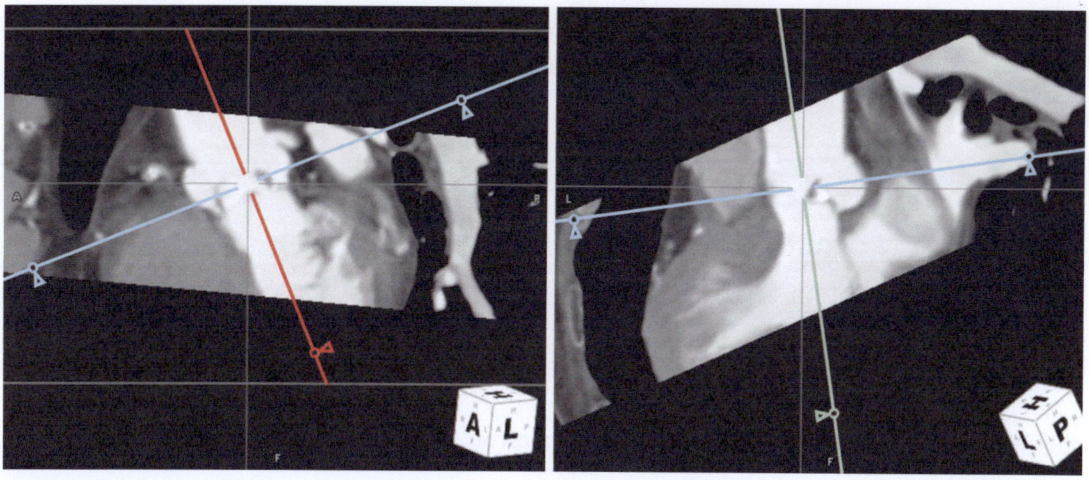

Fig. 4.3 Multi-planar reconstruction (MPR) display procedure. The movement of the aortic valves is displayed by MPR imaging, which is generally applied for the measurement of aortic sizing parameters

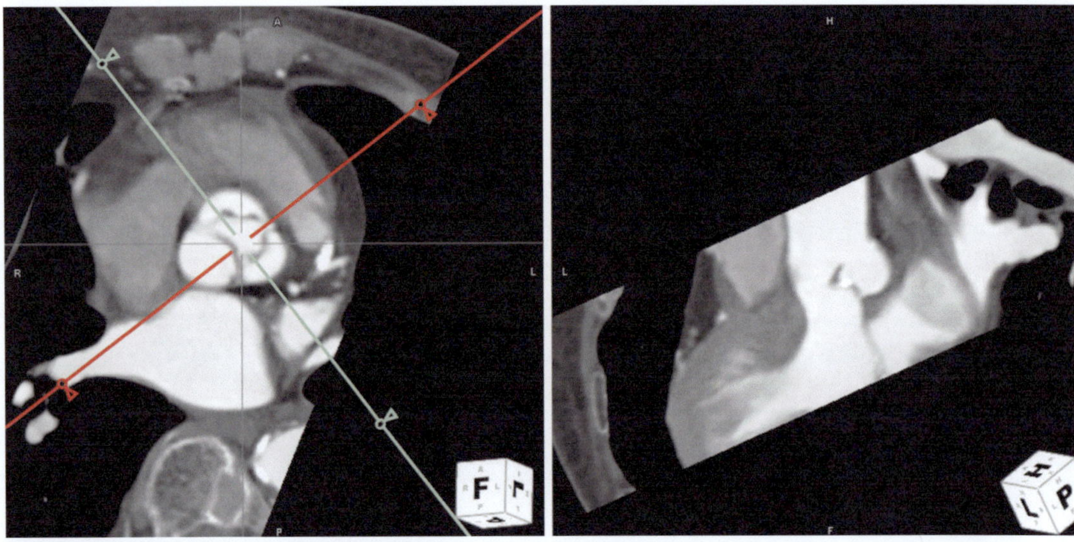

Fig. 4.3 (continued)

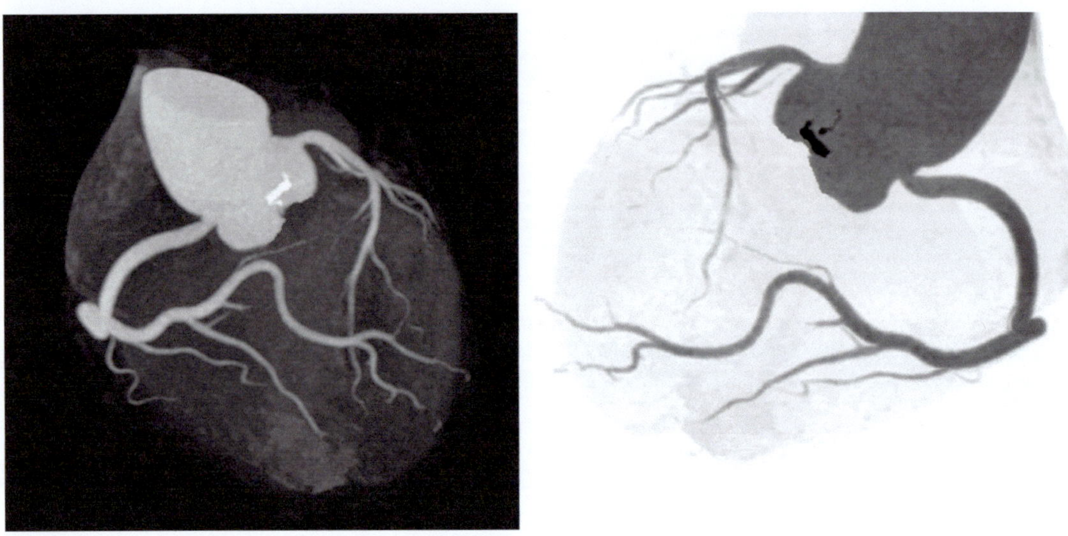

Fig. 4.4 Maximum intensity projection display procedure. Maximum intensity projection imaging can display images that imitate invasive coronary angiography and efficiently visualize calcification, which, when the image is converted into a 3D image, enables the easy assessment of aortic root calcification

4.3 Aortic Valve Scanning Procedure (Scanning Apparatus, Scanning Timing, and Image Reconstruction Procedure)

Scanning Equipment

Aortic valves move rapidly. Thus, high temporal resolution (high shutter speed) is required to observe and measure them. Temporal resolution depends on the rotational speed of the gantry, and a dual-source detector type is advantageous compared to the single-source type. To supplement inferior aspects of hardware by software, it may be necessary to devise a reconstruction method to increase temporal resolution. Also, to decrease motion artifacts, it is important to consider such aspects as securing the thoracic area with bands and having the patient practice proper breath-holding techniques.

Imaging and Reconstruction Procedures

To create high-quality CT images, determination of the appropriate cardiac phase is required. Procedures include determining the optimal phase before scanning by aiming for the end-diastolic phase, for example, by using prospective ECG gating, and, alternatively, determining the optimal phase after scanning (retrospective ECG gating). To decrease the radiation dose, the former protocol is appropriate, but in cases in which both the systolic and diastolic phases need to be scanned, the latter protocol must be used. At the author's facility, retrospective ECG gating is essentially applied in cases of aortic valve assessment, and 4-dimensional (4D) imaging is provided if necessary. However, to decrease the amount of radiation exposure, we use a lower tube voltage and high-sensitivity detector or an iterative reconstruction algorithm.

4.4 Measurements Required for Aortic Valve Surgery

Until now, structural assessment and observation of aortic valves was mainly carried out with echocardiography. However, as the performance of transcatheter aortic valve implantation (TAVI) has increased, CT measurements of the aorta and aortic valve are now regarded as essential.

Standard Measurement Criteria

The diameters of the aortic annulus, sinus of Valsalva, sinotubular junction (STJ), and ascending aorta are required. Normally, it is ideal to use the imaging plane that it is perpendicular to the axis of the aorta for these measurements (Fig. 4.5). Furthermore, in the case of TAVI, there is a procedure for measurement of the aortic annulus diameter that is recommended based on expert consensus

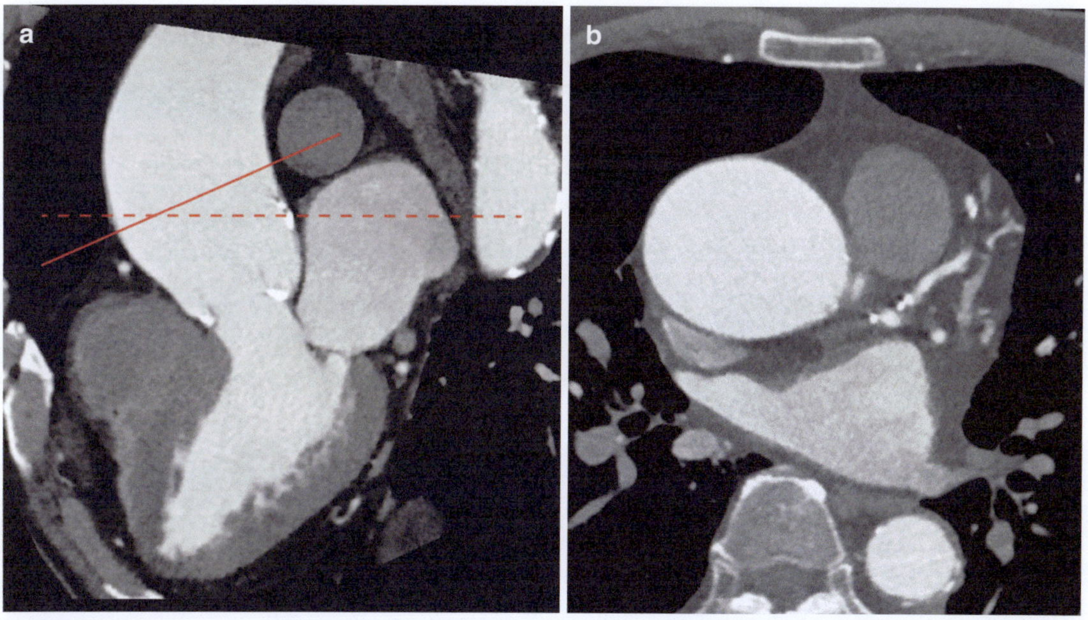

Fig. 4.5 Measurement of aortic diameter. Measurement of the aortic diameter is required when preparing for surgery. However, (**a**) when measuring the diameter of an enlarged ascending aorta, it is ideal to obtain the cross-sectional plane that is perpendicular to the aortic axis. (**b**) The minimum diameter of the aorta cannot be measured but can be overestimated during normal assessment via axial imaging

from the Society of Cardiovascular Computed Tomography [3]. The annulus, which is the narrowest part of the aortic root, consists of a virtual basal ring connecting the hinge points of the three leaflets. Measurement is carried out by determining the hinge point of each leaflet by using the transverse section, sagittal section, and coronal section acquired by MPR and tracing the annulus after confirming the hinge points (Fig. 4.6). The annulus diameter is estimated by measuring the major and minor axes of this virtual basal ring along with the circumferential length and area. However, the tracing procedure is difficult and can vary between measurers. Therefore, to eliminate inter-observer error, the full width at half maximum procedure for tracing the annulus is recommended (Fig. 4.7). The annulus is not a perfect

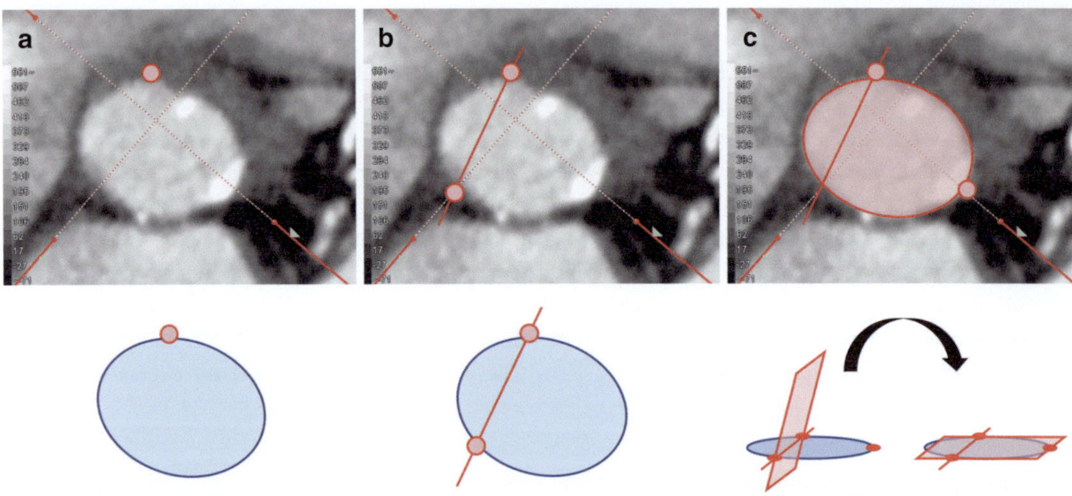

Fig. 4.6 Measurement of annulus diameter by application of MPR imaging. Preoperative measurement of the annulus diameter is essential, especially for TAVI. The method for determining the aortic annular plane including the hinge points of the three leaflets is shown. First, (**a**) the hinge point of one of the leaflets is determined; then (**b**) the line that passes through the hinge point of another leaflet is determined; and finally, (**c**) the plane including the hinge point of the third leaflet is determined and the annulus is traced following this plane

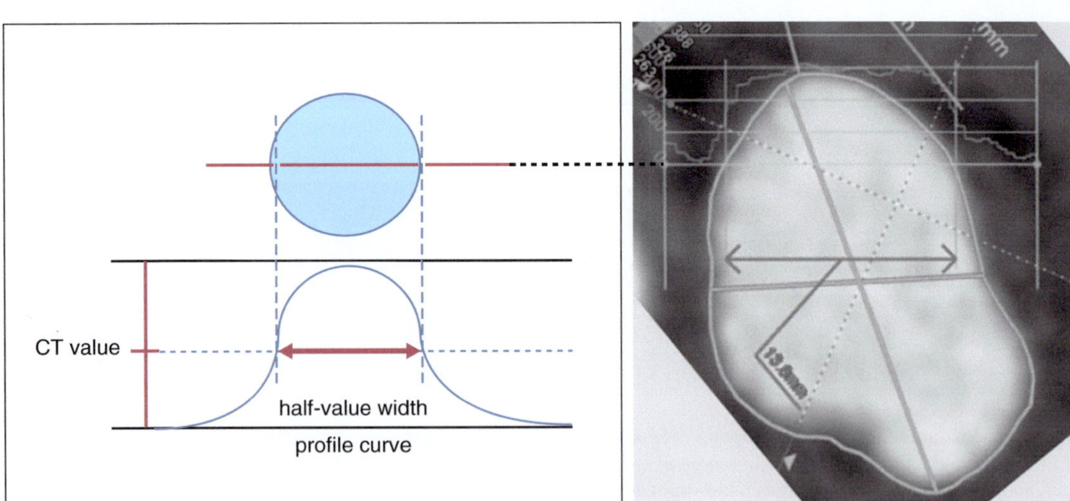

Fig. 4.7 Tracing procedure using the half-value width. The contrast and brightness of MPR imaging may be affected by the window level, and traces may vary among different analyzers. Therefore, the full width at half maximum procedure is recommended

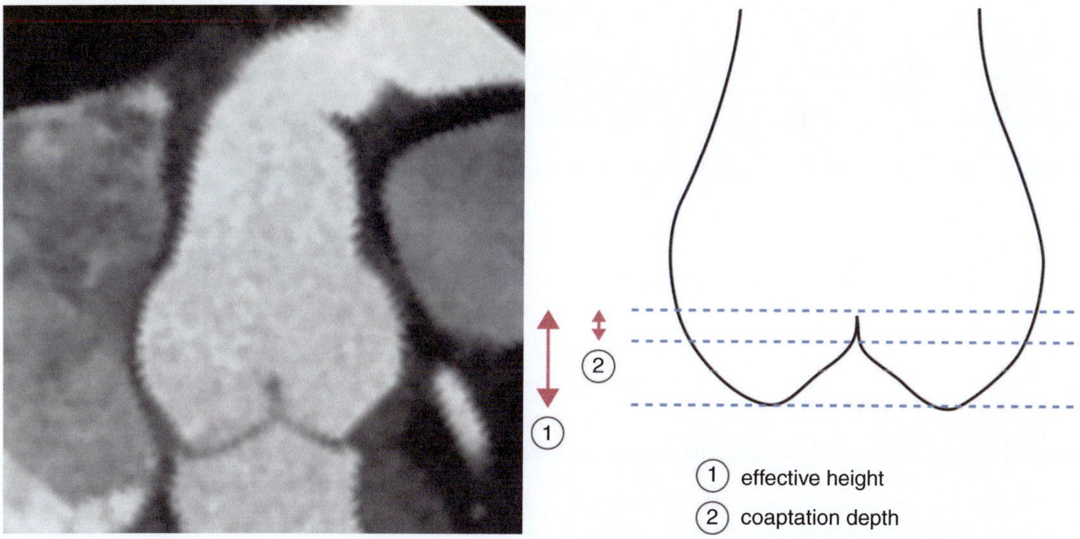

Fig. 4.8 Postoperative MPR CT imaging after an aortic root remodeling procedure and geometric measurement of the leaflets

circle but is an ellipse, and its shape becomes the largest and the closest to a perfect circle in the early systolic phase. For this reason, the image from the systolic phase is needed to measure the maximum annulus diameter. However, in the case of aortic regurgitation, it is essential to obtain a structural assessment and measurements in the diastolic phase, and therefore, as mentioned earlier, the retrospective gating procedure should be used. Furthermore, images must be obtained from the optimal cardiac phase depending on the purpose. Measurements of the sinus of Valsalva and the diameter of the STJ are similarly performed. Because the size of the three cusps is different, there is no correct way to measure the diameter of the sinus of Valsalva, and we use the cross-sectional image obtained at the highest valvular leaflet to measure the diameter of the STJ.

Determination of Effective Height and Coaptation Depth

The measurements of effective height and coaptation depth are essential for aortic valve repair, and these measurements are possible by applying MPR imaging in the longitudinal direction of each cusp after determining the basal ring. Especially, MPR is considered essential as a predictive factor for postoperative durability [4] and is also used for postoperative CT assessment (Fig. 4.8). In contrast, the leaflet size (length) is highly important for valve-sparing aortic root replacement such as aortic root remodeling surgery, but in which the size of each leaflet generally differs. The diameter of the deepest part of the leaflet can be used as a parameter for sizing the leaflets; however, this is impossible to show using only one 2D MPR image because aortic valves are generally tricuspid valves. Therefore, we tend to use three separate MPR images to confirm the maximum leaflet length for each leaflet (Fig. 4.9).

4.5 3D and 4D Imaging

Generally, 4D images are not applied to cardiac CT imaging. However, the impact of 4D-CT imaging though recent innovations in the spatial and temporal resolution of CT scanning is considered to be enormous (Fig. 4.10). To prepare 4D images, the data for one cardiac cycle is required. Thus, the increase in radiation exposure and the amount of data obtained arise as problems. To reduce the dose of radiation exposure, it is now possible to scan at a much lower exposure level

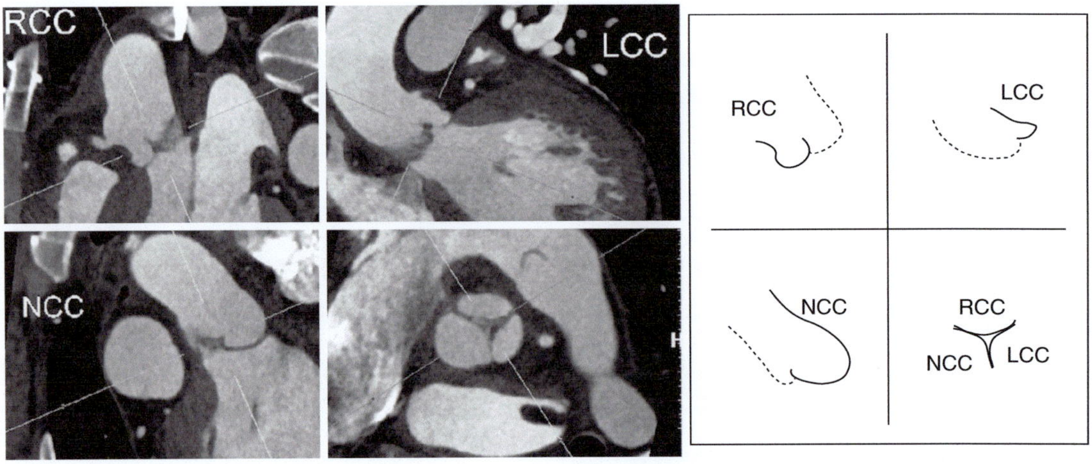

Fig. 4.9 Preoperative measurement of leaflet length in a case of aortic regurgitation with leaflet prolapse. It is difficult to obtain the plane enabling the measurement of leaflet length that passes the deepest part of each leaflet of the tricuspid valve. At our facility, three MPR images that pass through the deepest part of each leaflet are provided. *RCC* right coronary cusp, *LCC* left coronary cusp, *NCC* non-coronary cusp

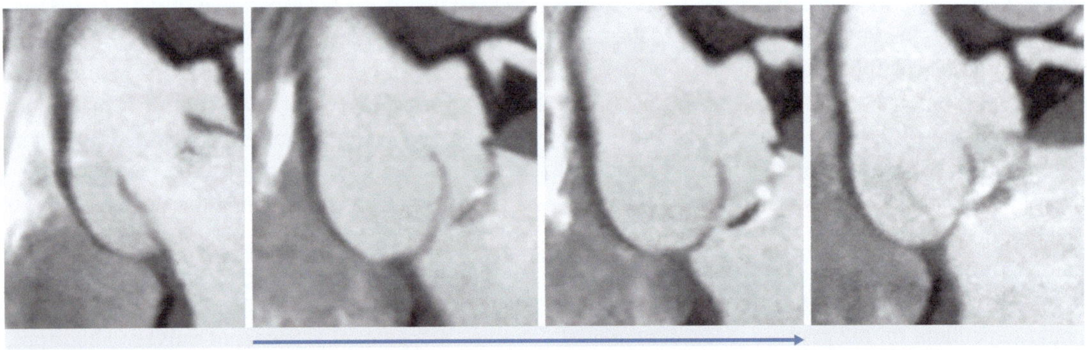

Fig. 4.10 A 4D image using MPR imaging in a case of aortic regurgitation due to bicuspid valve prolapse. The actual movement and flexibility of the leaflets are easier to observe when viewed with 4D imaging

than ever before thanks to improvements in reconstruction techniques gained by an iterative algorithm and the breakthrough development of high-sensitivity detectors. Also, considering the importance of performing safer surgeries with high accuracy, higher-precision 4D imaging should be aggressively applied. Furthermore, new software has recently been developed that can enable not only smooth 4D images prepared by editing with the software but also even clearer 4D images through recent noise reduction technologies. Although the title of this chapter relates to CT measurement, visual diagnosis of the precise movement of the aortic valves in one cardiac cycle and the surrounding environment is considered to be equal to or more important than the measurements themselves. Additionally, adapting voxel-tracking technology allows the quantitative evaluation of movement, and our facility is intending to quantitatively evaluate the changes in the area and diameter of the annulus during one cardiac cycle (Fig. 4.11). With this method, display of the elasticity of the tissue in a quantitative manner is expected.

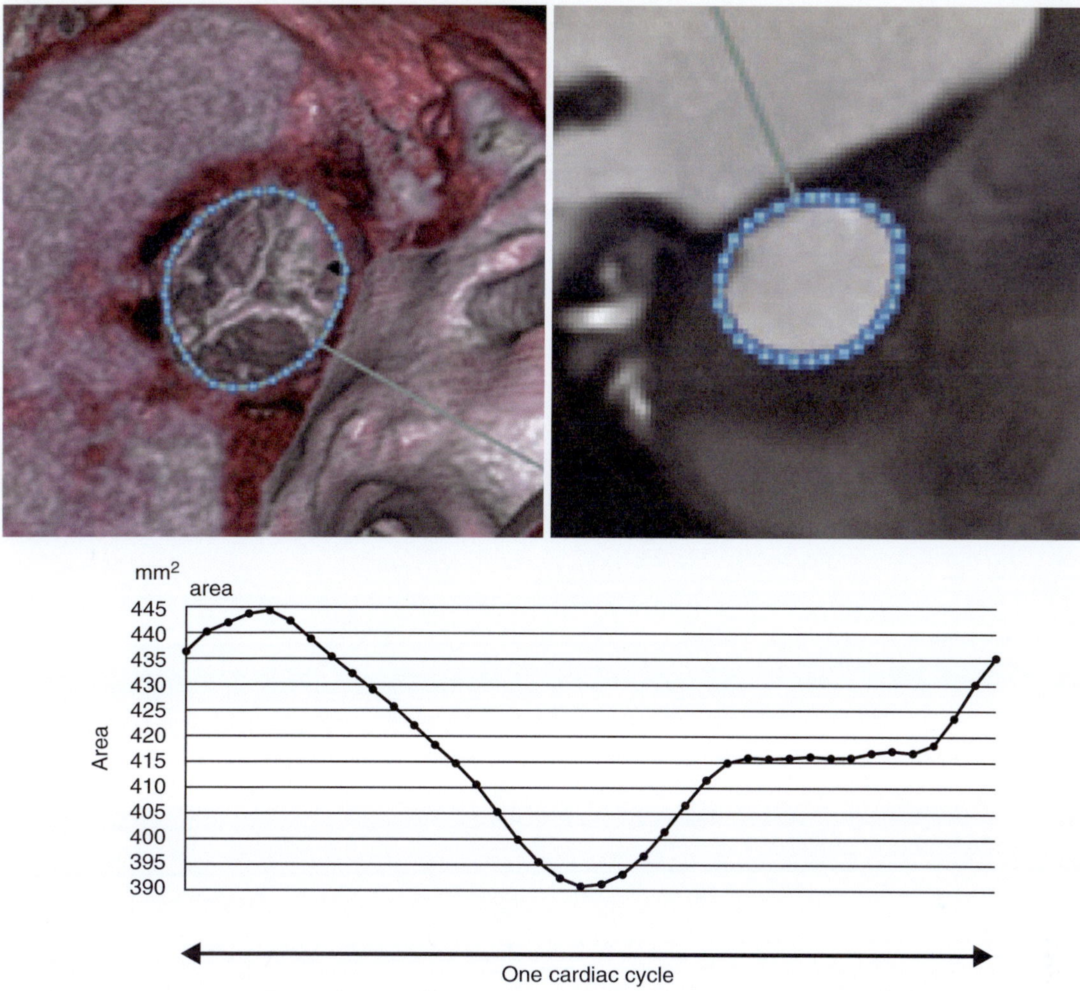

Fig. 4.11 Changes in the annular ring during the cardiac cycle. Use of the voxel tracking method enables dynamic evaluation of the annulus during one cardiac cycle

4.6 Conclusion

In this chapter, we described the usefulness of 3D-CT measurement to perform aortic valvuloplasty. Especially, positive application of 4D imaging will lead to further analysis of physiological aortic valve motion and the surrounding structures 3-dimensionally and dynamically, and it is expected that this method will become a necessary tool for surgeons. Also, the realization of "preoperative simulation by CT" in the future is expected if image processing on the workstation becomes easier with further innovations in imaging technology.

References

1. Hoffman EJ, Huang SC, Phelps ME. Quantitation in positron emission computed tomography: 1. Effect of object size. J Comput Assist Tomogr. 1979;3:299–308.
2. Joseph PM, Spital RD. The effects of scatter in x-ray computed tomography. Med Phys. 1982;9:464–72.
3. Achenbach S, Delgado V, Hausleiter J, Schoenhagen P, Min JK, Leipsic JA. SCCT expert consensus document on computed tomography imaging before transcatheter aortic valve implantation (TAVI)/ transcatheter aortic valve replacement (TAVR). J Cardiovasc Comput Tomogr. 2012;6:366–80.
4. Pethig K, Milz A, Hagl C, Harringer W, Haverich A. Aortic valve reimplantation in ascending aortic aneurysm: risk factors for early valve failure. Ann Thorac Surg. 2002;73:29–33.

5 ONE-POINT ADVICE: Optimizing Aortic Valve Repair Techniques with Computational Models

Gil Marom, Karin Lavon, Rami Haj-Ali, and Ehud Raanani

5.1 Background

During aortic valve repair procedures, surgeons improve the function of the valve by modifying its anatomy. Such improvements are aimed at achieving sufficient coaptation area and effective height, two parameters that were identified as indicators for the long-term function of repaired aortic valves [1]. Valve-sparing procedures, in which the aneurysmatic aortic root is replaced with a graft while retaining the native valve, give surgeons the freedom to choose both the sinotubular and aortoventricular sizes and the height of the commissures [2]. Other types of valve repairs that involve cusp interventions also directly influence the final anatomy of the cusps. The size of the cusp needs to be chosen for various valve types and prolapse corrections [3], and the desired inter-commissural angle of the bicuspid aortic valve (BAV) should be decided during reimplantation [4] and sinus plication [5] procedures. Numerical models can be used as a predictive tool to estimate the mechanical performance of valves with various geometrical configurations. In this chapter, we review our numerical studies of aortic valve repair techniques and the clinically relevant conclusions that they provide.

5.2 Physical and Numerical Models

Various geometries of tricuspid aortic valves and roots were reconstructed using parametric geometric relationships [6] and were based on mechanical models that simulated the stretching of the leaflets and root. Figure 5.1 shows 16 geometries from one of the parametric studies with aortoventricular annulus diameters (d_{AVA}) between 22 and 28 mm and sinotubular diameters (d_{STJ}) between $0.8{\cdot}d_{AVA}$ and $1.4{\cdot}d_{AVA}$ [7]. Similar methods were used to generate geometries for various cusp sizes by modifying the geometric height (h_G), i.e., the length of the cusp symmetry line [8]. The BAV cases were created with asymmetric cusps and sinuses, and the fused cusps were created by connecting the two smaller identical cusps [9]. These described geometries were used as the initial configurations of the valve and root by assuming that the tissues were stress free and that the aortoventricular and sinotubular annuli were stationary. The mechanical models

G. Marom (✉) · K. Lavon · R. Haj-Ali
Faculty of Engineering, School of Mechanical Engineering, Tel Aviv University, Tel Aviv, Israel
e-mail: maromgil@tau.ac.il

E. Raanani
Cardiac Surgery and Leviev Cardiothoracic and Vascular Center, Sheba Medical Center, Tel Hashomer, Israel

T. Kunihara, S. Takanashi (eds.), *Aortic Valve Preservation*, https://doi.org/10.1007/978-981-13-2068-2_5

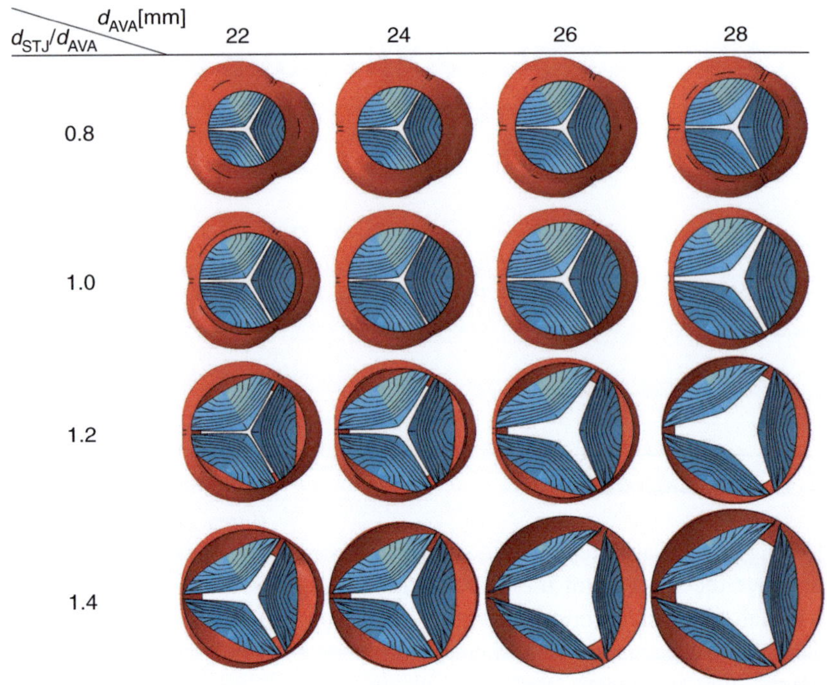

Fig. 5.1 Views from the aorta of the 16 representative geometries of models with various values of d_{AVA} and d_{STJ}. (Adapted from Marom et al. [7] with permission)

included collagen fibers to represent the anisotropic tissue. A non-frictional contact was defined between the cusps. The meshes of the tissue parts contained more than 14,000 elements in each of the models. Physiologic pressure waveforms were employed at the left ventricular and ascending aorta boundaries. The blood domain was discretized with a mesh of approximately 700,000 cells, and dynamic mesh refinement was used near the walls. The structural problem was solved by finite element analysis in Abaqus (Simulia, Providence, RI, USA), and FlowVision (Capvidia, Leuven, Belgium) was the flow solver and managed the coupling between the codes.

5.3 Effect of Cusp Size on Coaptation and Mechanical Stress

The influence of cusp size was evaluated by comparing valves with h_G between 15.4 and 18.9 mm [8]. Cross-sections of the deformed valves in their diastolic positions (Fig. 5.2) show that the coaptation height (h_C) increases with the increase of h_G. A comparison of mechanical stresses showed that the common case (h_G = 16.2 mm) had the lowest stress levels, whereas the case with the smallest h_G, in which the valve was not fully closed, had the highest levels. The effective height (h_E), defined as the vertical distance between the midpoint of the free edge and the aortoventricular annulus, and the average coaptation height ($\overline{h}_C$), defined as the coaptation area to free edge length ratio, were calculated for each case. The graphs in Fig. 5.2 show that both h_E and $\overline{h}_C$ increase with h_G. Also, the common case has higher h_E and $\overline{h}_C$ values than can be expected from the other cases.

5.4 Effect of Aortoventricular Diameter on Coaptation and Mechanical Stress

Six additional cases with d_{AVA} between 20 and 30 mm, but with the same d_{STJ} and h_G values (26.4 and 16.2 mm, respectively), were compared [10]. The cross-sections in Fig. 5.3 show that h_C decreases with the increase of d_{AVA} and that the partially opened valves ($d_{AVA} \geq 28$ mm) are prolapsed into the ventricle with a distinctive 'belly

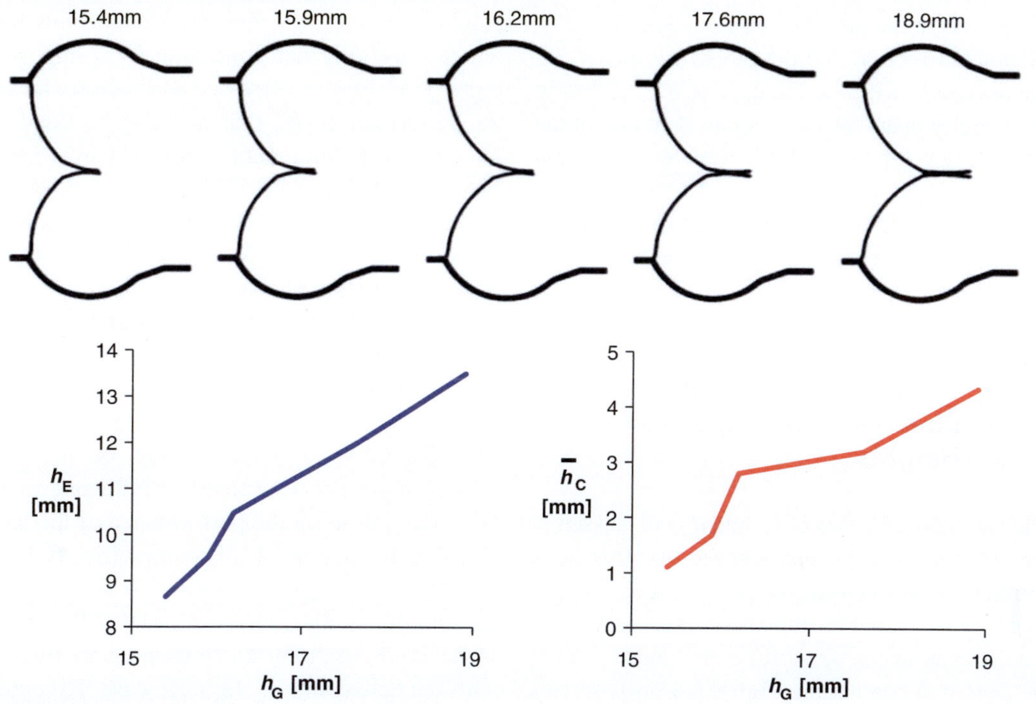

Fig. 5.2 Top: Cross-sections of diastolic aortic valves with various values of h_G. The valve is not closed in the 15.4-mm valve, even though this view does not depict this fact. Bottom: h_E and $\bar{h}_C$ as a function of h_G. (Adapted from Marom et al. [8] with permission)

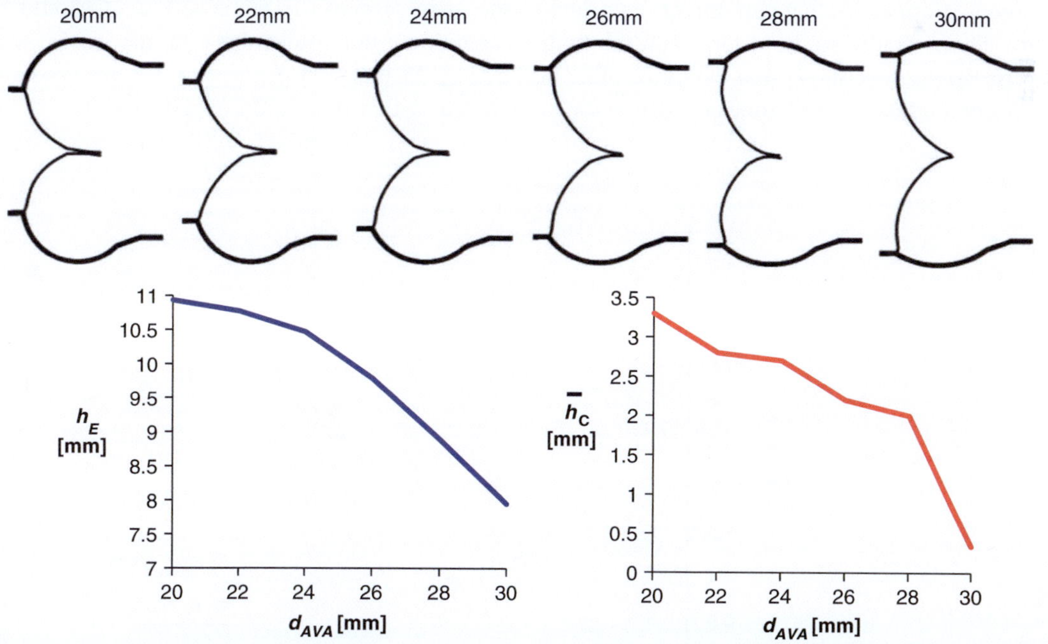

Fig. 5.3 Top: Cross-sections of diastolic aortic valves with various values of d_{AVA}. The valves with $d_{AVJ} \geq 28$ mm are not closed, even though this view does not depict this fact. Bottom: h_E and $\bar{h}_C$ as a function of d_{AVA}. (Adapted from Marom et al. [10] with permission)

region'. As in the previous section, there is a correlation between h_E and the global parameter $\bar{h}_C$ that decreases with the increase of d_{AVA}. Stress in the partially open valves is higher than that in the fully closed valves on both the free edge and symmetry lines, whereas the model with a d_{AVA} of 22 mm has the lowest magnitude of stress. For all cases, the highest stress level is found on the free edge near the commissures.

5.5 Correlation Between Effective and Coaptation Heights

The parametric studies of h_G and d_{AVA} discussed in the two previous sections showed that there is a correlation between h_E and $\bar{h}_C$. Because h_E can be easily measured during valve repair surgeries, this correlation can be useful in helping to predict the degree of coaptation. Figure 5.4 presents this relationship between $\bar{h}_C$ and h_E in all ten models presented in the above sections along with their linear correlation [8]. The three cases with $h_E < 9$ mm, in which the valves were not fully closed, exhibited regurgitation and were exposed to higher stress levels that can impair their durability. These results are in accord with the findings of Bierbach et al. [1] that the range of h_E in the normal adult is 7–12 mm and that 96% of patients with moderate or severe aortic insufficiency had an $h_E < 9$ mm. The conclusions from our findings are that improving h_E during valve repair may lead to increased coaptation and better performance and that this can be done not only by cusp intervention but also by focused reduction of d_{AVA}.

5.6 Optimization of the Sinotubular Junction to Aortoventricular Diameters Ratio

The previous parametric study of d_{AVA} was expanded to also examine the influence of the d_{STJ} to d_{AVA} ratio on the performance of the valve [7]. The 16 models of this parametric study are presented in Fig. 5.1. Similar to the previous parametric studies, cross-sections of the diastolic configurations are presented in Fig. 5.5 with the calculated $\bar{h}_C$ for each case. Except for the case with d_{STJ}/d_{AVA} = 1.2, the cases with d_{AVA} = 24 mm have the largest $\bar{h}_C$ relative to the other cases with equal d_{STJ}/d_{AVA}. In addition, $\bar{h}_C$ increases with the decrease of d_{STJ}/d_{AVA} for $d_{AVA} \geq 24$ mm but not for $d_{AVA} = 22$ mm, in which the cusp prolapse is more severe. It should be mentioned that the valves in the cases with $d_{AVA} \geq 26$ mm and $d_{STJ}/d_{AVA} \geq 1.2$ are not fully closed, a fact that could explain the low $\bar{h}_C$ in these cases. The models in this parametric study

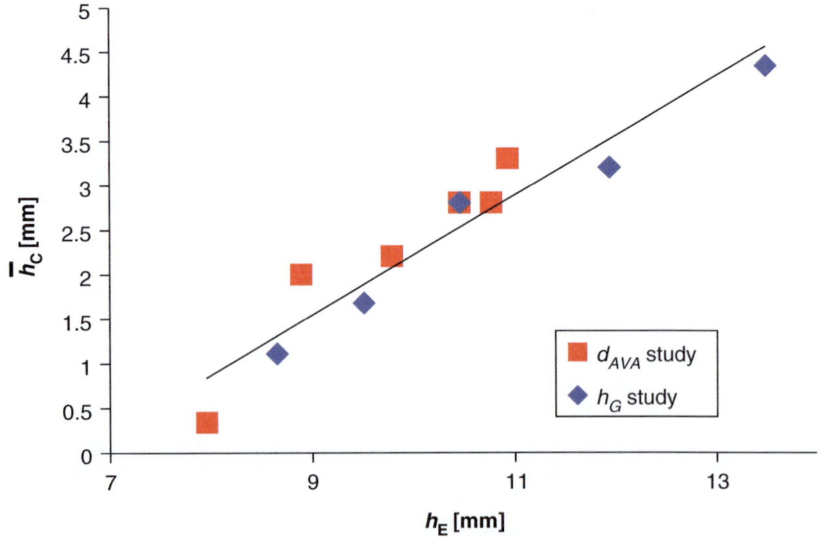

Fig. 5.4 $\bar{h}_C$ as a function of h_E. (Adapted from Marom et al. [8] with permission)

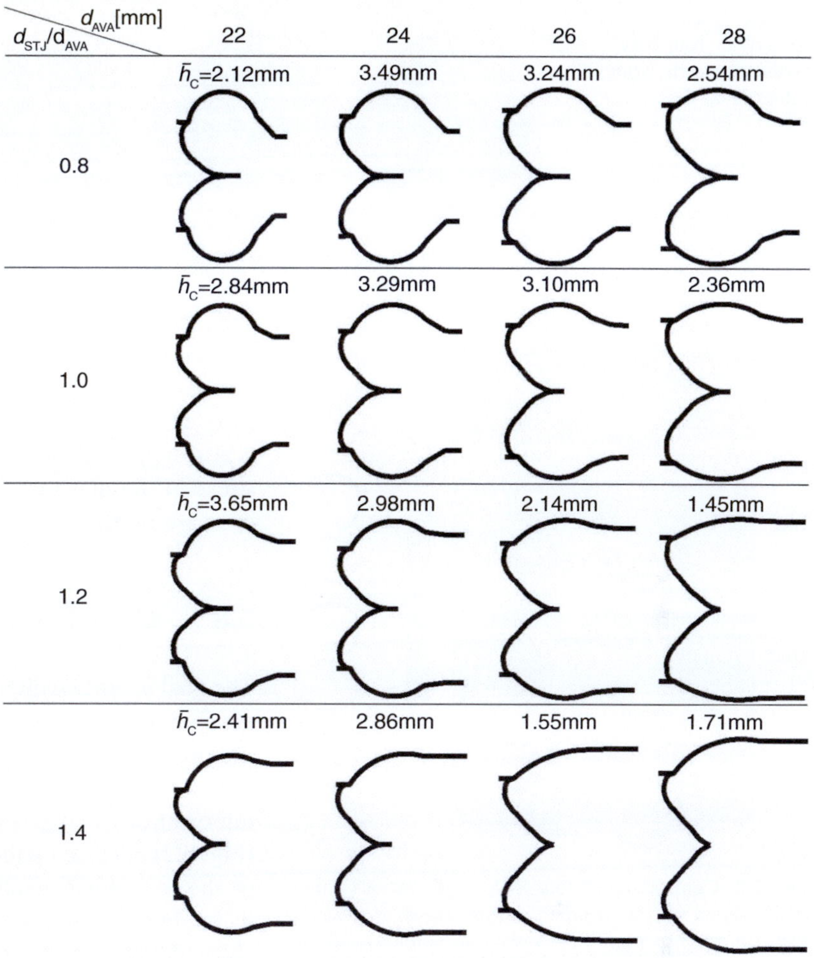

Fig. 5.5 Cross-sections of diastolic aortic valves with various values of d_{AVA} and d_{STJ}/d_{AVA}. The valves with $d_{AVA} \geq 26$ mm and $d_{STJ}/d_{AVA} \geq 1.2$ are not closed, even though this view does not demonstrate this fact. The $\bar{h}_C$ is marked above each cross-section. (Adapted from Marom et al. [7] with permission)

included fiber bundles that were not accounted for in the previously described studies, and maximum magnitudes of stress were found in these fibers. In the cases in which the valves were not fully closed, the fibers carry even larger stress relative to their surroundings. The five cases with the 'best' coaptation ($\bar{h}_C > 3$ mm) have similar distributions of stress and magnitudes.

5.7 Effect of Inter-Commissural Angle in BAVs on Valve Functionality

In this section, four models of BAV with fused cusps (type 1) and an inter-commissural angle (θ_{IC}) between 120° and 180° were compared. Figure 5.6 shows the initial geometries of the four models. Unlike the models presented in the previous section, the collagen fiber bundles that were used here are based on an averaged network map from porcine valves [11]. The effect of θ_{IC} on the flow regime is shown in the left column of Fig. 5.7 for the instance of peak systole. The jet flow is affected by the shape and location of the valve opening. In the 120° case, the opening is wider but is located closer to the non-fused sinus. This asymmetry leads to a jet flow that is directed toward the non-fused sinus. Larger θ_{IC} have narrower elliptic openings (the so-called 'fish-mouth'), but they are located closer to the center of the root and the jet is not directed towards the aortic walls. Although the jets in larger θ_{IC} have higher magnitudes of velocity, it appears that the smaller θ_{IC} might have a higher probability for vessel wall injury in the region hit by the blood jet. During peak systole, the highest stress values were found in the raphe region in all four cases.

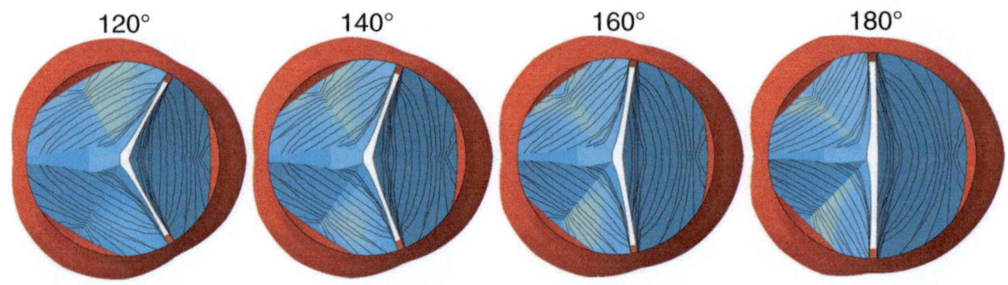

Fig. 5.6 Views from the aorta of the four BAV geometries with various values of θ_{IC}

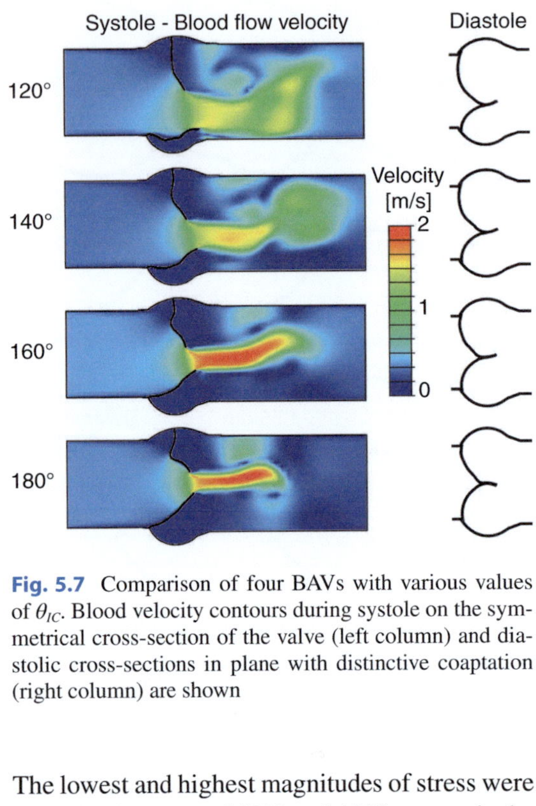

Fig. 5.7 Comparison of four BAVs with various values of θ_{IC}. Blood velocity contours during systole on the symmetrical cross-section of the valve (left column) and diastolic cross-sections in plane with distinctive coaptation (right column) are shown

The lowest and highest magnitudes of stress were found in the cases of 120° and 180°, respectively, but no difference was found in the magnitude values of the 140° and 160° cases.

The diastolic configurations of the valves were also compared in similar cross-sections to the previous parametric studies (right column of Fig. 5.7). The plane is located at a distance of 0.6 cm from the center where the non-fused and fused cusps have an almost symmetric section and the coaptation is more visible than in the raphe region. The coaptation heights are comparable, but the larger fused cusps (lower θ_{IC}) tend to prolapse more into the ventricle. The highest stress levels were found in the raphe in all cases, and the magnitude of stress in this region increased with the decrease of θ_{IC}. This result indicates that in lower θ_{IC}, the fused cusps need to carry a larger portion of the load. This conclusion is also supported by the fact that the magnitude of stress in the non-fused cusp decreases with the decrease of θ_{IC}.

5.8 Clinical Implications

The goal in aortic valve repair surgeries is to create a completely closed valve with large coaptation to prevent regurgitation. In this chapter, we showed that $\overline{h}_C$ can be controlled not only by interventions that change the size of the cusp (Fig. 5.2) but also by those that change the shape of the root, for example, by changing d_{AVA} and d_{STJ} (Figs. 5.3 and 5.5). More importantly, we showed that h_E, an easily measured height during the procedural routine, is correlated with $\overline{h}_C$ as presented in Fig. 5.4. In this graph and in agreement with Bierbach et al. [1], the cases with $h_E < 9$ mm were not fully closed during diastole. In valve-sparing procedures, a higher h_E can be achieved by reducing d_{AVA}. The d_{STJ}/d_{AVA} study also shows that all valves with various ratios and $d_{AVA} \leq 24$ mm were fully closed, indicating that this is the desired range of d_{AVA}. The BAV parametric study showed that for the studied configurations, in which a lower θ_{IC} results in a more eccentric opening, a larger θ_{IC} is preferable because the associated jet flow is more central and not directed towards the aortic wall. In addition, this parametric study showed that a larger θ_{IC} is preferable because it results in smaller fused cusps and therefore less prolapse into the left ventricle.

References

1. Bierbach BO, Aichera D, Issaa OA, Bomberga H, Gräber S, Glombitza P, Schäfers HJ. Aortic root and cusp configuration determine aortic valve function. Eur J Cardiothorac Surg. 2010;38(4):400–6. https://doi.org/10.1016/j.ejcts.2010.01.060.
2. David TE, Feindel CM, David CM, Manlhiot C. A quarter of a century of experience with aortic valve-sparing operations. J Thorac Cardiovasc Surg. 2014;148(3):872–9. https://doi.org/10.1016/j.jtcvs.2014.04.048.
3. Aicher D, Langer F, Adam O, Tscholl D, Lausberg H, Schafers HJ. Cusp repair in aortic valve reconstruction: does the technique affect stability? J Thorac Cardiovasc Surg. 2007;134(6):1533–8. https://doi.org/10.1016/j.jtcvs.2007.08.023.
4. Kari FA, Kvitting JP, Stephens EH, Liang DH, Merk DR, Fischbein MP, Mitchell RS, Miller DC. Tirone David procedure for bicuspid aortic valve disease: impact of root geometry and valve type on mid-term outcomes. Interact Cardiovasc Thorac Surg. 2014;19(3):375–81. https://doi.org/10.1093/icvts/ivu123.
5. Schneider U, Schmied W, Aicher D, Giebels C, Winter L, Schafers HJ. Sinus plication to improve valve configuration in bicuspid aortic valve repair-early results. Ann Thorac Surg. 2016; https://doi.org/10.1016/j.athoracsur.2016.06.064.
6. Haj-Ali R, Marom G, Ben Zekry S, Rosenfeld M, Raanani E. A general three-dimensional parametric geometry of the native aortic valve and root for biomechanical modeling. J Biomech. 2012;45(14):2392–7. https://doi.org/10.1016/j.jbiomech.2012.07.017.
7. Marom G, Halevi R, Haj-Ali R, Rosenfeld M, Schafers HJ, Raanani E. Numerical model of the aortic root and valve: optimization of graft size and sinotubular junction to annulus ratio. J Thorac Cardiovasc Surg. 2013;146(5):1227–31. https://doi.org/10.1016/j.jtcvs.2013.01.030.
8. Marom G, Haj-Ali R, Rosenfeld M, Schafers HJ, Raanani E. Aortic root numeric model: correlation between intraoperative effective height and diastolic coaptation. J Thorac Cardiovasc Surg. 2013;145(1):303–4. https://doi.org/10.1016/j.jtcvs.2012.08.043.
9. Lavon K, Halevi R, Marom G, Ben Zekry S, Hamdan A, Schafers HJ, Raanani E, Haj-Ali R. Fluid-structure interaction models of bicuspid aortic valves: the effects of nonfused cusp angles. J Biomech Eng. 2017; 140(3):031010. https://doi.org/10.1115/1.4038329.
10. Marom G, Haj-Ali R, Rosenfeld M, Schafers HJ, Raanani E. Aortic root numeric model: annulus diameter prediction of effective height and coaptation in post-aortic valve repair. J Thorac Cardiovasc Surg. 2013;145(2):406–411.e1. https://doi.org/10.1016/j.jtcvs.2012.01.080.
11. Marom G, Peleg M, Halevi R, Rosenfeld M, Raanani E, Hamdan A, Haj-Ali R. Fluid-structure interaction model of aortic valve with porcine-specific collagen fiber alignment in the cusps. J Biomech Eng. 2013;135(10):101001–6. https://doi.org/10.1115/1.4024824.

6 Aortoscopy to Evaluate Cusp Configuration After Aortic Valvuloplasty

Takashi Kunihara

6.1 Introduction

Aortic valve repair is an attractive option for patients with aortic insufficiency, especially in the young. However, it has not yet become widely accepted (see Chap. 9 by Arimura) [1]. Why has aortic valve repair been performed so infrequently in contrast with mitral valve repair? There are some anatomical and technical reasons; however, the lack of direct intraoperative evaluation of aortic regurgitation (AR) after repair may be the greatest reason. Generally, the cusp configuration should be assessed using two or three traction sutures fixed at each commissure with the same tension and in a symmetric direction. This cannot always be realized, however, in the clinical setting. Furthermore, this evaluation technique does not imitate diastolic pressure. Therefore, unexpected AR can occasionally be observed after aortic unclamping even if the repair seems appropriate visually. This could be avoided if we could assess the cusp configuration exactly under the condition of physiological pressure.

T. Kunihara (✉)
Department of Cardiac Surgery, The Jikei University School of Medicine, Tokyo, Japan
e-mail: kunihara@jikei.ac.jp

6.2 History of Aortoscopy

Aortoscopy to evaluate cusp geometry after aortic valve repair under a physiological (pressurized) condition was already proposed by Itoh et al., one of the pioneers of valve-preserving root replacement in Japan (see column Itoh), two decades ago [2]. Then, they introduced endoscopy for 17 patients both before and after valve-sparing root replacement and successfully reduced postoperative AR. They emphasized that the pre-procedural endoscopic assessment could clarify indications and limitations of the valve-preserving procedure [3]. Since then, endoscopic evaluation of the aortic valve has not received much attention [4, 5]. However, as experience with aortic valve repair has increased, experts in this field have recognized the importance of the physiological assessment of cusp geometry. The Essen group revived the use of aortic valve angioscopy and reported their experience with 26 patients who underwent aortic valve repair in 2014 and found consistency with the transesophageal echocardiographic findings [6]. As the editorial commentary for this report, Sievers clearly showed that the morphologic appearance of leaflets became unpredictably irregular without the presence of diastolic pressure, making the assessment difficult (Fig. 6.1) [7]. However, Okita et al. advocated checking the valve from the left ventricular side using a flexible videoscope (Fig. 6.2) [8]. This allows

T. Kunihara, S. Takanashi (eds.), *Aortic Valve Preservation*,
https://doi.org/10.1007/978-981-13-2068-2_6

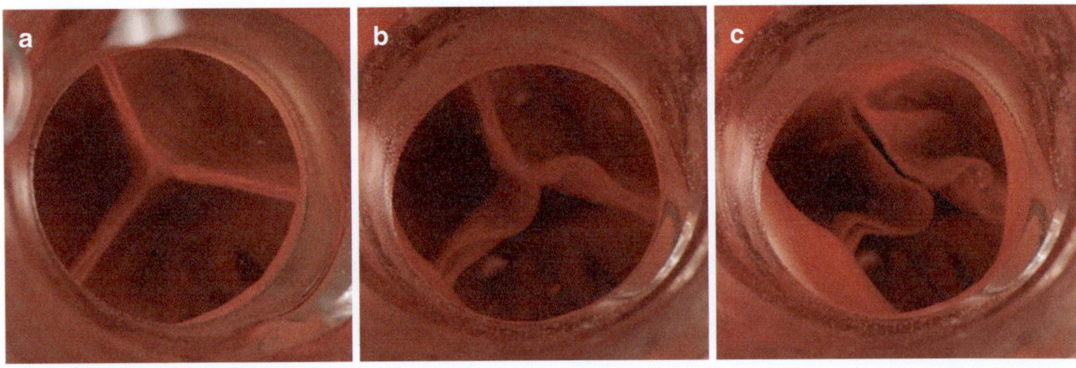

Fig. 6.1 Endoscopic view of the normal aortic root at 80 mmHg (**a**), 40 mmHg (**b**), and 0 mmHg (**c**). Leaflet coaptation area appears straight in panel **a** but becomes irregular at the lower diastolic pressures, making the assessment of the leaflet configuration difficult

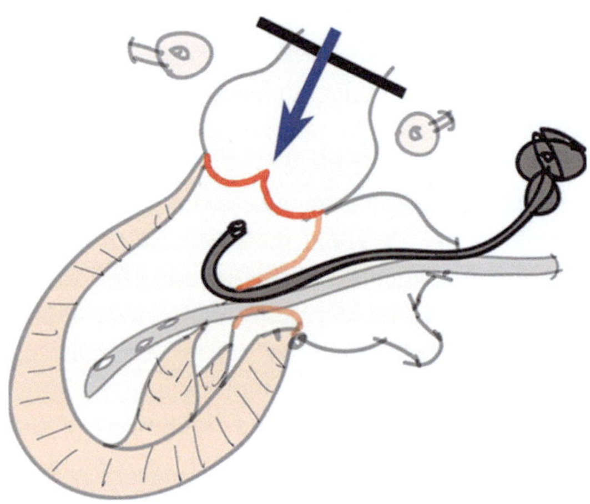

Fig. 6.2 Videoscopic assessment of the aortic valve from the left ventricular side

easy observation of regurgitant flow, but it cannot disclose the etiology of the failure.

6.3 Our Experience

Since receiving approval of our institutional ethical committee for use of aortoscopy (The Cardiovascular Institute, Tokyo, Japan), we have applied it in 25 consecutive patients who have undergone aortic valve repair or valve-sparing root replacement since December 2015. Following the anastomosis between the vascular prosthesis and the aortic root, a rigid 10-mm endoscope is inserted into the prosthesis, the end of which is temporally closed. Crystalloid cardioplegic solution is applied to the prosthesis at a perfusion pressure of 50–60 mmHg. The cusp configuration is observed on a wide-screen monitor, and the coaptation of each cusp is assessed. Additional cusp repair is undertaken if necessary, which is then checked again with the endoscope.

Here, we compare seven consecutive patients who had undergone an elective isolated aortic root remodeling procedure with external suture annuloplasty using CV-0 suture and without complex cusp repair such as the use of the pericardial patch and were evaluated with aortoscopy with ten similar previous patients who did not undergo aortoscopic evaluation. Aortic cross-clamping time was significantly longer with the use of aortoscopy (126 ± 20 min) than without (107 ± 13 min) ($P < .01$). Cardiopulmonary bypass time was also significantly longer with the use of aortoscopy (156 ± 22 min) than without (127 ± 13 min) ($P = .03$) (Fig. 6.3). The preoperative AR grade was less in the patients with aortoscopy (2.4 ± 1.9) than in those without (3.4 ± 0.8) ($P = .15$) when the AR grade (1–4) was considered as a continuous value. The postoperative AR grade almost disappeared in the patients with aortoscopy (0.1 ± 0.4), whereas mild AR was seen in those without (0.7 ± 0.6), although the difference was not significant ($P = .08$) (Fig. 6.4).

There was no need for re-exploration for bleeding, and there was no mortality. Additional cusp repair was performed in two patients after aortoscopic assessment. No second aortic cross-clamping was required in either patient series. Two patients without aortoscopy underwent reoperation due to suture dehiscence and cusp perforation on the 1st and 15th postoperative days, respectively. Both of these causes were unrelated to cusp prolapse and would have been difficult to predict by aortoscopy. No reoperations were performed during a mean follow-up period of 25 ± 10 months.

A representative patient in whom aortoscopy was very useful is shown in Fig. 6.5. This patient with right coronary cusp (RCC) prolapse underwent central plication of the RCC and the effective heights of all cusps appeared to be 10 mm at this step. However, aortoscopy after sinotubular junction remodeling indicated a redundant left and non-coronary cusp (LCC, NCC) (Fig. 6.5a). Central plication was also performed for the LCC and NCC, but the LCC continued to be redundant (Fig. 6.5b). After additional plication of the LCC, all three cusps were at an identical height (Fig. 6.5c). Postoperative echocardiography showed no AR with ideal cusp configuration.

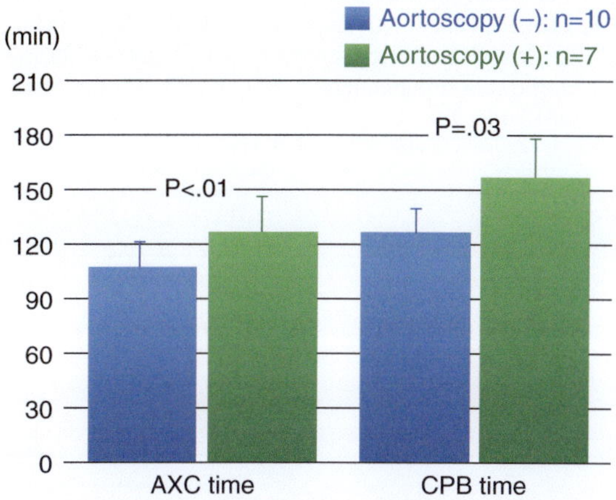

Fig. 6.3 Aortic cross-clamping (AXC) time and cardiopulmonary bypass (CPB) time in patients who underwent an elective isolated aortic root remodeling procedure with external suture annuloplasty and without complex cusp repair (i.e., the use of a pericardial patch) evaluated with or without aortoscopy

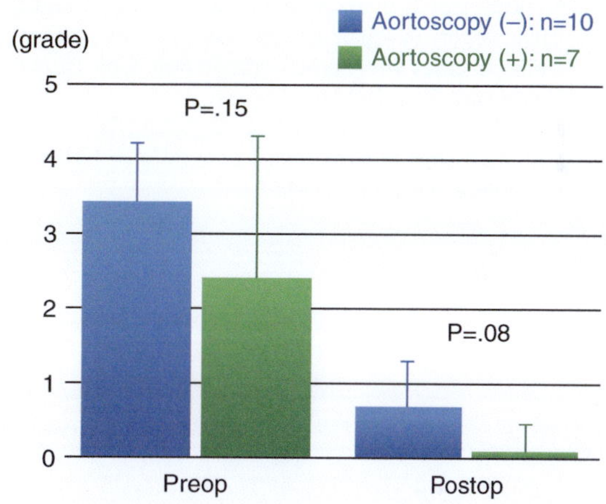

Fig. 6.4 Pre- and postoperative aortic regurgitation grades in patients who underwent an elective isolated aortic root remodeling procedure with external suture annuloplasty and without complex cusp repair (i.e., the use of a pericardial patch) evaluated with or without aortoscopy

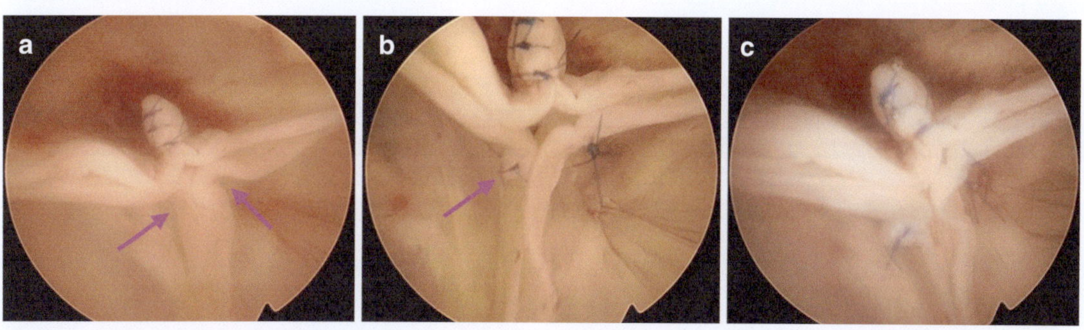

Fig. 6.5 Aortoscopic assessment of the cusp configuration. After central plication of the right coronary cusp (RCC), aortoscopy indicated a redundant left and noncoronary cusp (LCC, NCC) (arrows) (**a**). Central plication was also performed for the LCC and NCC, but the LCC was still redundant (arrow) (**b**). Additional plication of the LCC brought all three cusps to an identical height (**c**)

6.4 Conclusion

Aortoscopy increases procedural time but does not appear to increase operative risk. It seems useful to enhance the accuracy of repair, and it can possibly prevent a second operation by indicating the need for additional maneuvers. Of course, long-term follow-up with a sufficient case volume is mandatory to confirm these findings.

References

1. Arimura S, Seki M, Sasaki K, Takai H, Matsuhama M, Kunihara T, et al. A nationwide survey of aortic valve surgery in Japan: current status of valve preservation in cases with aortic regurgitation. Gen Thorac Cardiovasc Surg. 2017;65:429–34.
2. Itoh T, Ohtsubo S, Furukawa K, Norita H. Aortic root endoscopy in valve-sparing operations. J Thorac Cardiovasc Surg. 1997;114:141–2.
3. Ohtsubo S, Itoh T, Natsuaki M, Furukawa K, Yoshikai M, Suda H, et al. Successful valve-sparing in aortic root reconstruction under endoscopic guidance. Eur J Cardiothorac Surg. 2000;17:420–5.
4. Meunier JP, Berkane N, Lopez S, El Ghobary T, Teboul J, Malzac B, et al. Traumatic aortic regurgitation: aortic valvuloplasty controlled by aortoscopy. J Heart Valve Dis. 2001;10:784–8.
5. Iida H, Sudo Y, Sunazawa T, Ukita H. Endoscopic observation following aortic cusp plication. Gen Thorac Cardiovasc Surg. 2007;55:425–7.
6. Tsagakis K, Benedik J, El Khoury G, Jakob H. Aortic valve repair: intraoperative evaluation of valve geometry by angioscopy. J Thorac Cardiovasc Surg. 2015;149:1666–8.
7. Sievers HH. Better seeing is more believing: angioscopy in aortic valve repair. J Thorac Cardiovasc Surg. 2015;149:1668–9.
8. Okita Y, Oka T, Miyahara S, Okada K. Direct visualization of the aortic cusp from the left ventricle during aortic root reimplantation. J Thorac Cardiovasc Surg. 2012;144:981–2.

7 Indications and Contraindications for Aortic Valve Repair

Tatsuhiko Komiya

7.1 Surgical Indications for Aortic Regurgitation

Various guidelines address the surgical indications for aortic regurgitation (AR) (Table 7.1) [1–3]. When the regurgitation has progressed and symptoms are present, surgical indications need to be considered. Even if symptoms are absent, in Europe, surgical treatment is recommended when either of the following exist: the left ventricular ejection fraction (LVEF) is <50% or left ventricular dilatation (left ventricular end-systolic diameter [LVDs] >50 mm, or LVDs/body surface area ratio >25 mm/m^2 [Class IIa], or left ventricular end-diastolic diameter [LVDd] >65 mm [Class IIb]). Left ventricular dilatation in Japanese patients is precisely classified and defined by guidelines, but considering the difference in physique between European and Japanese patients, it is appropriate to apply values corrected by body surface area. For a patient with body surface area of 1.5 m^2, a LVDs >37.5 mm is indicated for surgical intervention. It is important to note that surgical treatment is recommended in the early stage of left ventricular dilatation compared to the previous guidelines and that the LVDs has become the important indicator.

T. Komiya (✉)
Institute of Cardiovascular Surgery, Kurashiki Central Hospital, Okayama, Japan
e-mail: komiya@kchnet.or.jp

These guidelines were written on the assumption that aortic valve replacement will be performed with a prosthetic valve. Surgery in the early stage is recommended for the mitral valve as the efficiency of valve repair over valve replacement has already been established. However, adequate evidence for valve repair has not yet been obtained for aortic valves. Considering both the necessity of lifetime anticoagulant treatment in the case of a mechanical valve and the durability of the bioprosthesis, aortic valve repair in adolescent patients could be valid. In the report by Aicher et al., the mortality within 30 days in aortic valve repair was 3.4% in 640 patients with an average age of 56 ± 17 years, and most of the mortalities occurred in elderly patients who underwent simultaneous coronary artery bypass surgery. The 10-year survival rate was 80%. The 10-year freedom from reoperation for tricuspid valves (N = 411) was 93% and that for bicuspid valves (N = 205) was 81%, indicating a slightly poorer result for bicuspid valves. The primary reasons for reoperation were progression of leaflet prolapse and dehiscence of sutures in most of the cases, and the secondary reasons were infectious endocarditis, regression of leaflets, and secondary annulus enlargement [4]. In the report by Price et al., the 30-day mortality for aortic valve repair was 0.8%, and the 10-year survival rate was 73% in 475 patients with an average age of 53 ± 16 years. The 10-year freedom from reoperation was 86%, and there

T. Kunihara, S. Takanashi (eds.), *Aortic Valve Preservation*,
https://doi.org/10.1007/978-981-13-2068-2_7

Table 7.1 Surgical indications of aortic valve replacement for severe aortic regurgitation

	USA	Europe	Japan
Symptom	Symptomatic	Symptomatic	Symptomatic: Class I
Left ventricular ejection fraction	EF < 50%: Class I	EF < 50%: Class I	EF < 50%: Class I EF < 25%: Class II b
Left ventricular dilatation	ESD > 50 mm or ESD > 25 mm/m^2: Class II a EDD > 65 mm: Class II b	ESD > 50 mm or ESD > 25 mm/m^2: Class II a EDD > 70 mm: Class II a	ESD > 55 mm or EDD > 75 mm: Class I ESD > 50 mm or EDD > 70 mm: Class IIa ESD > 45 mm or EDD > 60 mm: Class II b
Concomitant cardiac surgery	Yes: Class I (moderate AR: Class IIa)	Yes: Class I	Yes: Class I

was no significant difference between the tricuspid and bicuspid cases. The annual occurrences of valve-related events were 1.1% for embolism, 0.23% for hemorrhage, and 0.19% for infectious endocarditis [5]. In the Mayo Clinic report, the operative mortality for aortic valve repair without root replacement was 0.6% in 331 patients with an average age of 53 ± 17 years, and 1% of the patients required reoperation in the early stage. The 10-year survival rate was 81%, and the risk factors were left ventricular dilatation (LVDs >50 mm) and a decrease in LVEF to <50%. The 10-year freedom from reoperation was 79%, and advanced preoperative AR and mild AR at hospital discharge were the risk factors for reoperation. A bicuspid aortic valve proved to be no risk factor for recurrence [6].

Although valve repair for young patients with a bicuspid valve is promising, neither the optimal surgical technique to obtain favorable results at all facilities nor the durability of a repaired valve compared to a bioprosthesis has yet been confirmed. In the Mayo Clinic report, 50% of the patients (average age, 41 years old) who underwent valve repair required aortic valve replacement within 10 years, but when compared with matched patients who underwent aortic valve replacement with a bioprosthesis, the 10-year freedom from reoperation for valve repair was 72% and that for valve replacement was 64%, which seems relatively equal [7]. de Kerchove et al. reported that the addition of root replacement to valve repair improved the 6-year reoperation-free rate to 100% [8]. Aicher et al. reported that the 10-year reoperation-free rate for bicuspid valve repair was 82% in 559 patients [9], but the addition of annuloplasty might have decreased the number of reoperations [10].

In patients with the typical fusion structure occurring in bicuspid valves, a central angle of the commissure of close to 120° carries the risk of causing stenosis due to the excessive leaflet plication required. Also, there are several reported cases of a unicuspid valve diagnosed preoperatively as a bicuspid valve. Furthermore, a patch may be required in cases of calcification of the raphe. To secure the quality of the plasty, a precise preoperative diagnosis is crucial, and careful consultation regarding the application and timing of the valve repair is necessary.

In cases of AR caused by fragility of the valve itself, the valve repair method is not successful. This same apprehension originally held for mitral valves as well, but the favorable long-term results of mitral valve repair have shown this apprehension to be groundless. There is no doubt that annuloplasty using an artificial ring contributed to this result. Although this is not yet considered the same for aortic valve repair, it is believed that better results could be established with annulus stabilization. In addition, adequate coaptation is necessary to obtain long-term stability of the aortic valve. It is essential to diagnose not only the presence of AR but also the structure of the valves and the depth of coaptation using intraoperative 3-dimensional echocardiography.

7.2 Surgical Treatment in Patients with Aortic Root Enlargement

The prevention of AR is expected by valve-sparing root replacement for aortic root enlargement even when AR is not present, and the application of this surgery is discussed in terms of the diameter of the aorta [1–3, 11] (Table 7.2). According to the guidelines, replacement is performed when the aortic root diameter is 5 cm or greater (Class IIa) for a bicuspid valve or 4.5 cm or greater (Class IIa) in patients requiring aortic valve surgery. For tricuspid valves, valve-sparing root replacement is recommended even in the absence of AR for diameters of 5 cm or greater (Class I), and root replacement needs to be considered when the root size is 4.5 cm or greater in patients with connective tissue disease such as Marfan syndrome, and 4 cm or greater in women who wish to become pregnant (Class IIa). For patients without connective tissue disease, root replacement is suitable when the aortic root is 4.5 cm or greater if significant AR exists, but this type of surgery could be performed in facilities with a high experience level even in patients with a root diameter under 4.5 cm. In patients with type A acute aortic dissection, when intimal dissection reaches the right or left coronary sinus or the root enlarges beyond 4.5 cm, root replacement is required although preservation of leaflets may be difficult (Class I).

David, the pioneer of valve-sparing root replacement, has reported favorable late results. The operative mortality rate was 1.1% in 371 patients (reimplantation rate was 80%) including 12% with type A acute aortic dissection. The addition of plication of the leaflet free edge was performed in 37% of the patients and reinforcement of the leaflet free edge in 24%. There were 10 cases of reoperation. The 18-year reoperation-free rate was 95%, and the 18-year freedom from greater than or equal to moderate AR was 78%. Although there are no predictive factors for AR recurrence, if a patient shows clear-cut valve degeneration, valve-preservation is not thought to be indicated [12]. Thus, it appears that the long-term follow-up results for valve-sparing root replacement were favorable for root enlargement accompanied by slight valvular degeneration. Regarding postoperative recurrent AR at 1 year after the David-V operation, mild AR was present in 43%, moderate AR in 5%, and severe AR in 2% of the patients. At a median of 28 months,

Table 7.2 Surgical treatment in patients with aortic root enlargement

	USA	Europe	Japan
Marfan syndrome	Aortic diameter > 45 mm + family history: Class I Aortic diameter > 40 mm + desire for pregnancy: Class II a	Aortic diameter > 45 mm + risk factor[a]: Class II a	Aortic diameter > 45 mm: Class II a Aortic diameter > 40 mm + desire for pregnancy: Class II a
Bicuspid valve	Aortic diameter > 55 mm: Class I Aortic diameter > 50 mm + risk factor[b]: Class II a Aortic diameter > 45 mm + severe AS or AR: Class II a	Aortic diameter > 50 mm + risk factor[c]: Class II a	Aortic diameter > 45 mm: Class I Aortic diameter > 40 mm: Class II a
With surgical indication for aortic valve		Aortic diameter > 45 mm: Class II a	Aortic diameter > 50 mm: Class I
Other situations	Aortic diameter > 50 mm: Class I	Aortic diameter > 55 mm: Class II a	Aortic diameter > 50 mm: Class II b

[a]A family history with aortic dissection, a growth rate of more than 2 mm/year, or desire for pregnancy
[b]A family history with aortic dissection or a growth rate of more than 5 mm/year
[c]Aortic coarctation, hypertension, a family history with aortic dissection, or a growth rate of more than 2 mm/year

mild AR had progressed to moderate AR in 12% of the patients, but as there was no further progression, no reoperations were necessary, indicating that postoperative mild AR may be an acceptable condition [13].

The report from the Emory group regarding the application of valve-sparing root replacement using the David-V technique included 78 patients in the expanded group (29 patients with acute aortic dissection, 53 with equal to or greater than grade 3 AR, and 14 patients with reoperation) and 72 patients in the traditional group. Only three cases of operative death occurred in the expanded group, but the long-term moderate AR-free rate was similar between the two groups at 91% and 95% [14]. A follow-up report indicated a 4.7% rate of operative death, 14% of the patients required leaflet repair, and 83% of the intraoperative AR was limited to less than grade 1 in 43 cases of valve-sparing root replacement for type A acute aortic dissection. There were no late reoperations for aortic valve replacement, and the occurrence of AR was limited to equal to or less than grade 1 in 94% of the patients [15].

7.3 Conclusion

Recently, surgical treatment at the early stage for asymptomatic mitral valve regurgitation has been recommended by the guidelines because of the favorable long-term follow-up results revealed for mitral valve repair. Stable surgical results can be obtained by high-volume centers due to the establishment of a reproducible repair technique. The development of several types of annuloplasty rings has enhanced these results. In contrast, the superiority of aortic valve repair over valve replacement has not yet been established. Thus, there is no evidence of aortic valve repair in the early stage of AR. At this point, the indications for aortic valve replacement, namely, asymptomatic cases with decreased LVEF and moderate left ventricle dilatation, is equally applied to aortic valve repair. In the case of a bicuspid valve, the long-term follow-up results are favorable with the addition of root replacement or annuloplasty. Thus, it may be possible to recommend an early-stage operation. Furthermore, even for tricuspid valves with root enlargement, beneficial long-term follow-up results have been reported with the valve-sparing root replacement method when performed before further progression of cusp pathology. As is the case with mitral valves, in these aortic lesions, valve repair is expected to be highly reliable; therefore, it may be possible to prove its efficiency as an early-stage operation.

Aortic valve repair is gaining more and more attention and is being performed in an increasing number of facilities. If progress is made in the development of the surgical method and annuloplasty rings through the accumulation and analysis of operative data, and if multiple insights into the selection of appropriate patients can be gained, it may be possible to recommend the operation at the early stage similarly to that with mitral valves. Adequate experience is required to determine whether valve repair or replacement is appropriate, and it is also clear that a learning curve is involved in improving the quality of the plasty technique [16]. Depending on the condition of the leaflets, the possibility of applying aortic valve replacement is not small at the moment. Therefore, verification at experienced facilities is crucial to expand the indications for aortic valve repair.

References

1. Nishimura RA, Otto CM, et al. 2014 AHA/ACC Guideline for the management of patients with valvular heart disease. A report of the American College of Cardiology/American Heart Association Task Force on practice guidelines. Circulation. 2014;129:e521–643.
2. Vahanian A, Alfieri O, et al. European guidelines on the management of valvular heart disease (version 2012): the joint task force on the management of valvular heart disease of the European Society of Cardiology (ESC) and the European Association for Cardio-Thoracic Surgery (EACTS). Eur J Cardiothorac Surg. 2012;42:S1–44.
3. Okita Y, Okada Y, Otsuji Y, Komeda M, Nakatani S, Matsuzaki M, et al. Guidelines for surgical and interventional treatment of valvular heart disease (JCS 2012). http://www.j-circ.or.jp/guideline/pdf/jcs2012_ookita_h.pdf.

4. Aicher D, Fries R, et al. Aortic valve repair leads to a low incidence of valve-related complications. Eur J Cardiothorac Surg. 2010;37:127–32.
5. Price J, De Kerchove L, et al. Risk of valve-related events after aortic valve repair. Ann Thorac Surg. 2013;95:606–12.
6. Sharma V, Suri RM, et al. Expanding relevance of aortic valve repair—is earlier operation indicated? J Thorac Cardiovasc Surg. 2014;147:100–8.
7. Ashikhmina E, Sundt TM 3rd, et al. Repair of the bicuspid aortic valve: a viable alternative to replacement with a bioprosthesis. J Thorac Cardiovasc Surg. 2010;139:1395–401.
8. de Kerchove L, Boodhwani M, et al. Valve sparing-root replacement with the reimplantation technique to increase the durability of bicuspid aortic valve repair. J Thorac Cardiovasc Surg. 2011;142:1430–8.
9. Aicher D, Schneider U, et al. Early results with annular support in reconstruction of the bicuspid aortic valve. J Thorac Cardiovasc Surg. 2013;145:S30–4.
10. Schneider U, Hofmann C, Aicher D, Takahashi H, Miura Y, Schäfers HJ. Suture annuloplasty significantly improves the durability of bicuspid aortic valve repair. Ann Thorac Surg. 2017;103:504–10.
11. Svensson LG, Adams DH, et al. Aortic valve and ascending aorta guidelines for management and quality measures: executive summary. Ann Thorac Surg. 2013;95:1491–505.
12. David TE, Feindel CM, et al. A quarter of a century of experience with aortic valve-sparing operations. J Thorac Cardiovasc Surg. 2014;148:872–9.
13. Stephens EH, Liang DH, et al. Incidence and progression of mild aortic regurgitation after Tirone David reimplantation valve-sparing aortic root replacement. J Thorac Cardiovasc Surg. 2014;147:169–78.
14. Leshnower BG, Guyton RA, et al. Expanding the indications for the David V aortic root replacement: early results. J Thorac Cardiovasc Surg. 2012;143:879–84.
15. Leshnower BG, Myung RJ, et al. Midterm results of David V valve-sparing aortic root replacement in acute type a aortic dissection. Ann Thorac Surg. 2015;99:795–801.
16. Malas T, Saczkowski R, Sohmer B, Ruel M, Mesana T, de Kerchove L, El Khoury G, Boodhwani M. Is aortic valve repair reproducible? Analysis of the learning curve for aortic valve repair. Can J Cardiol. 2015;31:1497.e15–22.

ONE-POINT ADVICE: Significance of Aortic Valvuloplasty in the Valve-in-Valve Era

8

Kentaro Hayashida

8.1 Introduction

Transcatheter aortic valve implantation (TAVI) was developed as a therapeutic option for those patients who are deemed to be at high risk for surgical aortic valve replacement or inoperable. After the first case was performed by Professor Cribier from the Department of Cardiology, Rouen University in France in 2002 [1], this therapeutic option received the CE Mark in Europe in 2007, and approval from the U.S. FDA was granted to the SAPIEN valve from Edward Lifesciences in 2011 and the CoreValve from Medtronic in 2014. Presently, over 150,000 patients have been treated with this technique worldwide, and it is rapidly improving and prevailing around the world. In October 2013, it finally received insurance reimbursement in Japan. Since then, over 8000 patients have been treated, and the number of facilities approved to perform the procedure is increasing.

Currently in Europe, TAVI is successfully performed even for disease that is not applicable in Japan. As an example, TAVI for degenerative surgical bioprostheses, the "valve-in-valve" (VIV) method, is performed as a part of daily clinical practice (Fig. 8.1). Therefore, as a form of treatment for degenerative surgical bioprostheses without thoracotomy, it is a significantly beneficial treatment for patients at high risk. However, the methods used in this procedure are difficult, and there is also room for further improvement.

In this article, it is assumed that the VIV method will be allowed as the latest form of TAVI treatment in Japan. The significance of surgical aortic valvuloplasty and further development are also discussed.

8.2 Current Status of VIV

Currently, VIV is gradually spreading mainly in Europe and the U.S.A., and a global multicenter registry was reported in *JAMA* in 2014 as the largest report [2]. Its focus was 459 cases of VIV performed in 55 facilities in Europe and the U.S.A. from 2007 to 2013. Thirty-day mortality was 7.5%, and the major stroke rate was 1.7%. In addition, although the 1-year survival rate was 83.2%, of special importance, the 1-year survival rate for VIV for small valves of 20 mm or less was 74.8%, which was significantly lower. Moreover, "bioprosthesis size of 21 mm or less" was identified as an independent predictor of mortality (hazard ratio 2.04: 95% confidence interval 1.14–3.67, $p = 0.02$).

Furthermore, there was a difference in the residual pressure gradient depending on the type

K. Hayashida (✉)
Department of Cardiology, Keio University School of Medicine, Tokyo, Japan
e-mail: k-hayashida@umin.ac.jp

T. Kunihara, S. Takanashi (eds.), *Aortic Valve Preservation*,
https://doi.org/10.1007/978-981-13-2068-2_8

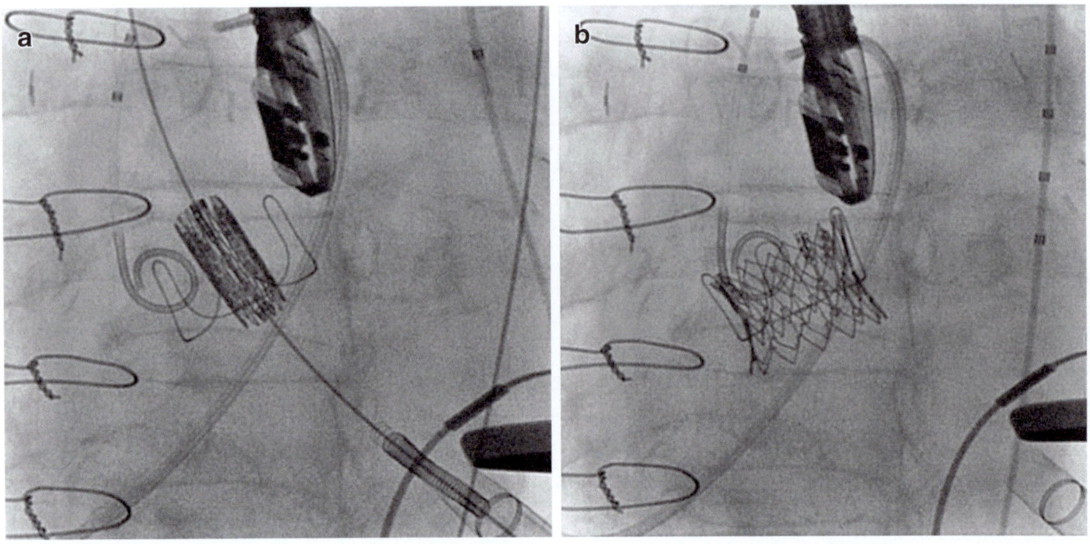

Fig. 8.1 Valve-in-valve method for a degenerative bioprosthetic valve with a SAPIEN XT. (**a**) Application of the trans-apical approach after careful determination of the positioning for deployment. (**b**) Final findings of TAVI

of TAVI valve used, and the probability of the mean pressure gradient remaining at 20 mmHg or more was approximately 25% for the CoreValve, whereas the probability rose significantly to approximately 40% for the SAPIEN valve. The reason for this is that with the SAPIEN, the TAVI valve is positioned at the intra-annular position, and therefore it has more influence on a narrow annulus. In contrast, because the functional part of the CoreValve is located at the supra-annular position, it is thus less affected by a narrow annulus than is the SAPIEN valve.

Actually, the sewing ring is a part of the surgical bioprosthesis, and thus the true internal diameter is smaller than the manufacturer-reported valve size. Therefore, a pressure gradient will remain in valves sized less than 21 mm, and this may cause patient-prosthesis mismatch. Especially in Japan, as a surgical bioprosthesis larger than 21 mm is not frequently implanted in the aortic position, there is a high possibility of the VIV procedure being difficult in the future.

Currently, two nonrandomized prospective VIV studies using either the SAPIEN valve [3] or CoreValve [4] have already been reported with improved outcomes. The PARTNER 2 VIV registry to test the SAPIEN valve revealed 30-day mortality of 2.7%, a major stroke rate of 2.7%, and 1-year mortality of 12.4% [3]. Similarly, the CoreValve U.S. Expanded Use Study showed 30-day mortality of 2.2%, a major stroke rate of 0.4%, and a 1-year mortality of 14.6% [4]. Further improved outcomes might be expected with further advancements in modalities.

8.3 Expectations for Aortic Valvuloplasty

Based on the above, it is clear that the results of future VIV procedures may become more unfavorable if a surgical bioprosthesis sized less than 21 mm is implanted. Therefore, considering the future VIV procedure, an operative method should maintain an annulus size as large as possible. Because aortic valvuloplasty can eliminate a sewing ring and thus keep the annulus size large and also maintain the anatomical features of the sinus of Valsalva, its role will become more important in the future.

Next, from the perspective of a future VIV procedure, aortic valvuloplasty is expected to maintain a larger aortic annulus that will not result in a significant pressure gradient after a future VIV procedure. In patients with short leaflets, annuloplasty is often added to ensure sufficient leaflet coaptation depth, but it should be performed only to a marginal degree.

Moreover, during TAVI, the sinus of Valsalva functions as a storage site for calcification attached to the leaflets, and thus, maintaining its larger size will reduce the risk of coronary artery occlusion during the VIV procedure. Therefore, during root replacement, the remodeling method would appear to be more appropriate than the reimplantation method, and even if the reimplantation method is performed, it is necessary to use a graft with sinuses.

Also, it must be noted that extremely long cusps after repair are associated with an increased risk of coronary artery occlusion. From this perspective, it is predicted that future VIV will be difficult if all three cusps are substituted with long autologous pericardial patches. Thus, aortic valvuloplasty will remain as a significant procedure. However, if short leaflets are extended by autologous pericardium, it is essential to keep the extensions as short as possible.

To fix both the current SAPIEN valve and CoreValve in place, calcification of the native valve is necessary. Therefore, it is thought that when the valve deforms and deteriorates after valvuloplasty, it will become difficult to keep it in place without the presence of calcification. TAVI is a procedure that is mainly applied in elderly patients with aortic valve stenosis, but it can also be applied for aortic regurgitation (AR). However, in this case, the risk of migration is considered to be high with the currently available devices [5]. Therefore, the Jana Valve was developed as a second-generation device that can also be adapted to AR (Fig. 8.2). This valve has a clip-like structure that pinches and fixes itself to the leaflets and therefore can function even if there is only slight calcification. It acquired the CE Mark for use in AR in 2013 [6]. A recent meta-analysis including 237 cases concluded that TAVI for pure AR is technically feasible and associated with an acceptable risk of early mortality (7%) without cerebrovascular events [7]. In the future, such devices may be appropriate for VIV procedures after aortic annuloplasty.

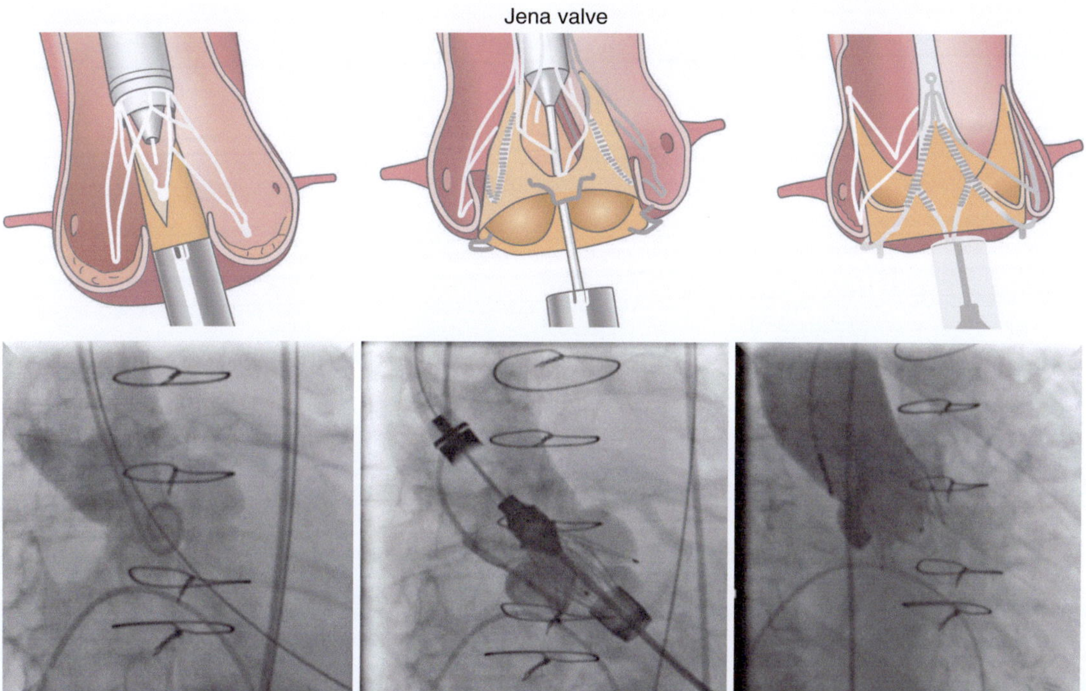

Fig. 8.2 Deployment of the Jena valve in a patient with AR. Left: The aortic valve showing AR. Middle: Positioning for deployment of the Jena valve. Right: AR disappeared after deployment of the Jena valve

8.4 Conclusion

The expectations for aortic valvuloplasty in the VIV era were outlined. In Japan, there are many patients with a small aortic annulus. From the perspectives of future VIV, aortic valvuloplasty should be performed by taking the abovementioned problems into account especially in young people. Further developments are expected for this surgical method.

References

1. Cribier A, Eltchaninoff H, Bash A, Borenstein N, Tron C, Bauer F, et al. Percutaneous transcatheter implantation of an aortic valve prosthesis for calcific aortic stenosis: first human case description. Circulation. 2002;106:3006–8.
2. Dvir D, Webb JG, Bleiziffer S, Pasic M, Waksman R, Kodali S, Valve-in-Valve International Data Registry Investigators, et al. Transcatheter aortic valve implantation in failed bioprosthetic surgical valves. JAMA. 2014;312:162–70.
3. Webb JG, Mack MJ, White JM, Dvir D, Blanke P, Herrmann HC, et al. Transcatheter aortic valve implantation within degenerated aortic surgical bioprostheses: PARTNER 2 valve-in-valve registry. J Am Coll Cardiol. 2017;69:2253–62.
4. Deeb GM, Chetcuti SJ, Reardon MJ, Patel HJ, Grossman PM, Schreiber T, et al. 1-year results in patients undergoing transcatheter aortic valve replacement with failed surgical bioprostheses. JACC Cardiovasc Interv. 2017;10:1034–44.
5. Roy DA, Schaefer U, Guetta V, Hildick-Smith D, Möllmann H, Dumonteil N, et al. Transcatheter aortic valve implantation for pure severe native aortic valve regurgitation. J Am Coll Cardiol. 2013;61:1577–84.
6. Taramasso M, Pozzoli A, Latib A, La Canna G, Colombo A, Maisano F, et al. New devices for TAVI: technologies and initial clinical experiences. Nat Rev Cardiol. 2014;11:157–67.
7. Franzone A, Piccolo R, Siontis GC, Lanz J, Stortecky S, Praz F, et al. Transcatheter aortic valve replacement for the treatment of pure native aortic valve regurgitation: a systematic review. JACC Cardiovasc Interv. 2016;9:2308–17.

Trends in Aortic Valve-Sparing Surgery

9

Satoshi Arimura and Takashi Kunihara

9.1 Introduction

Currently, aortic valvuloplasty (AVP) and valve-sparing root replacement (VSRR) are increasingly being performed in many facilities (Fig. 9.1) [1]. However, a detailed nationwide survey of aortic valve-sparing surgery is lacking. This chapter reviews the current trends in aortic valve-sparing surgery worldwide.

9.2 Surveys of Aortic Valve-Sparing Operations

According to the Euro Heart Survey on valvular heart disease conducted by the European Society of Cardiology in 92 centers from 25 countries in 2001, AVP was applied in only 1.7% of aortic valve procedures performed for aortic regurgitation (AR) [2]. However, only 119 patients with AR were investigated in this survey.

The annual updated registry of the German Society for Thoracic and Cardiovascular Surgery (GSTCVS) in 2015 reported 11,307 isolated aortic valve surgeries and 2100 aortic root surgeries performed in Germany during 2015. AVP was applied in 124 (1.0%) of the aortic valve procedures, and VSRR was applied in 603 (23.7%) of the aortic root procedures. Of the 603 VSRRs, 89 (15%) were for aortic root remodeling (hereinafter referred to as remodeling) and 514 (85%) were for aortic valve reimplantation (hereinafter referred to as reimplantation) [3].

A recent report from the Society of Thoracic Surgeons database study in the US revealed that 13,743 aortic root surgeries were performed from 2004 to early 2010, and VSRR was applied in 1918 (14%) of the procedures [1]. Distinct from other surveys, this report showed the annual trend for each type of aortic root surgery. VSRR had increased steadily from 2004 to 2007, but it plateaued from 2007 to 2009. Future trends will be of great interest.

The Japanese Association for Thoracic Surgery has conducted annual surveys of thoracic surgery throughout Japan [4]. It reported that 13,260 aortic valve surgeries and 1064 aortic root surgeries were performed in Japan during 2014. Only 397 (3.0%) of the aortic valve surgeries were aortic valve repair surgeries and 236 (34%) of the aortic root surgeries were VSRRs; however, the details of the techniques used or their outcomes were not clarified. In addition, except for the Euro Heart Survey, the etiologies of the aortic valve disease were not reported in the previous surveys.

S. Arimura
Department of Cardiovascular Surgery, The Cardiovascular Institute, Tokyo, Japan

T. Kunihara (✉)
Department of Cardiac Surgery, The Jikei University School of Medicine, Tokyo, Japan
e-mail: kunihara@jikei.ac.jp

T. Kunihara, S. Takanashi (eds.), *Aortic Valve Preservation*, https://doi.org/10.1007/978-981-13-2068-2_9

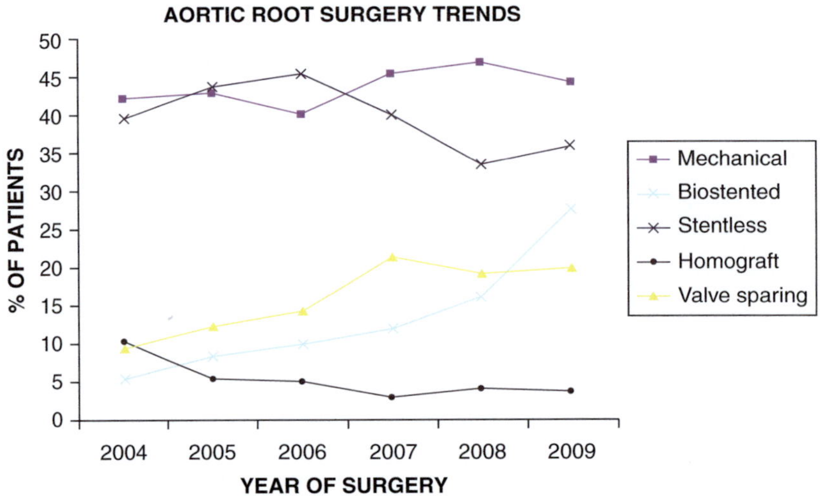

Fig. 9.1 Trends in the choice of aortic root replacement prosthesis by year of surgery [1]

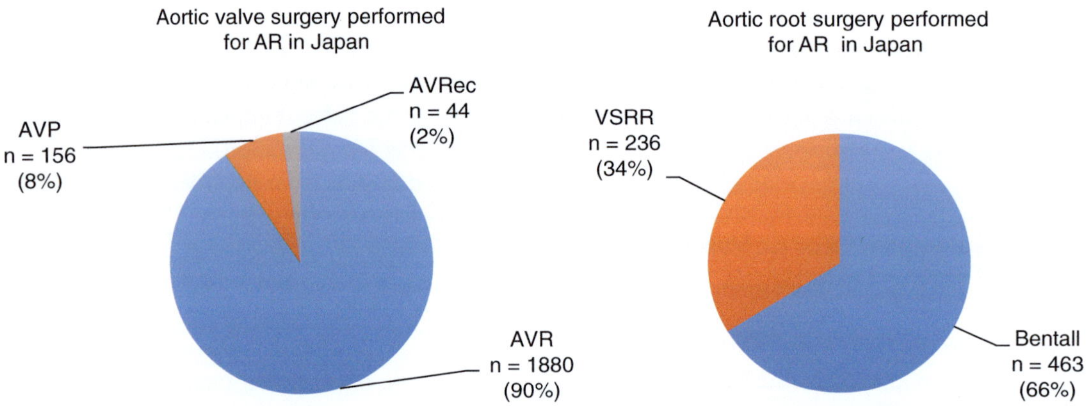

Fig. 9.2 Numbers and percentages of aortic valve and aortic root surgeries performed for aortic regurgitation (AR) in 2014. *AVP* aortic valvuloplasty, *AVRec* aortic valve reconstruction (with autologous pericardium), *AVR* aortic valve replacement, *VSRR* valve-sparing root replacement [5]

9.3 Our Questionnaire-Based Nationwide Survey

Therefore, we conducted a survey to clarify the current status and details of aortic valve-sparing operations (AVSOs) in Japan [5]. We defined AVP and VSRR collectively as AVSOs. Our questionnaire-based survey represents the first attempt to collect and analyze the current status of AVSOs in Japan. Of the 508 institutions contacted, 250 (49%) returned the initial questionnaire, and 57 (11%) of the 250 responding institutions returned the secondary questionnaire focused specifically on AVSOs. Our analysis of the data showed that AVP was applied in only 8% of aortic valve procedures performed for AR, and VSRR was applied in 34% of aortic root surgeries performed for AR (Fig. 9.2). Of the VSRRs, 27% were for remodeling and 73% were for reimplantation. Our survey also allowed us to clarify the status of AVSOs in Japan. AVSO was performed in only a limited number of facilities and, therefore, for a limited

Table 9.1 Institutions classified according to the number of AVSOs performed in Japan

No. of operations performed annually	No. of institutions	Total no. of AVSOs
1–4	48	109 (46%)
5–9	4	25 (11%)
10 or more	5	99 (42%)
Total	57	233

AVSO aortic valve-sparing operation

number of patients. The number of AVSOs performed per facility in Japan was small, with only 9 (3.6%) facilities performing more than 5 such surgeries per year (Table 9.1).

This survey data accounted for 59% (7859/13,260) of the aortic valve operations and 72% (771/1064) of aortic root operations performed in Japan in 2014. Aortic valve replacements and Bentall operations performed for AR totaled 1880 and 463 in this survey, respectively. Therefore we can estimate that (1880 × 100/59) + (463 × 100/72) = 3829 patients with AR underwent aortic valve replacement with or without root replacement in Japan per year. In an experienced center, approximately 30% of surgical cases with AR are assigned to aortic valve replacement due to unsuitable cusp pathology (unpublished data). So we speculate 3829 × 0.7 = 2680 cases are potential candidates for AVSO but assigned to aortic valve replacement in Japan per year.

The average age of these patients was around 55 years, which might make the role of AVSOs more relevant with regard to avoiding prosthesis-related complications [6]. We found the rates of 30-day mortality and reoperation for AR after AVP, remodeling, and reimplantation in Japan to be 1%, 0%, and 1% and 3%, 3%, and 1%, respectively. Operative outcomes of aortic root replacement are generally better in high-volume institutions [7], and AVSO appears to have a learning curve of approximately 40–60 cases [8]. Although the majority of institutions are low-volume centers, our study showed excellent early outcomes of AVSO performed in Japan [5], which seems similar to the findings of previous reports. Operative mortality after AVP, reimplantation, and remodeling were reported to be 4%, 1.6%, and 3.4%, respectively, in Germany [2]. In the US, lower operative mortality was observed in VSRRs (1.88%) compared with root reconstruction with a valve conduit (5.0%) [1].

There are also few reports comparing the types of VSRRs performed globally. Our survey data showed that reimplantation was more frequently performed than remodeling in Japan, as in Germany. Whether these trends will change in the future remains to be seen.

9.4 Conclusion

AVSOs have been performed in Japan for limited patients with the majority being performed in institutions with limited experience but with excellent early outcomes. As a previous study shows, AVSOs have a definite learning curve [8]. For a better long-term outcome, further clinical research and standardization of the procedures are essential.

References

1. Stamou SC, Williams ML, Gunn TM, Hagberg RC, Lobdell KW, Kouchoukos NT. Aortic root surgery in the United States: a report from the Society of Thoracic Surgeons database. J Thorac Cardiovasc Surg. 2015;149:116–22.e4.
2. Iung B, Baron G, Butchart EG, Delahaye F, Gohlke-Bärwolf C, Levang OW, Tornos P, Vanoverschelde JL, Vermeer F, Boersma E, Ravaud P, Vahanian A. A prospective survey of patients with valvular heart disease in Europe: the euro heart survey on valvular heart disease. Eur Heart J. 2003;24:1231–43.
3. Beckmann A, Funkat AK, Lewandowski J, Frie M, Ernst M, Hekmat K, Schiller W, Gummert JF, Welz A. German heart surgery report 2015: the annual updated registry of the German society for thoracic and cardiovascular surgery. Thorac Cardiovasc Surg. 2016;64:462–74.

4. Committee for Scientific Affairs, The Japanese Association for Thoracic Surgery, Masuda M, Okumura M, Doki Y, Endo S, Hirata Y, Kobayashi J, Kuwano H, Motomura N, Nishida H, Saiki Y, Saito A, Shimizu H, Tanaka F, Tanemoto K, Toh Y, Tsukihara H, Wakui S, Yokomise H. Thoracic and cardiovascular surgery in Japan during 2014: annual report by The Japanese Association for Thoracic Surgery. Gen Thorac Cardiovasc Surg. 2016;64:665–97.
5. Arimura S, Seki M, Sasaki K, Takai H, Matsuhama M, Kunihara T, Okita Y, Takanashi S, Komiya T, Yaku H, Okabayashi H, Takemura H, Arai H, Sawazaki M, Matsui Y, Shiiya N. A nationwide survey of aortic valve surgery in Japan: current status of valve preservation in cases with aortic regurgitation. Gen Thorac Cardiovasc Surg. 2017;65:429–34.
6. Hammermeister K, Sethi GK, Henderson WG, Grover FL, Oprian C, Rahimtoola SH. Outcomes 15 years after valve replacement with a mechanical versus a bioprosthetic valve: final report of the Veterans Affairs randomized trial. J Am Coll Cardiol. 2000;36:1152–8.
7. Hughes GC, Zhao Y, Rankin JS, Scarborough JE, O'Brien S, Bavaria JE, Wolfe WG, Gaca JG, Gammie JS, Shahian DM, Smith PK. Effects of institutional volumes on operative outcomes for aortic root replacement in North America. J Thorac Cardiovasc Surg. 2013;145:166–70.
8. Malas T, Saczkowski R, Sohmer B, Ruel M, Mesana T, de Kerchove L, El Khoury G, Boodhwani M. Is aortic valve repair reproducible? Analysis of the learning curve for aortic valve repair. Can J Cardiol. 2015;31:1497.e15–22.

Part II
Concepts and Approaches

Bicuspid Aortic Valve 10

Norihiko Shiiya

10.1 Introduction

Although valve repair for aortic regurgitation (AR) has gained attention and the application of individual procedures is becoming standardized according to the pathophysiology of regurgitation, repair techniques for the bicuspid aortic valve (BAV) have not yet been standardized. The main reason for this is the diversity of BAV phenotypes. Even considering just the cusps, the level of diversity in the BAV is great as one must consider the presence/absence of a raphe, the types of fused cusps, and the orientation of the commissures. In addition, BAV/AR is frequently associated with dilatation of the aortoventricular junction (AVJ), Valsalva sinus, sinotubular junction (STJ), and the ascending aorta. Thus, there are rather few cases that can be managed well simply by treating the cusps alone. In this article, taking these factors into account, the BAV phenotype, its clinical significance, various repair techniques, and problems specific to BAV are discussed.

N. Shiiya (✉)
First Department of Surgery, Hamamatsu University School of Medicine, Hamamatsu, Japan
e-mail: shiyanor@hama-med.ac.jp

T. Kunihara, S. Takanashi (eds.), *Aortic Valve Preservation*,
https://doi.org/10.1007/978-981-13-2068-2_10

10.2 Historical Evolution

The history of BAV/AR repair is long, and free margin plication near the commissure was already reported in the 1960s. The origin of the current concept can be found from the AATS (American Association for Thoracic Surgery) lecture the "French correction" presented by Carpentier in 1983 [1]. The procedure applied was correction of the free margin length by triangular resection of the prolapsing cusp and plication of the aortic annulus (In this chapter, this term is assumed to denote the crown-shaped three-dimensional valve insertion line) by circular horizontal mattress suture. Concerning BAV, Cosgrove et al. [2] reported early outcomes in 21 of 28 cases (75%) of aortic valve repair in 1991. Technically, the procedure was a combination of raphe resection and triangular resection-suture of the fused cusp with Cabrol's subcommissural annuloplasty [3]. These procedures are performed to repair a BAV as a bicuspid valve, and their basis remains the same although some modification has been added. However, the importance of intervention to AVJ dilatation has been reported from recent studies on long-term results [4–6], and several new strategies have been introduced [7, 8], including aggressive adaptation of valve-sparing aortic root replacement (VSARR) [9]. Quite recently, Schäfers' group has reported that adding external suture annuloplasty to BAV repair improves freedom from reoperation at

5 years up to 93% compared with that of 73% in their early series [10].

In contrast, various techniques of tricuspidization have also been reported by several surgeons. Unlike the method to repair a BAV as a bicuspid valve, tricuspidization does not sacrifice the orifice area even if cusp plication is added to secure an effective height (eH). For this reason, there is room for consideration when the free margin length of the fused cusp is considerably longer than the non-fused cusp. Because another chapter discusses the procedure of tricuspidization, this article describes the techniques used to repair the BAV as a bicuspid valve.

10.3 Basis for Selecting the Operative Method

El Khoury's classification [11] in accordance with Carpentier's classification in mitral valves is effective for understanding the pathophysiology and selection of the operative method (see page 24 (Chap. 3)). For BAV, it is also necessary to understand the various phenotypes to logically select a surgical method. The phenotype is related not only with hemodynamics but also with genetics [12].

Cusp Morphology

The most convenient classification for the surgeon is that of Sievers and Schmidtke [13] (Fig. 10.1), which includes unicuspid valves. In this classification, the presence or absence and the number of raphes are indicated by type (0 means no raphe, 2 means a unicuspid valve), the fused cusp by a combination of L/R/N (left/right/non-coronary cusp), and the hemodynamic condition by S/I/B (stenosis/insufficiency/both). The most common is type 1 L/R, which includes two thirds of all cases, whereas the incidence of Type 0, which indicates a pure bicuspid valve configuration, is as low as 7%. This tendency is the same when dealing only with regurgitant valves.

Sabet et al. [14] refer to the spatial orientation of the commissures. The arrangement of 180/180° is found in 5% of commissures, and 1/3 of them have no raphe. However, only 2% have an arrangement of 120/240°. The most common is the so-called 150/210° configuration, which accounts for 92%. In a study simulating the stress on the cusps according to the cusp configuration [15], stress on the 180/180° Sievers type 0 valve was shown to be lower than that on the 150/210° type 1 L/R valve. The average age at the time of BAV/AR surgery is younger than that for BAV/AS [14, 16], and the frequency of calcification is also reported to be lower in BAV/AR [14]. As the degree of cusp calcification depends upon the stress and time elapsed, such knowledge about stress is important not only for estimating the natural history of the BAV but also for considering the prognosis of the repaired valve. Aicher et al. reported that the long-term durability of the repaired BAV is favorable when the smaller angle of the commissures is more than 160° [4].

Aortopathy

Otto and colleagues [17] examined the relation between aortic shape and aortic valve morphology, which was based on the conventional classification of BAV: the anterior-posterior (type 1)

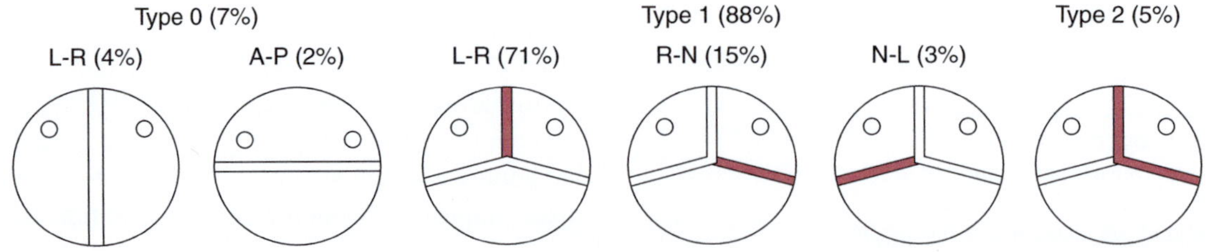

Fig. 10.1 The Sievers classification

cusp orientation, in which the right and the left cusps were fused, and the right-left cusp orientation. They classified the latter further into type 2, in which the right and the non-coronary cusps were fused, and the rarer type 3, in which the left and the non-coronary cusps were fused. The shape of the aorta was classified into N (normal), in which the STJ exists and the sinus is larger than the ascending aorta, A (ascending dilatation), in which the ascending aorta is larger than the sinus, and E (sinus effacement), in which the STJ is not present. Type 1 represents 80% of BAV, and 60% of them have an N-shaped aorta, whereas in type 2, the A shape comprises more than half. For both types 1 and 2, the E-shape aorta is rare (Table 10.1). In contrast, Fazel et al. [18] classified the pattern of aortic dilatation into four clusters: aortic root alone (cluster I, 13%), tubular ascending aorta alone (cluster II, 14%), tubular portion and transverse arch (cluster III, 28%) and aortic root and tubular portion with tapering across the transverse arch (cluster IV, 45%). The important thing here is that dilatation of the aortic root was present in up to 60% of cases, and a bovine arch was found in one third of them. This means that the N shape of Otto and colleagues does not indicate an aorta without root dilatation but only shows that the aortic root is larger than the ascending aorta.

Changes in the aortic annulus accompanying the aortopathy also differ greatly between aortic stenosis (AS) and AR among BAV. Sabet et al. [14] reported that annular dilatation (possibly indicating AVJ dilatation) in AR was recognized in approximately half of the cases, which was higher than that in AS (11%). Sadee et al. [16] reported that root dilatation was recognized in about 1/3 of their cases, and its presence increased the risk of the occurrence of AR by a factor of 4. Thus, aortopathy is closely involved in the occurrence of BAV/AR.

Table 10.1 Phenotype of aortopathy (Otto)

	N	A	E	Subtotal/ total
R-L orientation Type 1	86 (60%)	50 (35%)	8 (5%)	144/152
A-P orientation Type 2	12 (32%)	20 (54%)	5 (14%)	37/39
Type 3				/1

10.4 Decision Making in BAV Repair

Root Replacement or Not

Ascending aortic dilatation in BAV aortopathy is thought to be associated with hemodynamic factors and tissue vulnerability including a gene-related problem. For this reason, the threshold diameter for therapeutic intervention has been set smaller than that for a tricuspid aortic valve, and in the ESC (European Society of Cardiology) guideline [19], it is 45 mm at the time of aortic valve surgery. However, a recent study has reported that the diameter of the ascending aorta at the onset of aortic dissection was 10 mm larger in the BAV [20], and the validity of early surgical intervention was reconsidered. Also for the aortic root, analysis of long-term prognosis after aortic valve replacement and separate repair of the ascending aorta without root replacement has shown the stability of the remaining native aortic root [21]. However, the phenotype of BAV was not considered in these reports. More recently, Sievers et al. [22] reported that in stenotic BAVs, aortic dilatation was more localized to the ascending aorta, whereas BAVs with AR were associated with a more extensive aortopathy involving the root.

From the viewpoint of the long-term durability of valve repair, the importance of intervention to AVJ dilatation has been pointed out [4–6], and VSARR tends to be aggressively implemented even for lesions that do not meet the diameter-based criteria [9]. In VSARR, unlike various attempts to reduce and stabilize the AVJ without root replacement, the spatial orientation of the commissures can be freely modified, which may be another benefit of VSARR. However, surgical stress on the patients is greater than that of ascending aorta replacement, and the validity of the “unnecessary” intervention to the small root has been argued.

Patient Selection

In the long-term follow-up of a BAV that is repaired as a bicuspid valve, an increase in the pressure gradient can be a problem [8], in addition to the recurrence of AR (see the next section of this article). In this respect, the presence of a pre-operative pressure gradient and a high degree of thickening/calcification of the cusps is not preferable. The latter also acts disadvantageously in cusp coaptation and reduces the geometric height (gH) from the fusion of transverse fine wrinkles of the cusp tissue. To solve the problem of cusp sclerosis and low gH, pericardium may be used to extend [23] or augment the cusps in addition to resection of the thickened part. However, the use of pericardium is a negative prognostic factor for the long-term durability of the repair [4]. Thus, it would be ideal to select lesions that do not have advanced sclerosis that restricts valve opening.

10.5 Problems Intrinsic to BAV Repair as a Bicuspid Valve

In repairing the BAV as a bicuspid valve, securing both an adequate valve orifice area and durability of the repair are incompatible. This is a unique problem not found in tricuspidization.

Effective Height

Aicher and colleagues showed the importance of eH in the long-term results of aortic valve repair and reported that a higher eH is necessary in the BAV than in the tricuspid aortic valve, and the reoperation-free rate was high when the eH was 9 mm or more [4]. To gain eH, central plication may also be needed for the non-fused cusp. In the case of the BAV, however, as the relative length of the cusp free margin to the STJ diameter becomes shorter, the opening of the cusp becomes increasingly restricted. In other words, securing both eH and an adequate valve orifice area is incompatible, and thus, it is important to determine the point of compromise. An appropriate value of eH depends on gH, and it should not be decided alone. Establishment of criteria that can be adapted even for Japanese, who are much smaller compared with Western people, will be appreciated. I personally set the target value of eH to be 45% of gH.

Spatial Orientation of the Commissures

Aicher and colleagues recommend placing commissures at 180/180° [4], the purpose of which is to improve the opening of the fused cusp. It may also be possible to alleviate secondary calcification of the cusp due to the reduction of stress. However, as the opening of the non-fused cusp is directed towards the restriction when converting 150/210° valves into 180/180° (simple mathematics), a question about the net effect on the valve orifice area is raised. Vallabhajosyula and colleagues [24] reported that the pressure gradient of a BAV repaired at 150/210° is lower than that at 180/180°. In the simulation by Jermihov et al. as well [15], the valve orifice area of a perfectly symmetrical 180/180° valve was smaller than that of a 150/210° valve. In addition, even if raphe excision and triangular resection were added to a Sievers type 1 valve, there are two nadirs in the fused cusp and a perfectly symmetrical valve is not formed. Stress on this type of valve has not been studied. To create a perfectly symmetric BAV, the method of Gleason [25] can be performed, in which the fused cusp is detached from the annulus, the raphe is resected, a symmetric cusp is reconstructed with pericardium, and the cusp is sutured deeper into the left ventricular outflow tract (Fig. 10.2). When the pericardial patch is used at the hinge part, however, due to the difference in mechanical properties between the pericardium and the cusp tissue, only the native cusp part may move, and the opening of the pericardial part may be restricted, which may further compromise the durability of the pericardial patch itself. Thus, the orientation of the commissures is also an unsolved problem inherent in the procedure of repairing the BAV as a bicuspid valve.

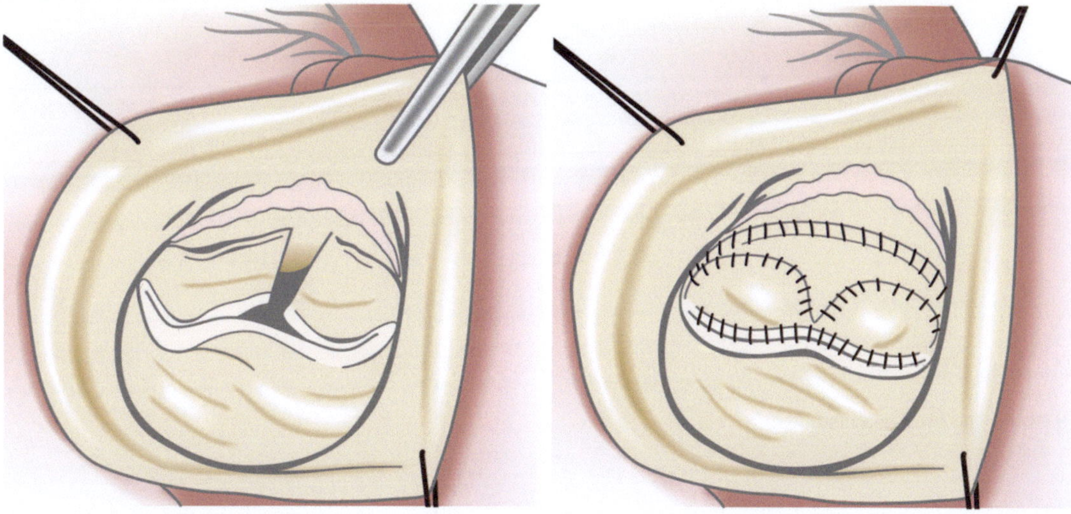

Fig. 10.2 The Gleason method

10.6 Operative Technique

Repair of the Fused Cusp

Because the fused cusp is usually redundant and prolapsed, the raphe that restricts the cusp motion is resected and a central plication is added to the free edge. I use 6-0 monofilament sutures and make the free margin length equal to that of the non-fused cusp. Each suture is placed to shorten the free margin by 2 mm. When large plication is required, triangular resection or plication [26] of the cusp body is required to correct the slackness of the cusp belly and achieve good coaptation. I add it when more than two stitches are required for central plication. When marked thickening and sclerosis of the fused part are present, triangular resection is better. It is desirable that the point of central plication faces the Arantius body of the non-fused cusp. Paracentral plication may also be used if central plication is impossible due to thickening of this part and resection of the thickened part will not leave enough free-margin length.

If the gH is not high enough, extension by pericardium [23] can also be added. Shaving the thickened cusp on the aortic surface may also gain approximately 2 mm of gH (I call this procedure "unrolling"). In the case of prolapse due to fenestration rupture, a pericardial patch is generally a preferred method of repair [27]. Free edge suspension by a continuous ePTFE (expanded polytetrafluoroethylene) suture [28] is currently used mainly to reinforce the fenestration, and its application to correct prolapse has become less frequent.

Treatment for the Non-fused Cusp

If the eH is low, central plication is added to achieve the target value. It is important to avoid symmetrical prolapse, especially when VSARR is performed.

Procedures for the Aortic Annulus and Root

Cabrol's subcommissural annuloplasty proved to be insufficient to ensure good long-term outcomes [4–6]. Circular plication of the AVJ using suture, a Dacron strip, or a specially designed ring and aggressive application of VSARR [9] are thus increasingly used. The former can be classified into internal and external methods, but the details are given in another chapter. Svensson

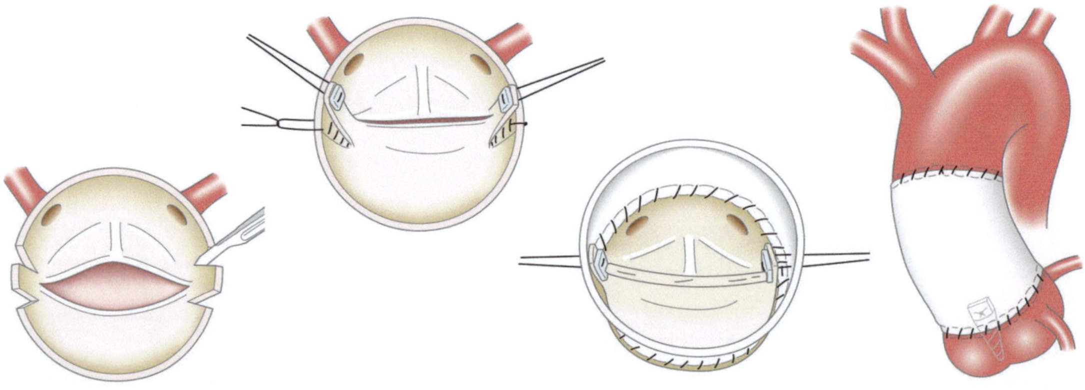

Fig. 10.3 The Svensson method

et al. [8] reported a method of root plication that detaches the commissures and fixes them at a higher level for patients with mild root dilatation (Fig. 10.3). Although the Cabrol method is not suitable for AVJ correction, it is useful to correct the commissural gap in conjunction with a figure-of-eight suture [8].

10.7 My Tips

The sequence of individual procedures is important in the repair of the BAV, and if there is enlargement of the aortic annulus, I will handle this first because the target value of eH is influenced by the AVJ diameter (and also by the changes in the shape of the sinus of Valsalva and the STJ diameter in the case of VSARR). When VSARR is not performed, I currently use an external Dacron strip for AVJ reduction. In doing so, I transect the aorta at the level of the STJ for dissection of the root down to the level of the AVJ. The target AVJ diameter is determined according to the gH, but at least 20 mm is secured. In actual practice, a 26-mm Dacron vascular prosthesis is most frequently used. Central plication of the non-fused cusp, if necessary, is then performed until the eH reaches the target value (gH—1/2AVJ or more). Using this as a reference, the central plication and triangular resection (or plication) of the fused cusp are performed. In the case of triangular plication, traction of the central plication suture facilitates determination of the triangular suture line. After placing several mattress sutures on the cusp body, a running suture is added up to the free edge, with resection of the excess cusp tissue performed when necessary (Fig. 10.4).

10.8 Results

As the current long-term performance of the tissue valve in the aortic position has continued to improve, valve repair must be evaluated by the long-term results. Ten-year results have only been reported by experts such as the Cleveland Clinic group [8], Mayo Clinic group [29], and the Schäfers [7] and El Khoury [30] groups. Although reoperation-free survival at 10 years is close to 90% for the El Khoury group and around 80% by for Cleveland Clinic and Schäfers groups, it is not necessarily ideal as indicated by the 49% rate from the Mayo Clinic group. Even in the David group's 8-year results [31], although their reoperation-free rate is 82%, the rate of freedom from AR of grade 3 or more is as low as 44%. These results are sufficiently compelling, however, for young people with poor long-term durability of tissue valves.

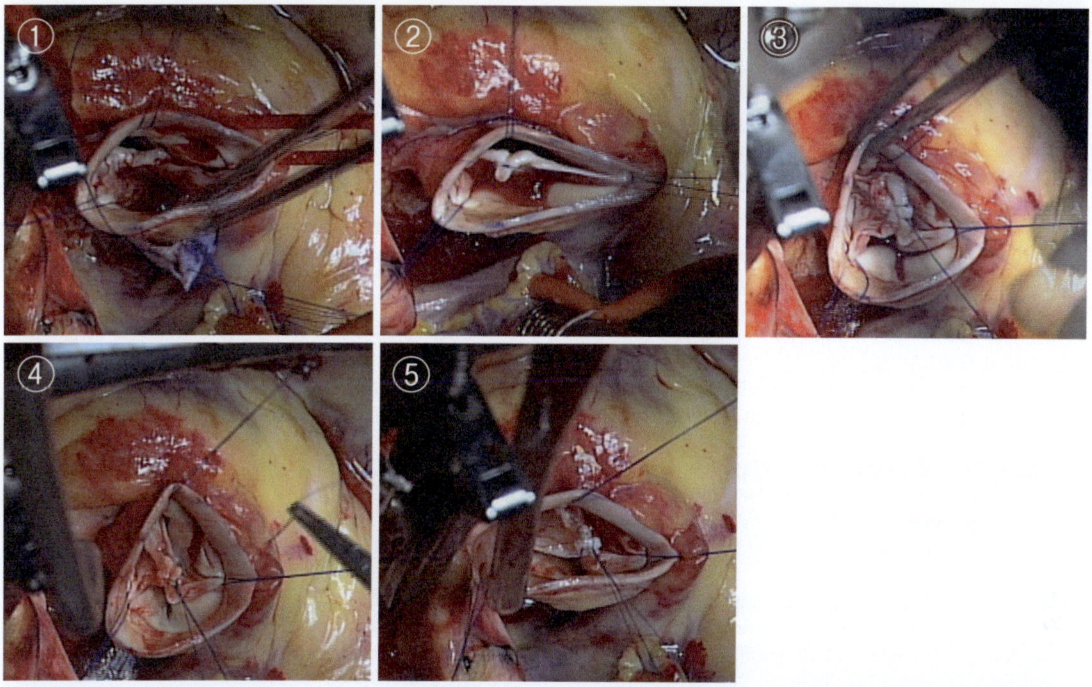

Fig. 10.4 A case of BAV repair without VSARR. (1) External Dacron strip for AVJ reduction/stabilization. (2) Adjustment of eH of the non-fused cusp with central plication. (3) Adjustment of free margin length of the fused cusp with central plication for correction of prolapse. (4) Triangular resection to remove thickened cusp tissue and to correct slackness of the cusp belly. (5) Suturing the cut end of the cusp body

10.9 Conclusion

Long-term outcomes of BAV repair still has room for improvement, and many innovative techniques or strategies are being introduced. It is expected that the effects of these innovations will be validated in further studies.

References

1. Carpentier A. Cardiac valve surgery—the "French correction". J Thorac Cardiovasc Surg. 1983;86:323–37.
2. Cosgrove DM, Rosenkranz ER, Hendren WG, Bartlett JC, Stewart WJ. Valvuloplasty for aortic insufficiency. J Thorac Cardiovasc Surg. 1991;102:571–6. discussion 76–7
3. Cabrol C, Cabrol A, Guiraudon G, Bertrand M. Treatment of aortic insufficiency by means of aortic annuloplasty. Arch Mal Coeur Vaiss. 1966;59:1305–12.
4. Aicher D, Kunihara T, Abou Issa O, Brittner B, Gräber S, Schäfers H-J. Valve configuration determines long-term results after repair of the bicuspid aortic valve. Circulation. 2011;123:178–85.
5. Navarra E, El Khoury G, Glineur D, Boodhwani M, Van Dyck M, Vanoverschelde JL, et al. Effect of annulus dimension and annuloplasty on bicuspid aortic valve repair. Eur J Cardiothorac Surg. 2013;44:316–22. discussion 22–3
6. Vallabhajosyula P, Komlo C, Szeto WY, Wallen TJ, Desai N, Bavaria JE. Root stabilization of the repaired bicuspid aortic valve: subcommissural annuloplasty versus root reimplantation. Ann Thorac Surg. 2014;97:1227–34.
7. Aicher D, Schneider U, Schmied W, Kunihara T, Tochii M, Schäfers H-J. Early results with annular support in reconstruction of the bicuspid aortic valve. J Thorac Cardiovasc Surg. 2013;145:S30–4.
8. Svensson LG, Al Kindi AH, Vivacqua A, Pettersson GB, Gillinov AM, Mihaljevic T, et al. Long-term durability of bicuspid aortic valve repair. Ann Thorac Surg. 2014;97:1539–47. discussion 48
9. de Kerchove L, Boodhwani M, Glineur D, Vandyck M, Vanoverschelde J-L, Noirhomme P, et al. Valve sparing-root replacement with the reimplantation technique to increase the durability of bicuspid aortic valve repair. J Thorac Cardiovasc Surg. 2011;142:1430–8.

10. Schneider U, Hofmann C, Aicher D, Takahashi H, Miura Y, Schäfers HJ. Suture annuloplasty significantly improves the durability of bicuspid aortic valve repair. Ann Thorac Surg. 2017;103:504–10.
11. Boodhwani M, de Kerchove L, Glineur D, Poncelet A, Rubay J, Astarci P, et al. Repair-oriented classification of aortic insufficiency: impact on surgical techniques and clinical outcomes. J Thorac Cardiovasc Surg. 2009;137:286–94.
12. Fernández B, Durán AC, Fernández-Gallego T, Fernández MC, Such M, Arqué JM, et al. Bicuspid aortic valves with different spatial orientations of the leaflets are distinct etiological entities. J Am Coll Cardiol. 2009;54:2312–8.
13. Sievers HH, Schmidtke C. A classification system for the bicuspid aortic valve from 304 surgical specimens. J Thorac Cardiovasc Surg. 2007;133:1226–33.
14. Sabet HY, Edwards WD, Tazelaar HD, Daly RC. Congenitally bicuspid aortic valves: a surgical pathology study of 542 cases (1991 through 1996) and a literature review of 2,715 additional cases. Mayo Clin Proc. 1999;74:14–26.
15. Jermihov P, Jia L, Sacks M, Gorman R, Gorman J III, Chandran K. Effect of geometry on the leaflet stresses in simulated models of congenital bicuspid aortic valves. Cardiovasc Eng Technol. 2011;2:48–56.
16. Sadee AS, Becker AE, Verheul HA, Bouma B, Hoedemaker G. Aortic valve regurgitation and the congenitally bicuspid aortic valve: a clinico-pathological correlation. Br Heart J. 1992;67:439–41.
17. Schaefer BM, Lewin MB, Stout KK, Gill E, Prueitt A, Byers PH, et al. The bicuspid aortic valve: an integrated phenotypic classification of leaflet morphology and aortic root shape. Heart. 2008;94:1634–8.
18. Fazel SS, Mallidi HR, Lee RS, Sheehan MP, Liang D, Fleischman D et al. The aortopathy of bicuspid aortic valve disease has distinctive patterns and usually involves the transverse aortic arch. J Thorac Cardiovasc Surg. 2008;135:901–7, 907.e1–2.
19. Vahanian A, Alfieri O, Andreotti F, Antunes MJ, Baron-Esquivias G, Baumgartner H, et al. Guidelines on the management of valvular heart disease (version 2012). Eur Heart J. 2012;33:2451–96.
20. Eleid MF, Forde I, Edwards WD, Maleszewski JJ, Suri RM, Schaff HV, et al. Type A aortic dissection in patients with bicuspid aortic valves: clinical and pathological comparison with tricuspid aortic valves. Heart. 2013;99:1668–74.
21. Park CB, Greason KL, Suri RM, Michelena HI, Schaff HV, Sundt TM 3rd. Fate of nonreplaced sinuses of Valsalva in bicuspid aortic valve disease. J Thorac Cardiovasc Surg. 2011;142:278–84.
22. Sievers HH, Stierle U, Hachmann RM, Charitos EI. New insights in the association between bicuspid aortic valve phenotype, aortic configuration and valve haemodynamics. Eur J Cardiothorac Surg. 2016;49:439–46.
23. Duran C, Kumar N, Gometza B, al Halees Z. Indications and limitations of aortic valve reconstruction. Ann Thorac Surg. 1991;52:447–53. discussion 53–4
24. Vallabhajosyula P, Szeto WY, Komlo CM, Ryan LP, Wallen TJ, Gorman RC, et al. Geometric orientation of the aortic neoroot in patients with raphed bicuspid aortic valve disease undergoing primary cusp repair and a root reimplantation procedure. Eur J Cardiothorac Surg. 2014;45:174–80. discussion 80
25. Gleason TG. Bicuspid aortic valve repair by complete conversion from "raphe'd" (type 1) to "symmetric" (type 0) morphology. J Thorac Cardiovasc Surg. 2014;148:2862–8.e1–2.
26. Boodhwani M, de Kerchove L, Glineur D, El Khoury G. A simple method for the quantification and correction of aortic cusp prolapse by means of free margin plication. J Thorac Cardiovasc Surg. 2010;139:1075–7.
27. Schafers HJ, Langer F, Glombitza P, Kunihara T, Fries R, Aicher D. Aortic valve reconstruction in myxomatous degeneration of aortic valves: are fenestrations a risk factor for repair failure? J Thorac Cardiovasc Surg. 2010;139:660–4.
28. David TE, Feindel CM, Webb GD, Colman JM, Armstrong S, Maganti M. Long-term results of aortic valve-sparing operations for aortic root aneurysm. J Thorac Cardiovasc Surg. 2006;132:347–54.
29. Ashikhmina E, Sundt TM 3rd, Dearani JA, Connolly HM, Li Z, Schaff HV. Repair of the bicuspid aortic valve: a viable alternative to replacement with a bioprosthesis. J Thorac Cardiovasc Surg. 2010;139:1395–401.
30. Price J, De Kerchove L, Glineur D, Vanoverschelde JL, Noirhomme P, El Khoury G. Risk of valve-related events after aortic valve repair. Ann Thorac Surg. 2013;95:606–12. discussion 13
31. Alsoufi B, Borger MA, Armstrong S, Maganti M, David TE. Results of valve preservation and repair for bicuspid aortic valve insufficiency. J Heart Valve Dis. 2005;14:752–8. discussion 58–9

11 ONE-POINT ADVICE: Tricuspidization of a Bicuspid Valve

Kohei Abe and Kohei Kawazoe

11.1 Introduction

Bicuspid valves are the most commonly seen condition in aortic dysplasia. Among young people, many valvular dysfunctions occur primarily due to an inability of the valve to close properly, and the availability of a long-lasting plasty technique is highly desirable.

11.2 History of the Operative Method

As a method of valve repair for a prolapsed bicuspid valve, triangular resection of the raphe of the fused leaflets and correction of the prolapse were reported by Cosgrove et al. in 1991 [1]. However, the stress applied to the fused leaflets was enormous, and most of the recurrences of AR were due to disruption at the plication, and freedom from reoperation was as low as 84% at 7 years. Therefore, tricuspidization was developed to equalize the stress between the leaflets and make them function more physiologically. When this technique was first developed, the annuloplasty was performed only at the commissures. However, recurrences due to dehiscence were observed, and the results were further stabilized after the subvalvular circular annuloplasty technique was adopted, which secures the entire annulus [2].

11.3 Indications and Contraindications

Cases in which degeneration of the aortic valve is small or limited to the raphe are good indications for tricuspidization. A 180° bicuspid valve without a raphe (Type 0) and highly degenerated and/or calcified leaflets are contraindications.

11.4 Advantages and Disadvantages

The advantages of this procedure, as previously described, are that the stress on each of the leaflets is even and the valve opening is more physiologic. By using the adjustable suspension method, it is possible to adjust the cusp height of the fused leaflets after cessation of cardiopulmonary bypass. However, the disadvantage is that if the aortic diameter where the raphe was lifted enlarges at a later date, the height of the lifted part will change, leading to the risk of recurrence of the aortic regurgitation (AR). Because the

K. Abe (✉)
Cardiovascular Center, St. Luke's International Hospital, Tokyo, Japan
e-mail: koabe@luke.ac.jp

K. Kawazoe
Cardiovascular Disease Center, Kansai Medical University Medical Center, Osaka, Japan

T. Kunihara, S. Takanashi (eds.), *Aortic Valve Preservation*,
https://doi.org/10.1007/978-981-13-2068-2_11

raphe is usually lifted to the height of the sinotubular junction, if enlargement is expected, this risk can be reduced by the simultaneous performance of aortic root replacement.

11.5 Procedures

Because a bicuspid valve with AR often involves widening of the annulus, an annuloplasty is performed for aortic valvuloplasty according to the size of the leaflets. These authors use the subvalvular circular annuloplasty method, in which a 5-mm-wide ring-shaped expanded polytetrafluoroethylene (ePTFE) sheet or tubular ePTFE graft is placed underneath the leaflets in the left ventricular outflow tract and is circumferentially fixed with pledgetted 5-0 polypropylene mattress sutures from the aortic side (Fig. 11.1).

First, the fused leaflet is folded using a 4-0 polypropylene double-braided suture with an ePTFE pledget to create an acute angle and coaptation at the raphe. Then, a Gore-Tex CV-6 suture is hooked on this pledget and drawn out of the aorta in a direction that does not distort the leaflet (usually in the direction of the sinus of Valsalva where the raphe adheres or is slightly higher than the other commissures). After closure of the aortotomy and cessation of cardiopulmonary bypass, the suture that was passed outside the aorta is adjusted and ligated under transesophageal echocardiographic monitoring of the leaflet coaptation status (Figs. 11.2 and 11.3).

11.6 My Tips

In cases in which strong thickening of the raphe portion is seen, the fused leaflets may not be able to be joined at an acute angle with pledgeted sutures alone. In this situation, it is very useful to make a small triangular excision and cut back on the raphe to obtain a good angle. If there is thickening in the non-fused leaflet around the Arantius body, active slicing of this area can obtain good coaptation.

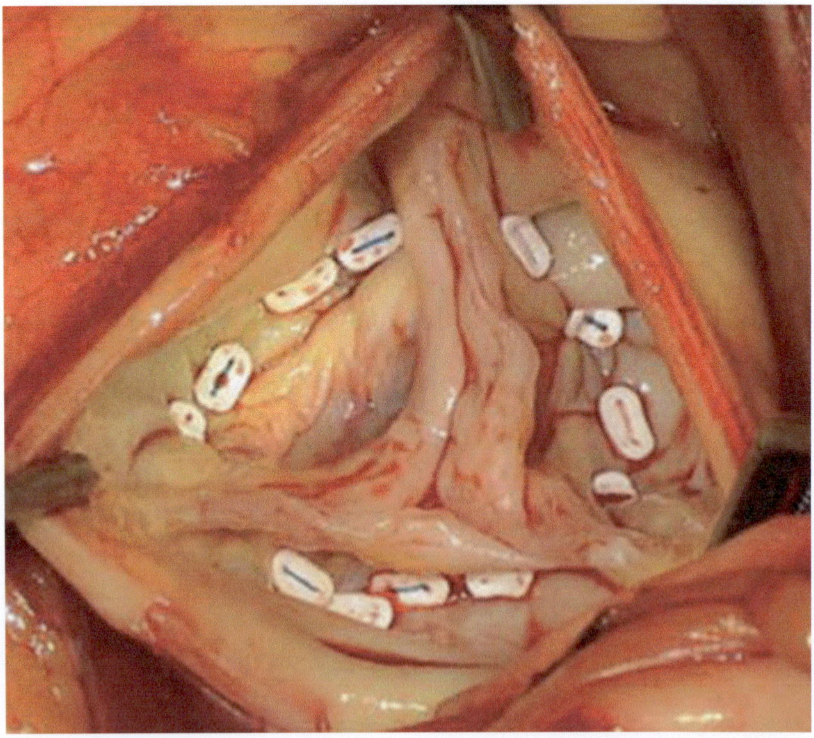

Fig. 11.1 Subvalvular circular annuloplasty seen from the aortic side. The pledgets are sutured onto the annulus, and a 5-mm-wide ePTFE sheet is fixed in place under the valve

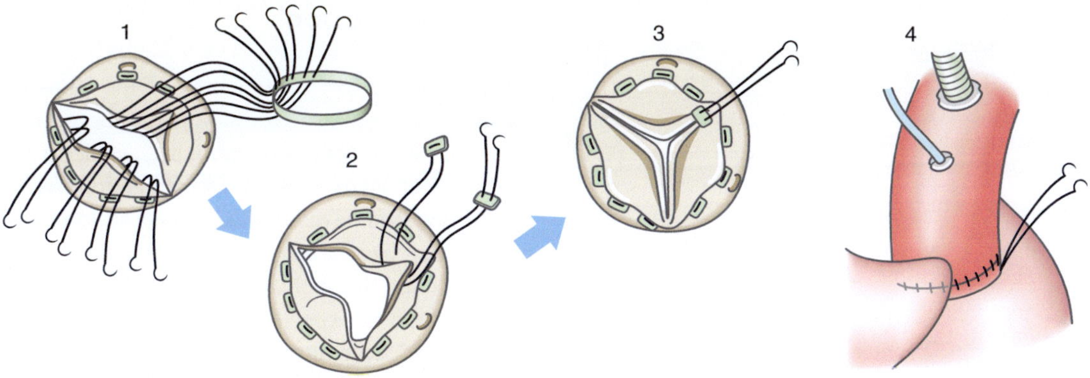

Fig. 11.2 Schema of subvalvular circular annuloplasty and tricuspidization. *1* Subvalvular circular annuloplasty with 5-0 polypropylene sutures with ePTFE pledgets on the aortic annulus. *2* Fixation of the raphe with ePTFE pledgets and a 4-0 polypropylene thread in the right and left coronary fused cusp. *3* A Gore-Tex CV-6 suture is hooked to the pledget on the raphe and is passed outside the aorta in a direction that results in good coaptation. *4* Image showing a Gore-Tex CV-6 suture led out of the aorta. Ligation is performed after adjusting the coaptation with the aid of transesophageal echocardiography

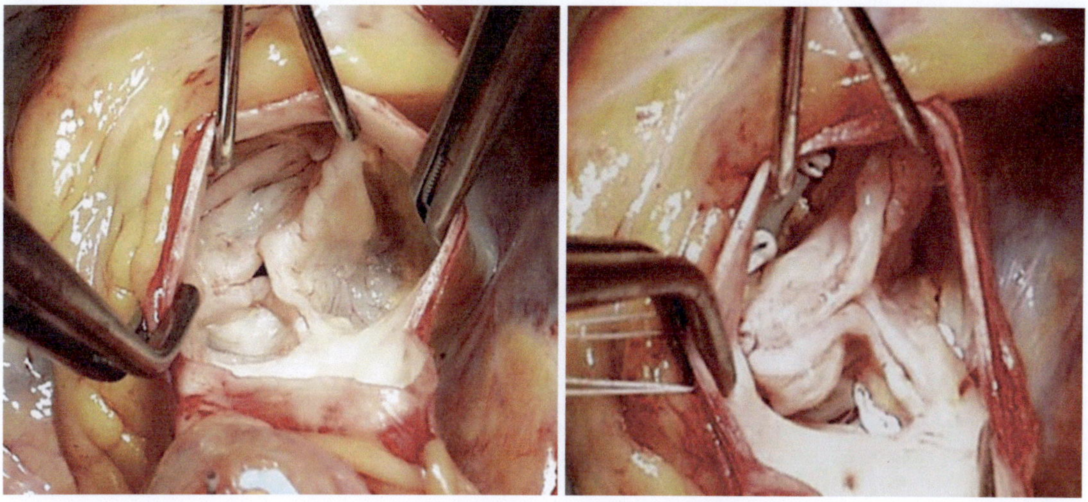

Fig. 11.3 Case in which the right and left coronary cusps are fused. The left image shows fusion of the right coronary cusp (upper left) and left coronary cusp (lower left), with the fused commissure (raphe) in between. The right image shows the subvalvular circular annuloplasty and tricuspidization that were performed, with a Gore-Tex suture for adjustment led out of the aorta to the left

11.7 Results

Since this technique was reported in 2003 [3], it has been applied to bicuspid valves mainly exhibiting AR. In reporting the long-term follow-up results in the European Association for Cardio-Thoracic Surgery annual meeting in 2014 [4], Mukaida et al. found that the overall rate of freedom from reoperation was 68.2% at 15 years (Fig. 11.4) and that after changing from annuloplasty to subvalvular circular annuloplasty, the rate improved to 92%, which proves the validity of this procedure in young people.

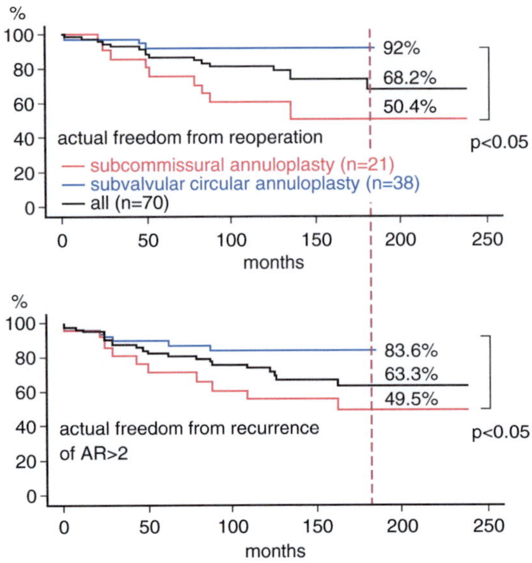

Fig. 11.4 Follow-up results after aortic valvuloplasty. Comparison between the group with subcommissural annuloplasty and that with subvalvular circular annuloplasty

11.8 Conclusion

Recently, the effect of widening of the sinus of Valsalva at long-term follow-up has become a concern, and thus concomitant aortic root replacement needs to be performed aggressively. In addition, we have adopted a method to determine plasty size by forming an ePTFE sheet into a ring shape for subvalvular circular annuloplasty, which is expected to further improve the results in the near future.

References

1. Cosgrove DM, et al. Valvuloplasty for aortic insufficiency. J Thorac Cardiovasc Surg. 1991;102:571–6.
2. Izumoto H, et al. Subvalvular circular annuloplasty as a component of aortic valve repair. J Heart Valve Dis. 2002;11:383–5.
3. Kawazoe K, et al. Tricuspidization of incompetent bicuspid aortic valve. J Thorac Cardiovasc Surg. 2003;126:908–10.
4. Mukaida K, et al. Aortic valvuloplasty for aortic insufficiency. Interact Cardiovasc Thorac Surg. 2014;19(Suppl. 1):S29.

Tricuspid Aortic Valve

12

Hitoshi Yaku, Kiyoshi Doi, Sachiko Yamazaki, and Satoshi Numata

12.1 Introduction

Aortic valve replacement (AVR) is applied as a surgical treatment for aortic valve regurgitation (AR), and if root enlargement is seen, aortic root replacement is performed. The results of these procedures are acceptable, but problems can arise from the implanted artificial valve. These problems include hemorrhagic complications caused by thromboembolism, infection and dysfunction of the artificial valve, and in the case of mechanical valves, warfarin administration, and all impart serious risk to the patient [1–3]. In a young population, exercise capability should be guaranteed, and body growth should be taken into account; therefore, an operation incorporating an artificial valve cannot be said to perfect.

Unfortunately, aortic valve repair is not yet a standard procedure, whereas valve repair for mitral regurgitation (MR) is performed as a standard surgical procedure. As with the mitral valve, the basic principles of aortic valve repair are thought to be (1) maintenance and restoration of leaflet mobility, (2) formation of a large coaptation area, and (3) fixation of the annulus (remodeling) [4]. However, due to the limitation of the amount of tissue present in the aortic valve leaflets, it is difficult to obtain a large coaptation area, and the best procedure for annulus remodeling has not been determined, which is why aortic valve repair is not yet accepted by a majority of surgeons. Recently, numerical values that can be used as indices for aortic valve repair, such as geometric height (gH) and effective height (eH), have been proposed, and these are contributing greatly to the standardization of aortic valve repair [5]. In this article, we explain the concept and the surgical technique for aortic valve repair of tricuspid leaflets and review the results from current reports.

12.2 History of Aortic Valve Repair

In the early stages of aortic valve repair, the main approach for AR was directed at the annulus or the commissure. In 1958, Taylor et al. had already applied external suture annuloplasty to 11 cases under beating-heart surgery [6], and in 1966, Cabrol et al. proposed subcommissural annuloplasty, which is the so-called "Cabrol stitch" [7]. Then, Carpentier et al. performed 95 cases of aortic annuloplasty surgery including interventions on the leaflets from 1971 to 1982, but the long-term follow-up results were disastrous and could not better those of valve replacement [8]. The main reason for this was the lack of an objective assessment index for aortic valve configuration, but since Schäfers et al. began to advocate the

H. Yaku (✉) · K. Doi · S. Yamazaki · S. Numata
Department of Cardiovascular Surgery, Kyoto Prefectural University of Medicine, Kyoto, Japan
e-mail: yakuh@koto.kpu-m.ac.jp

T. Kunihara, S. Takanashi (eds.), *Aortic Valve Preservation*,
https://doi.org/10.1007/978-981-13-2068-2_12

objective measurement of gH and eH in 2006 [5], aortic valve repair has emerged as a standardized and reproducible operative method, and it is currently spreading rapidly.

12.3 Indications and Contraindications

The surgical indications for aortic valve repair of the tricuspid aortic valve in AR are currently the same as those for AVR [9]. Worthy of special mention is that, unlike the guidelines for MR, the surgical indications are not determined only by the severity of AR but also by the presence of symptoms, enlargement of the left ventricle, or reduced heart function. However, Sharma et al. recommended surgery earlier than that for AVR in patients with a high possibility of aortic valve repair because of good early and long-term follow-up results of this procedure [10].

Thus, for what kinds of lesions is aortic valve repair possible? Technically, all types of AR can basically be considered as candidates. However, the success rate of repair largely depends on the quality and quantity of the leaflet tissue. A rheumatic etiology, infectious endocarditis, and calcification decrease the success rates of repair, and it is also difficult to repair a valve with cusp retraction because complicated procedures such as cusp extension with the pericardium are often required in such cases. Therefore, to estimate the possibility of repair, to some extent, preoperative evaluation is the key. Basically, evaluation of the cusp quality by 2- and 3-dimensional echocardiography and quantification by multiple detector computed tomography (MDCT) are suitable. In particular, it is important to accurately measure gH by MDCT, which will be further explained later [11].

12.4 Actual Operative Methods

Leaflet Repair

The bull's eye of leaflet repair is the correction of leaflet prolapse. In Type II dysfunction, because the length of the cusp free margin is longer than that of the corresponding annulus, excess movement of the leaflet occurs; thus, shortening of the free edges of the leaflets is the basic principle of the procedure. There are two methods, one by central plication and the other by resuspension.

Central Plication (Fig.12.1a)
At the center of the leaflet is the Arantius body, which is normally thickened. Also, as this is the point at which the least dynamic stress is applied, the application of central plication, which sutures this part, makes logical sense. This is performed with simple plication stitches with 6-0 polypropylene from the center. The free margin length is shortened with these stitches, and the prolapsing leaflet is raised in the Valsalva sinus.

The problem with this technique is in the extent of the suturing. In the case of a tricuspid valve, when one cusp is prolapsing, it is plicated to meet the height of the free edge of other two normal cusps. Also, when two cusps are prolapsing, they must be stitched to match the height of the free edge of the normal leaflet. In the rare case in which all three cusps are prolapsing, each free margin should be plicated to coapt them at the middle of the Valsalva sinuses [12]. Schäfers et al. have proposed suturing to create an eH of 8–9 mm or more [13].

Resuspension (Fig. 12.1b)
By applying expanded polytetrafluoroethylene (ePTFE) CV-6 suture, the cusp free margin is sutured and fixed at the commissure [14]. By pulling this thread, multiple small plications of the entire free edge are created. The extent to which the free edge is shortened is the same as that for central plication [15].

Patch Augmentation (Fig. 12.1c)
In the case of cusp retraction (Type III), augmentation is possible with the use of autologous pericardium. While the cusp free edge is maintained, an incision is made in a direction parallel to the annulus, and the leaflet is extended (upper row) by an elliptical pericardium patch. If the free edge is also retracted, the pericardium is trimmed into a rectangular shape with a width of 6–8 mm and is extended from the free edge (lower row). The length of the patch is adjusted to the distance between commissures, but it is normally 3–4 mm

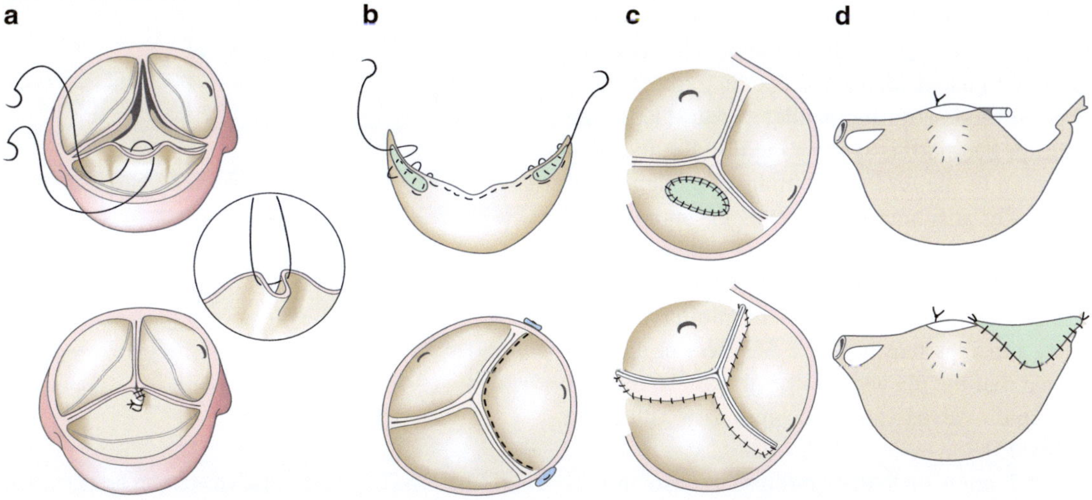

Fig. 12.1 Leaflet repair. (**a**) Central plication, (**b**) resuspension, (**c**) patch augmentation, (**d**) fenestration closure (Courtesy of Professor Yutaka Okita, Kobe University)

longer than 1/3 of the circumferential length of the aorta at the sinotubular junction (STJ) [4]. The autologous pericardium is generally treated with glutaraldehyde (0.6% for 10 min).

Fenestration Closure (Fig. 12.1d)
If the fenestration is in the part not involved in the leaflet coaptation, it may be left untreated, but if it is large, it should be closed with autologous pericardium.

Annuloplasty/Annular Remodeling

One of the reasons why aortic valve repair is not widely applied compared to mitral valve repair is that a simple and effective annuloplasty or remodeling method has not been established yet. Historically, subcommissural annuloplasty has been performed to suture the lower part of the commissure using mattress sutures [7]. Although this method is simple, its effect is limited [16]. Therefore, circular annular stabilization has been proposed, the details of which are given in other sections.

STJ Remodeling

When valve-sparing root replacement is performed, STJ remodeling will be performed with a vascular graft, but when isolated aortic valve repair is performed in the case of STJ enlargement, the ascending aorta is replaced with a vascular graft, resulting in reduction of the STJ size. Schäfers and colleagues suggest that STJ remodeling is necessary when the STJ is over 30 mm. Even in the case of mild enlargement that does not require replacement of the ascending aorta, it may be possible to prevent recurrent AR by reinforcement of the proximal side of the aortic incision line using a strip of a vascular graft to prevent further enlargement.

12.5 Our Tips

The principles of aortic valve repair are to restore the leaflets and the functional aortic annulus (STJ, aorto-ventricular junction; AVJ, and anatomic annulus) to their normal shape and size while maintaining normal motion of the leaflet cusps. The mobility of a leaflet is expressed as the ratio of the free margin length to the length of the leaflet attachment.

(Mobility of the leaflet) ≈ (free margin length)/(length of the leaflet attachment)

As this ratio increases, mobility of the leaflets becomes excessive, which will result in Type II dysfunction. Also, excessive annuloplasty can cause cusp prolapse. As this value decreases, the mobility of the leaflets becomes limited, which will result in Type III dysfunction. This is common in bicuspid valves and occurs in the case of over-correction during leaflet repair [17]. The concept behind this is explained by the fact that plication of the AVJ (shortening of the length of the leaflet attachment) improves the mobility of the leaflets, reduces the pressure gradient at the valve, and improves the leaflet coaptation. The leaflet size is important in determining whether valve repair is feasible, and Schäfers et al. suggested that the gH needs to be at least 16 mm for tricuspid valves and 20 mm for bicuspid valves [5].

Evaluation of leaflet prolapse is also important. A stay suture should be placed on the upper edge of each commissure and lightly lifted upward, away from AVJ. In the cases of STJ enlargement, it should be lifted slightly toward the inside assuming an appropriate inner diameter. For normal leaflets, the free edges run parallel at the same height and join at the center and approximately 1 cm above the nadir in the Valsalva sinus. When a specific leaflet prolapses, its free edge does not become parallel, and a transverse band is often found in the center of the body of the leaflet. Also, although rare, if all leaflets prolapse, the free edges are kept parallel and they join at the center, but their positions are low. For Japanese patients, leaflet repair is performed so that the eH becomes 8 mm or more [18].

Another important value is the coaptation height (cH), and it is reported that recurrence of AR after valve repair will increase if the cH is 4 mm or less. As a simulation of actual surgery, the calculation of one side of a right triangle as shown in Fig. 12.2 is helpful. When the gH is 17 mm and you want to change the eH to 9 mm and make the cH 4 mm, the following calculation can be performed: $(\text{target AVJ}/2)^2 = (\text{gH} - \text{cH})^2 - (\text{eH} - \text{cH})^2$. Thus, it is only necessary to make the annular diameter approximately 24 mm.

Another consideration of valve repair according to Rankin et al. is that the length of the free edge needs to be about 1.5 times longer than the annular diameter [19]. They plicate the annulus with subcommissural annuloplasty targeting a length of 19–20 mm, but at the same time, they do not make the free edge less than 26–30 mm. Also in their theory, it is assumed that the free margin length of the normal valve should be one half the circumferential length of the annulus; thus, the free margin is 3.14/2 when the annular diameter is 1. This is almost 1.5 times that of the annulus diameter. On the contrary, the annulus diameter, which is equal to the free margin length divided by 1.5, is appropriate to obtain good cusp coaptation [20].

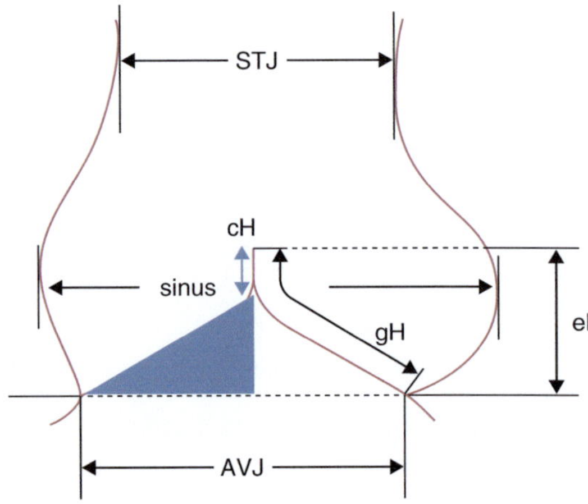

Fig. 12.2 The target annular diameter can be calculated as one side of a right triangle

Because of the extent of leaflet prolapse and the eH change after annuloplasty, it is thus important to ultimately perform leaflet repair. Therefore, the appropriate sequence of the aortic valve repair is (1) evaluation of the functional aortic annulus and leaflets, (2) plication of the AVJ, and (3) repair of the leaflets.

12.6 Surgical Results

Aortic Valve Repair Vs. AVR

The Brussels group compared the results of aortic valve repair versus replacement during the period from 1995 to 2012 [21]. After adjusting for risk in a comparison of 44 cases each, they reported that there was no statistical difference in the rate of operative mortality between aortic valve repair at 2% and replacement surgery at 5% ($p = 0.56$). The 9-year survival rate was significantly higher in valve repair vs. AVR (87% vs. 60%, p = 0.007). In a Cox proportional hazards analysis, the type of operation was an independent determinant of the postoperative survival rate. Valve repair had a slightly higher rate of reoperation, but the difference was not significant (8% vs. 2%, p = 0.35).

Early Results of Aortic Valve Repair

The Brussels group performed aortic valve repair in a series of 146 patients without a surgical death and only two cases of reoperation during hospitalization [22]. At the time of discharge from the hospital, the mean grade of valve regurgitation was 0.8 ± 0.7. The Homburg group reported a series of 640 cases of aortic valve repair with a total rate of hospital death of 3.4%, but in isolated aortic valve repair, the rate was reported to be 0.8% [23]. The Mayo group also reported operative mortality of 0.6% after aortic valve repair. All of these outcomes exceed those for AVR [10].

Long-Term Follow-Up Results of Aortic Valve Repair

In the report of the 640 cases of aortic valve repair from the Homburg group, the average patient age was 56 years, and the average follow-up period was 4.8 years [23]. The annual incidence of thromboembolism and infectious endocarditis were 0.2% and 0.16%, respectively. The 5- and 10-year rates of freedom from reoperation were 88% and 81% for bicuspid and 97% and 93% for tricuspid valves, respectively.

The Brussels group reported 475 cases of aortic valve repair with an average patient age of 53 years and average follow-up period of 4.6 years [24]. The 30-day mortality rate was 0.8%, the 10-year survival rate was 73.5 ± 5%, and the freedom from valve-related death was 90 ± 3%. The freedom from significant aortic regurgitation was 84 ± 3%, freedom from aortic valve reoperation was 86 ± 3%, and freedom from AVR was 90 ± 3%. Eight of 28 patients were able to undergo a re-repair operation. In addition, the incidences of thromboembolism, hemorrhage, and infectious endocarditis were 1.1%, 0.23%, and 0.19%, respectively. The 10-year freedom from valve-related events was 74 ± 3%.

The Mayo group reported 331 cases of aortic valve repair with an average patient age of 53 years and mean follow-up period of 5.8 years [10]. The hospital death rate was 0.6%, and the respective 5- and 10-year survival rates were 91% and 81%. Larger left ventricular end systolic diameter and lower left ventricular ejection fraction were the risk factors of long-term mortality. Incidences of reoperation at 5 and 10 years were 10% and 20%, respectively, and the preoperative degree of AR and residual regurgitation above a mild level at the time of discharge from hospital were risk factors for late reoperation.

Tricuspid Valve Vs. Bicuspid Valve

The Mayo group compared their long-term follow-up results at 10 years after aortic valve repair between patients with bicuspid and tricuspid valves [24]. The freedom from valve dysfunction, aortic valve reoperation, and AVR was not significantly different between the groups. The Homburg group also reported no significant difference in the freedom from recurrent AR between tricuspid and bicuspid valves at 10 years after aortic valve repair; however, in terms of freedom from reoperation, more reoperations were performed for bicuspid versus tricuspid valves [23]. However, freedom from AVR for bicuspid valves was equivalent to that for tricuspid valves, which indicates that re-repair was possible in many cases.

Plication Vs. Resuspension

The Brussels group reported the results due to differences in aortic valve repair [22]. Of 146 cases of valve repair, 76 were performed with only one procedure and 70 with two or more procedures. Resuspension was performed in 109 (75%), triangular resection/suture in 51 (35%), central plication in 47 (32%), and pericardial patch in 10 cases (7%). The 4-year freedom from recurrence of regurgitation (>2) was not different between the central plication vs. resuspension vs. combined procedures at 95 ± 8%, 83 ± 18%, and 100%, respectively (p = 0.37). However, rates were significantly worse for triangular resection versus pericardial patch unless resuspension was performed simultaneously. (82 ± 18% vs. 97 ± 4%, p = 0.026).

By univariate analysis, significant risk factors were lack of resuspension, preoperative NYHA class, single procedure for the prolapsing cusp, regurgitation ≥2 at the time of discharge from hospital, left ventricular end-diastolic diameter, and left ventricular end-systolic diameter. In a multivariate analysis, single procedure (p = 0.04) and left ventricular end-diastolic diameter (p = 0.02) remained as risk factors for the recurrence of regurgitation. From these results, the authors suggested that additional resuspension was acceptable when leaflet prolapse was prominent. Furthermore, it was reported that there was no evidence that resuspension using ePTFE sutures induced limited movement of the leaflets.

12.7 Conclusion

It would be difficult to say that aortic valve repair for AR is widely applied in the world or in Japan. Nevertheless, the concept of aortic valve repair is being widely shared, and it seems that surgery is progressing in the direction of standardization, and not just for the masters of this procedure. There is no doubt that advancements in preoperative evaluation by echocardiography and CT are also greatly influencing this progression [25]. The accumulation of long-term results of aortic valve repair in multiple centers across Japan is expected in the future.

References

1. Emery RW, Krogh CC, Arom KV, Emery AM, Benyo-Albrecht K, Joyce LD, et al. The St. Jude Medical cardiac valve prosthesis: a 25-year experience with single valve replacement. Ann Thorac Surg. 2005;79:776–82.
2. Forcillo J, Pellerin M, Perrault LP, Cartier R, Bouchard D, Demers P, et al. Carpentier-Edwards pericardial valve in the aortic position: 25-years experience. Ann Thorac Surg. 2013;96:486–93.
3. Anselmi A, Flécher E, Ruggieri VG, Harmouche M, Langanay T, Corbineau H, et al. Long-term results of the Medtronic Mosaic porcine bioprosthesis in the aortic position. J Thorac Cardiovasc Surg. 2014;147:1884–91.
4. Carpentier A, Adams DH, Filsoufi F, editors. Carpentier's reconstructive valve surgery from valve analysis to valve reconstruction. Philadelphia: Saunders; 2010.
5. Schäfers H-J, Bierbach B, Aicher D. A new approach to the assessment of aortic cusp geometry. J Thorac Cardiovasc Surg. 2006;132:436–8.
6. Taylor WJ, Thrower WB, Black H, Harken DE. The surgical correction of aortic insufficiency by circumclusion. J Thorac Surg. 1958;35:192–205.
7. Cabrol C, Cabrol A, Guiraudon G, Bertrand M. Treatment of aortic insufficiency by means of annuloplasty. Arch Mal Coeur Vaiss. 1966;59:1305–12.
8. Carpentier A. Cardiac valve surgery: the French correction. J Thorac Cardiovasc Surg. 1980;80:323–7.
9. Nishimura RA, Otto CM, Bonow RO, Carabello BA, Erwin JP III, Guyton RA, et al. 2014 AHA/ACC guideline for the management of patients with valvular heart disease: a report of the American College of Cardiology/American Heart Association Task Force on Practice Guidelines. Circulation. 2014;129:e521–643.
10. Sharma V, Suri RM, Dearani JA, Burkhart HM, Park SJ, Joyce LD, et al. Expanding relevance of aortic valve repair-is earlier operation indicated? J Thorac Cardiovasc Surg. 2014;147:100–7.
11. Komiya T. Aortic valve repair update. Gen Thorac Cardiovasc Surg. 2015;63:300–19.
12. Boodhwani M, de Kerchove L, Glineur D, El Khoury G. A simple method for quantification and correction of aortic cusp prolapse by means of free margin plication. J Thorac Cardiovasc Surg. 2010;139:1075–7.
13. Aicher D, Kunihara T, Issa OA, Brittner B, Graeber S, Schaefers H-J. Valve configuration determines long-term results after repair of the bicuspid aortic valve. Circulation 2011;123:178–85.
14. David TE, Armstrong S, Ivanov J, Webb GD. Aortic valve sparing operations: an update. Ann Thorac Surg. 1999;67(6):1840–2. discussion 1853–6
15. de Kerchove L, Boodhwani M, Glineur D, Poncelet A, Rubay J, Watremez C, et al. Cusp prolapse repair in trileaflet aortic valves: free margin plication and free margin resuspension techniques. Ann Thorac Surg. 2009;88:455–61. Discussion 461
16. de Kerchove L, Mastrobuoni S, Boodhwani M, Astarci P, Rubay J, Poncelet A, et al. The role of annular dimension and annuloplasty in tricuspid aortic valve repair. Eur J Cardiothorac Surg. 2016;49:428–37.
17. El Khoury G, de Kerchove L. Principles of aortic valve repair. J Thorac Cardiovasc Surg. 2013;145(3 Suppl):S26–9.

18. Miyahara S, Omura A, Sakamoto T, Nomura Y, Inoue T, Minami H, et al. Impact of postoperative cusp configuration on midterm durability after aortic root implantation. J Heart Valve Dis. 2013;22:509–16.
19. Rankin JS, Gaca JG. Techniques of aortic valve repair. Innovations. 2011;6:348–54.
20. Rankin RS, Bone MC, Fries PM, Aicher D, Schäfers H-J, Crooke PS, et al. A refind hemispheric model of normal human aortic valve and root geometry. J Thorac Cardiovasc Surg. 2013;146:103–8.
21. de Meester C, Pasquet A, Gerber BL, Vancraeynest D, Noirhomme P, El Khoury G, et al. Valve repair improves the outcome of surgery for chronic severe aortic regurgitation: a propensity score analysis. J Thorac Cardiovasc Surg. 2014;148:1913–20.
22. de Kerchove L, Glineur D, Poncelet A, Boodhwani M, Rubay J, Dhoore W, et al. Repair of aortic leaflet prolapse: a ten-year experience. Eur J Cardiothorac Surg. 2008;34:785–91.
23. Aicher D, Fries R, Rodionycheva S, Schmidt K, Langer F, Schäfers H-J. Aortic valve repair leads to a low incidence of valve-related complications. Eur J Cardiothorac Surg. 2010;37:127–32.
24. Price J, de Kerchove L, Glineur D, Vanoverschelde J-L, Noirhomme P, El Khoury G. Risk of valve-related events after aortic valve repair. Ann Thorac Surg. 2013;95:606–13.
25. le Polain de Waroux JB, Pouleur AC, Goffinet C, Vancraeynest D, Van Dyck M, Robert A, et al. Functional anatomy of aortic regurgitation: accuracy, prediction of surgical repairability, and outcome implications of transesophageal echocardiography. Circulation. 2007;120:I-120–6.

13 Others—Unicuspid Valve and Quadricuspid Valve

Hiroaki Takahashi

13.1 Introduction

A unicuspid aortic valve (UAV) is very rare, with a reported occurrence rate of just 0.02% [1]. However, it is also reported that in aortic valve replacement for aortic valve stenosis, a UAV is observed in about 5% of the cases [2], and it cannot be said to be a rare condition for cardiac surgeons. In addition, there are many cases diagnosed as a bicuspid aortic valve (BAV) not only on preoperative examination but also intraoperatively, and the actual frequency is thought to be higher than reported. Furthermore, the quadricuspid aortic valve (QAV) is an even rarer condition, the reported incidence by various researches is less than 0.01% [3]. In this chapter, an understanding of the anatomical knowledge of UAVs and QAVs and valvuloplasty other than mainstream aortic valve replacement and autologous pulmonary valve transplantation by Ross surgery are highlighted with an introduction to past reports and experiences at the facilities where the author used to work in.

13.2 History of the Operation

The timing of disease onset differs depending on the primary cause of the pathological condition resulting from a UAV. When aortic valve stenosis is regarded as the main lesion, onset is mainly from childhood to the 20s. Compared with that for a BAV, the timing for surgical intervention due to valve dysfunction is calculated to be about 10–20 years earlier. Furthermore, percutaneous balloon valvuloplasty is often performed in childhood. Of 143 patients with an average age of 26 years treated over 11 years at the author's previous institution, about 15% underwent percutaneous balloon valvuloplasty in childhood. Also, for patients with a UAV with aortic valve regurgitation as the main lesion, the time at which surgical intervention is required is mainly in the 30s to 40s, and the condition is often accompanied by aortic root and ascending aortic dilatation lesions.

Anderson's definition of the anatomical features of the UAV includes the acommissural type and unicommissural type [4]. However, most of the UAVs in regular biventricular cases are of the unicommissural type, and the commissure in the posterior position is in the normal location, whereas the two rudimentary commissures on the ventral side are fixed in a position lower than the origin of the right coronary artery (Fig. 13.1a, b) [5]. Very occasionally, there are cases in which three commissures are present at a low position, and this is called the acommissural type. In the echocardiographic short-axis image of the aortic valve, this type is characterized by an eccentric valvular orifice in systole and a single commissural attachment in the posterior position

H. Takahashi (✉)
Department of Cardiovascular Surgery, Kita-Harima Medical Center, Hyogo, Japan
e-mail: takahashi-cvs@hotmail.co.jp

T. Kunihara, S. Takanashi (eds.), *Aortic Valve Preservation*,
https://doi.org/10.1007/978-981-13-2068-2_13

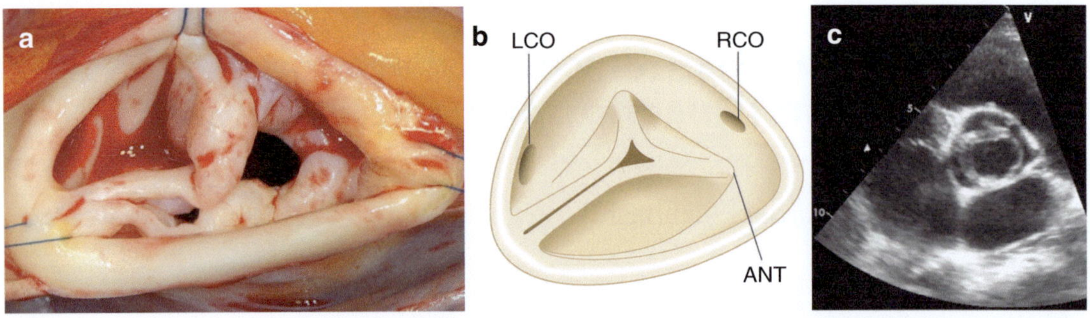

Fig. 13.1 A unicuspid aortic valve. (**a**) Intraoperative photograph, (**b**) quotation modified from reference 5 with permission, (**c**) transesophageal echocardiography. *ANT* anterior, *LCO* left coronary ostium, *RCO* right coronary ostium

(Fig. 13.1c) [1]. However, it is often difficult to evaluate this by preoperative echocardiography, and it is confirmed intraoperatively. Therefore, it is necessary that the cardiac surgeon performing the operation understands the anatomical features.

For a UAV, aortic valve replacement has mainly been performed due to the unique anatomical features described above. Except for tissue valve replacement for young women who wish to deliver a child in the future, mechanical valve replacement or Ross surgery are generally performed due to the more frequent occurrence in children and young people in their 20s to 30s. However, concerns such as size mismatch of mechanical valves in children, difficult postoperative anticoagulation therapy in children, and thromboembolism or hemorrhagic complications caused by anticoagulant therapy are indicated. Ross surgery with an autologous pulmonary valve is a technique that can solve these problems, but there are still several drawbacks such as surgical invasion for simultaneous double valve surgery, expansion of the aortic annulus over the long term, and reoperation at the pulmonary position. From these issues aortic valvuloplasty for UAV has been reported mainly from pediatric cardiac surgery centers.

In contrast, aortic valve replacement with a mechanical or biological valve has been performed for QAVs in a similar manner as that for UAVs. However, because aortic valve regurgitation is the main reason for QAV surgery, reports on valvuloplasty for a QAV have also been observed in recent years [6].

13.3 Indications and Contraindications

Calcification and shortening of the leaflets are often observed in the UAV, and hence valvuloplasty often requires removal of calcified leaflet tissue. At that time, precise assessment of the leaflet tissue is required, but if necessary, the effects of careful removal of the calcifications from the leaflet tissue on the mobility of the leaflets should be evaluated. In the author's previous facility, it is assumed that patients with a calcified area of leaflet tissue of about 50% or more are excluded from valvuloplasty. In patients in whom percutaneous balloon valvuloplasty was performed in childhood, it is often difficult to perform valvuloplasty due to the occurrence of leaflet destruction, and thus at the facility of d'Udekem et al., it is contraindicated to perform percutaneous balloon valvuloplasty for valve stenosis in childhood [7]. For aortic valve stenosis in childhood with potential risk of future valve dysfunction such as restenosis, not only valve replacement and Ross surgery but also a treatment plan including future aortic valvuloplasty should be discussed within the heart team.

In the report by Tutarel on QAVs, surgery was performed in about half of the cases, of which 75% were for isolated aortic valve regurgitation, and mechanical or tissue heart valve replacement was performed mainly for people in their 50s [8]. However, as mentioned above, valvuloplasty is also performed. There are also reports of aortic valve reimplantation procedure for lesions asso-

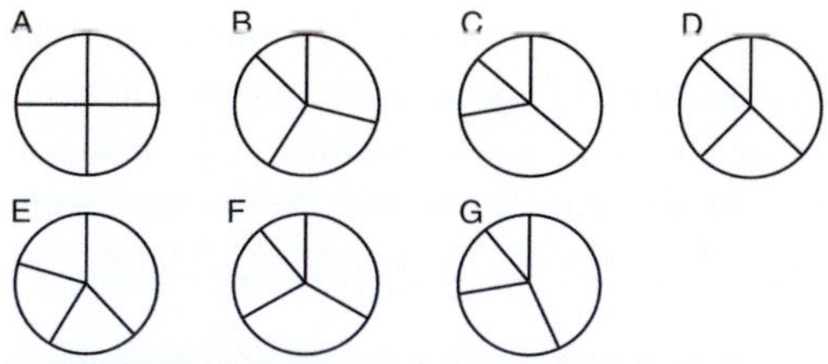

type of quadricuspid aortic valve

A : four equal cusps
B : three equal cusps and one smaller cusp
C : two equal larger cusps and two equal smaller cusps
D : one large, two intermediate and one small cusp
E : three equal cusps and one larger cusp
F : two equal larger cusps and two unequal smaller cusps
G : four unequal cusps

Fig. 13.2 Hurwitz and Robert's anatomical classification of QAVs

ciated with aortic root enlargement [6]. Hurwitz and Roberts devised a classification method based on seven subtypes (Fig. 13.2), and about 85% of cases are classified as Type A, B, or C [9]. Associated intracardiac lesions and abnormalities in the coronary artery stream are reported in 10–40% of cases, and therefore, care must be taken.

13.4 Advantages/Disadvantages

As mentioned earlier, surgical intervention in the case of a UAV is often required in patients from childhood to 20 to 30 years of age. The greatest merit of valvuloplasty for a UAV is that unlike mechanical valve replacement, the use of prosthetic materials can be avoided, so long-term anticoagulation therapy is unnecessary. Although Ross surgery using an autologous pulmonary valve is a technique that can solve these problems, in addition to the problems mentioned above, echocardiographic evaluation has recently shown a reduction in right heart function over the long term due to harvesting of the pulmonary autograft [10].

In the Melbourne report by d'Udekem et al., 142 aortic valvuloplasty procedures for patients under 20 years old were examined, and compared with bicuspid and tricuspid cases, a UAV would be a risk factor for reoperation [11]. In addition, in a comparison of 100 aortic valvuloplasty in patients 18 years old or younger, including those with UAVs, with 100 cases of Ross surgery, the freedom from reoperation at 5 years (including pulmonary valve re-replacement in the case of Ross surgery) was 87% vs. 86%, indicating almost no difference [7]. These findings indicate that valvuloplasty is aggressively performed for a UAV in these facilities as one option. However, there has been few report on the long-term outcomes of aortic valvuloplasty for UAVs, so surgical indication should deliberately determined. At the moment, aortic valvuloplasty is performed exclusively at a few limited experienced pediatric cardiac surgery centers and mainly for children to people in their 20s to 30s, including the implications of procrastinating the timing of Ross surgery as much as possible. However, when QAV cases are considered, valvuloplasty has an advantage in terms of reducing the risk of thromboembolism, hemorrhagic complications, or infective endocarditis that accompanies surgery with mechanical and tissue heart valves. However, biological valves offer better long-term results especially in elderly people aged 65 and older, and thus the implications should carefully be considered.

13.5 Actual Practice

As techniques of valvuloplasty for UAVs, the tricuspidization and bicuspidization have been introduced so far. Because the long-term performance of valvuloplasty using the pericardium is undesirable, many facilities perform the surgery leaving as much of the leaflet tissue as possible; however, to reconstruct the leaflets, materials such as the pericardium are required. As a supplementary material, the glutaraldehyde-treated autologous pericardium or xeno-pericardium are mainly used. Considering the prognosis of patients with a congenital BAV, it is thought that the tricuspidization is ideal from the aspect of valve function, but the tricuspidization using a pericardial patch requires advanced 3-dimensional technology, and intraoperative evaluation is difficult. Also, from their experiences, many surgeons likely assume that it is easier to perform aortic valvuloplasty for a BAV than for a tricuspid valve. At the author's previous institution, from the experience with aortic valvuloplasty so far, it is considered that surgery for a BAV is technically easier, and it is easy to evaluate the valve intraoperatively. Therefore, we have adapted the bicuspidization of a UAV. Initially, the fused cusp was incised in the direction of the anterior commissure, a new commissure was created at the same height as the normal commissure using the autologous pericardium [5]. However, the newly formed BAV was asymmetrical, and evaluation of the long-term performance of the valvuloplasty for BAV suggested that an asymmetric BAV with less than 160° commissure angle is at risk for reoperation. Also, there is a report that the efficiency of leaflet opening is best at 180° [12], and on this basis, we now create the new commissure on the opposite side at 180° and fill the open space with the autologous pericardium to form a symmetrical BAV (Fig. 13.3) [13]. For symmetrical bicuspidization of a UAV, echocardiographic evaluation has proved that valvular function is improved compared with that of an asymmetric BAV.

In children with stenosis of a UAV, there are cases involving narrowing of the left ventricular outflow tract, and additional procedures such as outflow tract enlargement may be necessary. However, aortic valve regurgitation is the main cause of adult cases, in which aortic annulus expansion may be confirmed. In this case, because the large aortic annulus diameter is a risk factor for reoperation, annuloplasty may be added. Various methods such as ring annuloplasty and suture annuloplasty have been reported, but the author's previous facilities have added suture annuloplasty using an expanded polytetrafluoroethylene (ePTFE) suture for patients with an annulus diameter exceeding 27 mm, mainly in adults. For patients with a body surface area of more than 2.0 m^2, the suture annuloplasty diameter is made to be 25 mm or if the body surface area is less, then a diameter of 23 mm is made by using a Hegar dilator.

Furthermore, surgical indication for accompanying lesions of aortic dilatation is fundamentally determined in accordance with that for a BAV. In the guidelines for Westerners with a body surface area of approximately 2.0 m^2, aortic root replacement and ascending aortic replacement are indicated for an aortic diameter of 45 mm or more during surgery on the aortic valve [14]. However, the risks of future aortic dilation and aortic dissection in patients with a UAV are higher than those for tricuspid and bicuspid valves, and their cut-off values need to be lowered slightly; at the author's previous facilities, it is set at 43 mm.

In contrast, a report of valvuloplasty for a QAV uses the bicuspidization or tricuspidization by eliminating the accessory cusp, and the pericardium is also used if necessary. At least two or more main leaflets are present for Types A, B, and C that are most frequently seen, so it is common to resect and re-suture the rudimentary commissure of small leaflet or to perform the tricuspidization by leaflet augmentation using the pericardium. It is thought that the bicuspidization is easier if a complicated form such as Type G is present.

13.6 My Tips

It is most important to correctly understand the anatomy of the UAV or QAV, to correctly interpret the leaflet orientation during the operation, and to carefully determine the surgical indication. In case of either a UAV or QAV, valvuloplasty is performed aiming to perform the bicuspidization or tricuspidization. However, in terms of the physique of adults, in Westerners, for example, the distance from the annulus to the leaflet free margin (geometric height) of less than 16 mm for a tricuspid and 19 mm or less for a bicuspid valve are risk factors for reoperation. Therefore, the geometric height of 17 mm or more in the case of a tricuspid and 20 mm or more for a bicuspid valve are requisite for valvuloplasty. Furthermore, the method used for evaluation after the valvuloplasty is also important. In the author's previous facilities, the height from the annulus to the leaflet free margin, the so-

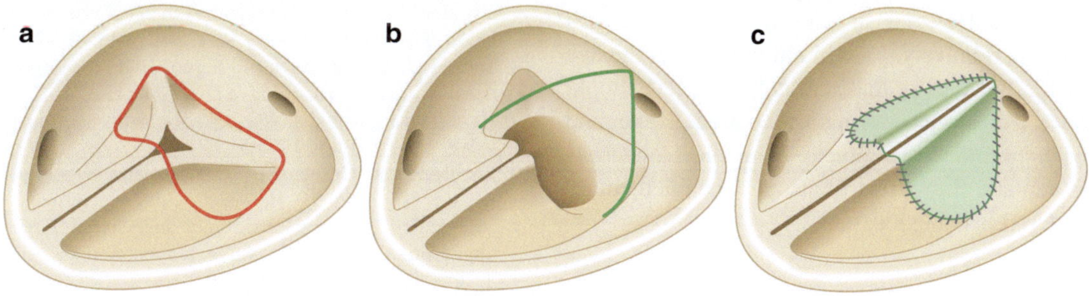

Fig. 13.3 Symmetric bicuspidization using the autologous pericardium. (**a**) Resection of the valve tissue on the right coronary artery side. (**b**) Set a new commissure of 180° on the opposite side. (**c**) Two symmetric bicuspid valves are prepared by compensating for the missing tissue with the autologous pericardium (modified from reference 13 with permission)

called effective height, is adjusted at 8–9 mm in children and 9–10 mm in adults.

13.7 Results

Although there are few reports on the long-term results of valvuloplasty for UAVs at the moment, we would like to introduce some data on 143 cases of valvuloplasty for a UAV performed at the author's previous facility [15]. During an average follow-up period of 4.6 years, when reviewing only children under 18, the 7-year freedom from reoperation was relatively good at 88%. In the patients 18 years of age or older, the results improved by changing the design of bicuspidization and the addition of suture annuloplasty in patients with an expanded annulus, but the 7-year freedom from reoperation was about 70% (the review may have been insufficient and is only a reference value). During the follow-up period, 26 of the 143 patients underwent aortic valve reoperation 1.5 years (median value) after the initial surgery, primarily for left ventricular outflow tract stenosis for children under 18, and for suture dehiscence between the pericardium and the leaflets and/or aortic wall in the patients 18 years and older.

Recently, the same institution published their experience of aortic root remodeling procedure for 25 young patients (mean age, 38 ± 12 years) with UAV [16]. Bicuspidization using the autologous pericardial patch with 180° commissure orientation was performed in all patients and a suture annuloplasty was added in the last 20 patients with annulus diameter over 25 mm. During mean follow-up period of 27 ± 18 months, three patients underwent reoperation (one replacement, two re-repair) due to endocarditis in one and limited suture dehiscence in two. Thus freedom from reoperation and aortic valve replacement at 5 years was 81% and 91%, respectively. They emphasized that none of the patients who underwent ePTFE suture annuloplasty had exhibited recurrent aortic regurgitation.

Although the results for QAV repair have been good up to now, these are results only for 2–3 years of postoperative follow-up. The long-term follow-up results are expected in the future, and multicenter studies will be necessary because it is a quite rare disease as mentioned earlier.

13.8 Conclusion

In young patients with a pressure gradient across the aortic valve, evaluation is necessary while keeping the possibility of a UAV in mind. Concomitant aortic dilated lesions should be treated according to or more aggressively than the indication for the BAV recommended by the guidelines. In addition, although there are few reports on the long-term performance of valvuloplasty for UAVs or QAVs at present, it is generally considered to be inferior to the results of valvuloplasty for BAVs, and therefore, the surgical indication should carefully be considered. Accordingly, the advantages of valvuloplasty as one of the options and the risk of the valve dysfunction after repair should thoroughly be informed. However, it is suggested that the outcome is relatively good in children under the age of 18, thus the optimal surgical procedure should be selected considering the patient's age and background. Development of medical materials to replace the pericardium as a supplementary material is being awaited.

References

1. Novaro GM, Mishra M, Griffin BP. Incidence and echocardiographic features of congenital unicuspid aortic valve in an adult population. J Heart Valve Dis. 2003;12:674–8.
2. Roberts WC, Ko JM. Frequency by decades of unicuspid, bicuspid, and tricuspid aortic valves in adults having isolated aortic valve replacement for aortic stenosis, with or without associated aortic regurgitation. Circulation. 2005;111:920–5.
3. Feldman BJ, Khandheria BK, Warnes CA, et al. Incidence, description and functional assessment of isolated quadricuspid aortic valves. Am J Cardiol. 1990;65:937–8.
4. Anderson RH. Understanding the structure of the unicuspid and unicommissural aortic valve. J Heart Valve Dis. 2003;12:670–3.
5. Schäfers HJ, Aicher D, Riodionycheva S, Lindinger A, Rädle-Hurst T, Langer F, et al. Bicuspidization of the unicuspid aortic valve: a new reconstructive approach. Ann Thorac Surg. 2008;85:2012–8.
6. Yamanaka K, Okada K, Okita Y. Aortic root replacement with a valve-sparing technique for quadricuspid aortic valve. Eur J Cardiothorac Surg. 2015;47:741–3.
7. d'Udekem Y, Siddiqui J, Seaman CS, Konstantinov IE, Galati JC, Cheung MM, et al. Long-term results of a strategy of aortic valve repair in the pediatric population. J Thorac Cardiovasc Surg. 2013;145:461–7.
8. Tutarel O. The quadricuspid aortic valve: a comprehensive review. J Heart Valve Dis. 2004;13:534–7.
9. Hurwitz LE, Roberts WC. Quadricuspid semilunar valve. Am J Cardiol. 1973;31:623–6.
10. Raedle-Hurst TM, Hosse M, Hoffmann S, Abdul-Khaliq H, Schäfers HJ. Ventricular performance assessed by 2-dimensional strain analysis after ross operation versus aortic valve reconstruction. Ann Thorac Surg. 2013;96:1567–73.
11. Tan Tanny SP, Yong MS, D'Udekem Y, Kowalski R, Wheaton G, D'Orsogna L, et al. Ross procedure in children: 17-year experience at a single institution. J Am Heart Assoc. 2013;2:e000153.
12. Aicher D, Kunihara T, Abou Issa O, Brittner B, Gräber S, Schäfers HJ. Valve configuration determines long-term results after repair of the bicuspid aortic valve. Circulation. 2011;123:178–85.
13. Aicher D, Bewarder M, Kindermann M, Abdul-Khalique H, Schäfers HJ. Aortic valve function after bicuspidization of the unicuspid aortic valve. Ann Thorac Surg. 2013;95:1545–50.
14. Vahanian A, Alfieri O, Andreotti F, et al. Guidelines on the management of valvular heart disease (version 2012): the joint task force on the management of valvular heart disease of the European Society of Cardiology (ESC) and the European Association for Cardio-Thoracic Surgery (EACTS). Eur Heart J. 2012;33:2451–96.
15. Takahashi H, Aicher D, Kunihara T, Schäfers HJ. Aortic valve repair in patients with unicuspid aortic valve by bicuspidization with augmentation using pericardium. Interact Cardiovasc Thorac Surg. 2013;17:S93.
16. Franciulli M, Aicher D, Rädle-Hurst T, Takahashi H, Rodionycheva S, Schäfers HJ. Root remodeling and aortic valve repair for unicuspid aortic valve. Ann Thorac Surg. 2014;98:823–9.

ONE-POINT ADVICE: The Limitations and Potential of MICS During Aortic Valvuloplasty

14

Toshiaki Ito

14.1 Introduction

Nowadays, when we consider the favorable long-term outcomes of biological valves, we automatically focus on young patients when discussing the main indications for aortic valvuloplasty (AVP). Many young patients, and particularly women, find the concept of minimally invasive cardiac surgery (MICS) desirable from a cosmetic perspective. When compared to midline incisions, MICS does not reduce the rates of mortality or major complications, so the main reasons for performing MICS are for cosmetic reasons and the need for early return to daily activities. As a rule, it is therefore desirable to determine the indications carefully.

There is already consensus that a right mini-thoracotomy is currently the best approach for mitral valve (MV) MICS. By comparison, there are several approaches for aortic valve (AV) MICS, and they cannot all be discussed in the same way. These procedures can be broadly classified into partial sternotomy [1], parasternal incision [2], anterior intercostal thoracotomy [3], and infra-axillary mini-thoracotomy [4] (Fig. 14.1) and are arranged in ascending order

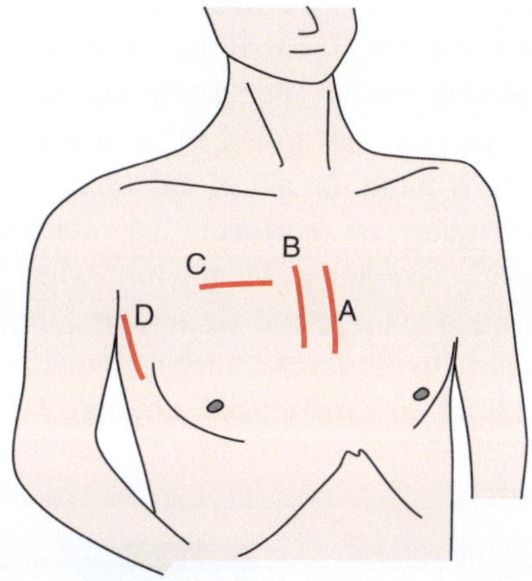

Fig. 14.1 Skin incisions for each type of MICS AV approach. *A* partial sternotomy, *B* parasternal incision, *C* anterior intercostal thoracotomy, *D* infra-axillary mini-thoracotomy

based on the distance to the AV. Conversely, from a cosmetic prospective, the first three approaches use a midline incision, so there are no major differences between them. Only intercostal thoracotomy offers cosmetic benefits equivalent to those seen after MV MICS. Procedures until anterior intercostal thoracotomy are the approaches that enable manual ligation procedures, and a knot pusher is required during lateral thoracotomy.

The author has currently performed aortic valve replacement (AVR) via axillary approach through the third intercostal space that are cosmetically superior from the perspective that the wound is

T. Ito (✉)
Department of Cardiovascular Surgery, Japanese Red Cross Nagoya First Hospital, Aichi, Japan
e-mail: cvs1@nagoya-1st.jrc.or.jp

T. Kunihara, S. Takanashi (eds.), *Aortic Valve Preservation*, https://doi.org/10.1007/978-981-13-2068-2_14

easily hidden anatomically [4]. Ten patients aged <40 years old also underwent this approach. From the cosmetic prospective, the patients appeared to be highly satisfied. However, I currently have no experience in performing aortic valvuloplasty by MICS approach. Accordingly, the following discussion will mainly be focused on the speculation of possible AVP by MICS based on my experience with AVR through a partial sternotomy, a parasternal incision, and an axillary incision, in addition to that with MV MICS.

First, valvuloplasty via a lateral thoracic approach, including an axillary incision, is considered to be quite difficult compared to that via a midline incision. The exposure itself enables a direct view of the AV (Fig. 14.2). However, fundamentally, it is performed by a surgeon independently without the aid of an assistant, and it is challenging to perform the complicated manipulations required. Meanwhile, when MICS is performed via a partial sternotomy, the exposure is close to the sternal midline incision, so in the hands of an experienced surgeon, I believe the procedure could be performed at this time. The same strategies used during MV MICS, listed below, can be applied when AVP is performed as MICS with a restricted field of view.

14.2 The Primary Targets of Valvuloplasty Should Be Easy, Simple Lesions

The etiology of AV lesions is classified as that of MV lesions [5]. Accordingly, the procedure is suitable for Type Ia lesions, which involve the sinotubular junction (STJ) enlargement alone, or type Id lesions, which are caused by perforation (see page 24, Chap. 3). Plication of the STJ or patch closure of the cusp perforation can probably be performed during MICS via a lateral thoracotomy approach. However, I believe that some experience is required to repair type II lesions, which are caused by cusp prolapse or to perform subcommissural annuloplasty.

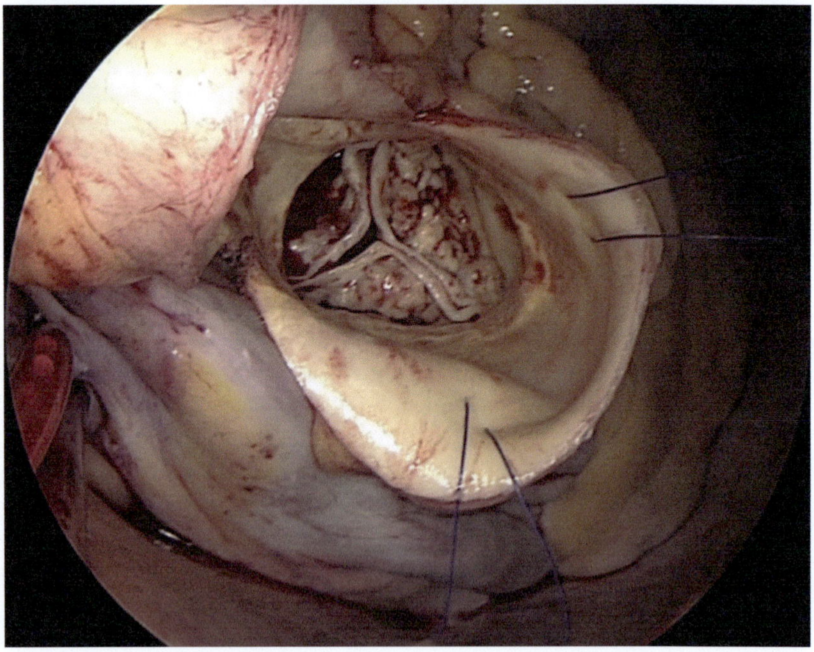

Fig. 14.2 AV viewed via an axillary incision approach. A thoracic approach via an axillary incision places the AV and incision along virtually the same axis, and it is possible to view the valve from directly above. However, the AV is ≥10 cm away from the axillary incision

14.3 Identification of the Lesion Site, Morphology, and Regurgitation Mechanisms, and Planning of the Valvuloplasty Technique Based on Preoperative Diagnosis

Because the operative procedure through limited visual field is time-consuming, it is preferable to perform the scheduled surgery exclusively according to the accurate preoperative diagnosis, planning valvuloplasty, and intraoperative reconfirmation of them. Contrast-enhanced CT and 3D-echocardiography are useful for this purpose. Contrast-enhanced CT has high spatial resolution, but cusp configuration will be poorly visualized in cases with thin cusps. Additional information about the regurgitant jet can be obtained with echocardiography, so the surgeon needs to integrate the information provided by both modalities. Surgeons have enough time available when valvuloplasty technique is definitively determined preoperatively, otherwise, AVP by MICS approach may be difficult.

14.4 Future Possibilities

AVP itself has not widely been performed, so I believe it will be possible by MICS approach when it can be popularized as routine surgery. There is already one report of surgery being performed to treat uncomplicated congenital heart disease in infant and pediatric patients via a right axillary incision and which also included simultaneous aortic valvuloplasty [6]. I suppose MICS approach will be indicated to the uncomplicated, simple AVP in the near future. However, I believe that it is dangerous to apply MICS approach to the complicated procedure at high risk of bleeding such as valve-sparing root replacement.

Mitral valve repair performed via a midline incision has increased in popularity since the 1990s, and nowadays it can reproducibly be performed via a MICS approach. When this history is reflected, I am certain that large part of AVP will be performed via a MICS approach. However, the AV has a more three-dimensional (3D) structure than the MV, and considering that AVP requires a relatively high degree of precision, preoperative evaluation should be performed using 3D imaging modalities, such as 3D-CT and 3D-echocardiography, and it would be useful to use 3D-endoscopes during MICS AVP surgery.

14.5 Conclusion

MICS AVP surgery may be possible for simple cases through a partial sternotomy approach, provided that the exact planning of the valvuloplasty technique based on preoperative precise diagnosis using 3D imaging modalities is made. 3D-endoscopes may facilitate MICS AVP surgery.

References

1. Furukawa N, Kuss O, Aboud A, Schönbrodt M, Renner A, Meibodi KH, et al. Ministernotomy versus conventional sternotomy for aortic valve replacement: matched propensity score analysis of 808 patients. Eur J Cardiothorac Surg. 2014;46:221–6.
2. Cosgrove DM 3rd, Sabik JF. Minimally invasive approach for aortic valve operations. Ann Thorac Surg. 1996;62:596–7.
3. Glauber M, Miceli A, Gilmanov D, Ferrarini M, Bevilacqua S, Farneti PA, et al. Right anterior minithoracotomy versus conventional aortic valve replacement: a propensity score matched study. J Thorac Cardiovasc Surg. 2013;145:1222–6.
4. Ito T, Maekawa A, Hoshino S, Hayashi Y. Right infraaxillary thoracotomy for minimally invasive aortic valve replacement. Ann Thorac Surg. 2013;96:715–7.
5. de Kerchove L, Glineur D, Poncelet A, Boodhwani M, Rubay J, Dhoore W, et al. Repair of aortic leaflet prolapse: a ten-year experience. Eur J Cardiothorac Surg. 2008;34:785–91.
6. Dave HH, Comber M, Solinger T, Bettex D, Dodge-Khatami A, Prêtre R. Mid-term results of right axillary incision for the repair of a wide range of congenital cardiac defects. Eur J Cardiothorac Surg. 2009;35:864–9.

15 History, Techniques, and Outcomes of the Reimplantation Method

Shunsuke Miyahara and Yutaka Okita

15.1 Introduction

Annuloaortic ectasia (AAE) mainly comprises diseases causing aortic root dilatation and presents various pathologies such as aortic aneurysm and aortic regurgitation. Particularly, the life expectancy of patients with Marfan syndrome depends highly on AAE accompanied by conditions such as aortic dissection and aortic regurgitation. Historically, full aortic root replacement using a composite valved conduit has generally been performed for this etiology. However, since its development, valve-sparing aortic root replacement surgery has been attracting attention as a surgical procedure that dramatically improves the quality of life of the patient. Of the two kinds of surgery, this paper focuses on the reimplantation method and outlines it with the experiences of the authors.

15.2 History of the Operation

Since 1968, when Bentall and De Bono first introduced the method of full aortic root replacement with a composite graft and reconstruction of the coronary arteries [1], the life prognosis of patients with Marfan syndrome has improved dramatically [2]. Thereafter, regardless of the presence of inherited connective tissue disorders, this method became a standard surgical procedure for lesions extending from the sinotubular junction (STJ) to the aortic annulus. The results of the Bentall operation were favorable, but the problems of anticoagulation therapy accompanying prosthetic valve replacement surgery and the prosthetic valve-related complications over the long term remained unresolved. For this reason, as a form of valve-sparing aortic root replacement surgery, Yacoub et al. devised the aortic root remodeling method (hereinafter referred to as remodeling) in 1979 [3]. In 1989, David launched the aortic valve reimplantation method (hereinafter referred to as reimplantation) [4]. Since then, the surgical procedure for these patient groups has shifted from the Bentall operation to valve-sparing aortic root replacement procedures. These surgical procedures have developed from the theoretical background that valve regurgitation occurs due to enlargement of the aortic annulus, sinuses of Valsalva, and the STJ and that valve regurgitation can be improved by correcting each lesion.

David et al. innovated a method of interpolating the aortic valve into a cylindrical vascular prosthesis inspired by the shape of the aortic root after excision of the Valsalva sinus, in the same manner as the subcoronary method using a stentless bioprosthesis [5]. The original method of

S. Miyahara · Y. Okita (✉)
Division of Cardiovascular Surgery, Department of Surgery, Kobe University Graduate School of Medicine, Kobe, Hyogo, Japan
e-mail: yokita@med.kobe-u.ac.jp

T. Kunihara, S. Takanashi (eds.), *Aortic Valve Preservation*,
https://doi.org/10.1007/978-981-13-2068-2_15

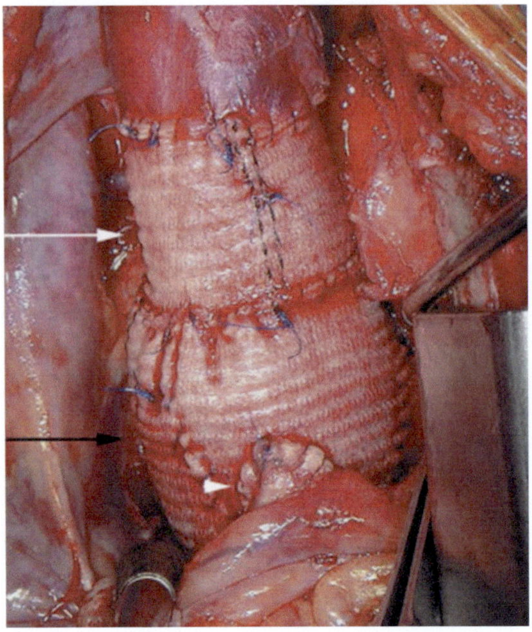

Fig. 15.1 The David V Stanford modification

reimplantation is called the David I procedure. In contrast, the remodeling method developed by Yacoub et al. and the operations with partial annular plication using a strip of Dacron fabric in addition to remodeling are called David II and David III, respectively [6]. David IV, in which the vascular graft is plicated at three locations at the level of the STJ and forms a bulge for the purpose of preserving the sinus of Valsalva, was adopted from the mid-1990s in the patient series of David et al. [7]. In addition, Miller et al. devised a technique to form the sinuses of Valsalva by using two vascular grafts with different diameters (David V: the Stanford modification). Since the diameter of the vascular graft used for the sinus portion of this method is 6–8 mm larger than that derived by the formula proposed by David et al. [8], not only the STJ but also the proximal edge of the vascular graft sutured to aorto-ventricular junction (AVJ) should be plicated (Fig. 15.1). The advantage of this technique is that the length of the sinus portion of the vascular graft can be decided after determining the location of the commissure, and since a large prosthesis is used for the sinus area, space for the surgical operation is sufficiently secured [9]. Furthermore, modification of the David V procedure has been reported from Japan [10], and the preservation of the physiological functions of the sinuses of Valsalva and the leaflets has been pursued through various improvement of surgical procedures. However, in 2000, a vascular graft with a sinus of Valsalva (Gelweave Valsalva: Sulzer Vascutek, Renfrewshire, Scotland) became commercially available and has been widely used due to its ability to obtain better physiological leaflet motion and the convenience of the procedure, and good long-term results have been reported [11, 12]. The drawback of this prosthesis is its tube-like configuration without a straight shape of the interleaflet triangles. Currently, a graft with both three distinct sinuses of Valsalva and straight interleaflet triangles is commercially available in Japan (J Graft SHIELD NEO VALSALVA; Japan Lifeline, Tokyo, Japan), which is expected to restore a near-normal root configuration and physiological leaflet motion (Fig. 15.2).

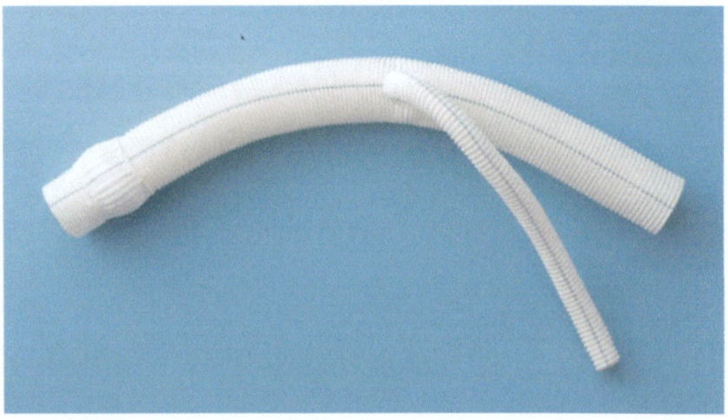

Fig. 15.2 A graft with three distinct sinuses of Valsalva and straight interleaflet triangles

15.3 Pros and Cons

Discussions on the advantages of reimplantation and remodeling were repeated from the latter half of the 1990s. The main differences between the two procedures include that (1) the AVJ is stabilized in the shape prescribed by the size of the vascular graft in reimplantation, whereas in remodeling, the AVJ is not supported unless annuloplasty is performed as an additional treatment, and (2) in the reimplantation method (especially in David I), the shape of the sinus of Valsalva disappears depending on the shape of the vascular graft, whereas in the remodeling method the shape is preserved. In David I, because the Valsalva sinuses are replaced by a cylindrical vascular graft, the physiological role of the original sinuses of Valsalva, such as forming a vortex flow in the sinus, is thought to be lost, whereas in the remodeling method, it is thought to be preserved. In the late 1990s, clinical data comparing remodeling and reimplantation were reported from these aspects, and the effect of preserving the geometry of the Valsalva sinuses was discussed. Leyh et al. compared the root distensibility and the leaflet motion between the two alternatives [13]. The remodeling method, which retains the form of the sinus of Valsalva, was found to provide more physiological opening and closing leaflet motion and sufficient root distensibility [13].

15.4 Actual Practice

The aortic incision is transversely placed 1–2 cm distal from the STJ so as not to deform the root dimension, and then a 5-0 polypropylene mattress stitch is placed in each commissure and the condition of each leaflet is observed (Fig. 15.3). In addition to the leaflet and root dimensions, the height from the AVJ to the apex of the noncoronary cusp (NCC)-left coronary cusp (LCC) commissure, called the Brussels height [14], is measured (Fig. 15.4). This will be a reference used in determining the size of the vascular graft, for which a graft with sinuses is used. The feature of its structure is the 1:1 ratio of the height in the longitudinal direction of the Valsalva sinus to the AVJ diameter. Because the height of the commissure part is often preserved in its normal form, the height of the commissure from the AVJ is optimal AVJ diameter = graft diameter [14]. When comparing a congenital bicuspid valve with a tricuspid valve, the AVJ and geometric height (gH) are often larger and the sinus of Valsalva diameter is smaller, so determination of the graft size also depends comprehensively on the height of the commissural part, gH, AVJ, and STJ (along the diameter of ascending aorta).

The aortic root is sharply dissected to reach the AVJ. The left- and non-coronary sinuses are dissected to the left atrial roof, and the right coronary sinus is dissected to the junction between the right ventricle/atrium and the aortic root. However, because the section of annulus between the right coronary cusp (RCC) and the LCC is equivalent to the muscular portion, dissection is required to partially cut out the right ventricular myocardium (2–3 mm). The right ventricular and right atrial muscles are thin and easily damaged,

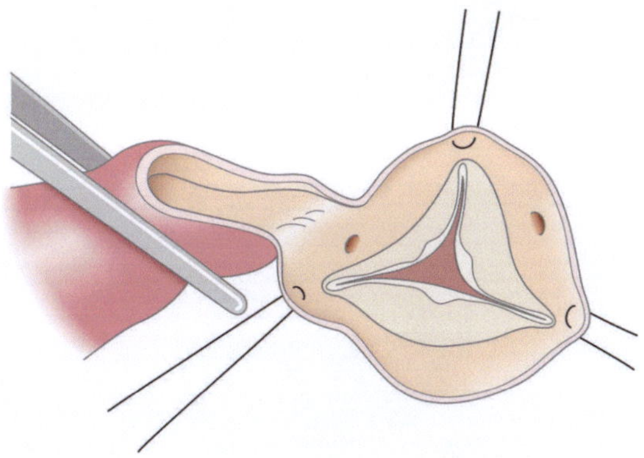

Fig. 15.3 Exposure of the aortic root. Following an aortotomy, the aortic root is exposed by applying traction on the commissures in the symmetric direction

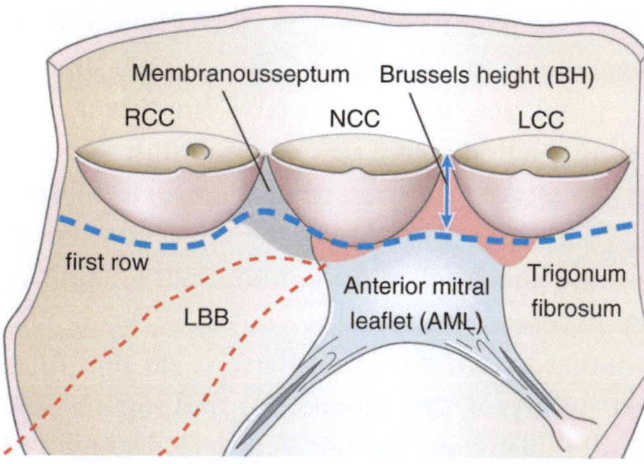

Fig. 15.4 Anatomy of the aortic root. *RCC* right coronary cusp, *LCC* left coronary cusp, *NCC* non-coronary cusp, *LBB* left bundle branch

so the use of a 22-mm suture needle with a tight curvature is recommended to easily pass through from the nadir of the RCC. The lower part of the RCC-LCC commissure forms aorto-pulmonary fibrous continuous tissue and prevents reaching the basal ring from the outside. In addition, the membranous septum is formed below the commissure of the RCC-NCC, and the left side of the heart conduction system lies on the surface of the muscular layer below the membranous septum (Fig. 15.4).

The aortic wall is cut off 5 mm away from the annulus, and as the first-row sutures, twelve 3-0 polyester mattress sutures with a spaghetti pledget are placed circularly around the annulus directly under it from the inside to outside. At this time, the suture line is at the level of AVJ, but due to the anatomical reasons mentioned earlier, the area beneath the commissure between the RCC and LCC is deviated 3–5 mm upward. Furthermore, because at the area between the RCC and NCC, a suture should be placed through the upper end of the membranous septum, it deviates 8–10 mm upward (Fig. 15.4).

These polyester sutures are passed through the lower end of the graft and tied, then the vascular graft is seated at the root externally. However, if the sutures are tightened strongly, the annulus may be deformed; thus, careful attention is required. Each commissure is then lifted upward with 5-0 polypropylene suture and fixed to the graft. At this time, it is important to apply sufficient tension to the commissure. Meanwhile, positioning of the commissure in the minor axis direction is also important, following the first suture row of the annulus so that the leaflets do not deform. When determining the commissure position in the minor axis, keep in mind that each inter-commissural length is not necessarily the same. After securing the commissure, confirm that there is no deformation in any of the leaflets. By pulling out the suction tube from the left ventricle through the aortic valve and aligning the junction of the leaflet tips, proper coaptation of the leaflets can be confirmed. In the case of a congenital bicuspid valve, two commissures may be fixed at 180° to clarify free margin length of each leaflet. This requires careful attention to prevent restricted leaflet motion. As in the case of a tricuspid valve, commissures are fixed at the position where they are lifted as much as possible in the long-axis direction, but in a case with a raphe, it will be fixed at a slightly lower position according to its height.

Attach the aortic remnant in the graft with the second row of continuous sutures using 5-0 polypropylene with a 17-mm 1/2 circle needle. Also, at this time, pay attention to avoid deforming the leaflets. Furthermore, to obtain a water-tight anastomosis, the width of each stitch is carefully maintained at 2–3 mm. The suture is passed from the inside of the aortic wall to the outside of the vascular graft, and the grip of the needle is reversed to reinsert the needle from the outside of the graft. This is intended to prevent distortion of the suture line and to ensure transmurality of the aortic wall (Fig. 15.5).

Cusp competency is assessed by the administration of cardioplegia solution following placement of the second-row sutures. Using a cardioplegia cannula, raise the internal circuit pressure to 200 mmHg to check for a sufficient degree of graft tightness and confirm that there is no aortic valve regurgitation. Transesophageal echocardiography will also show the aortic root

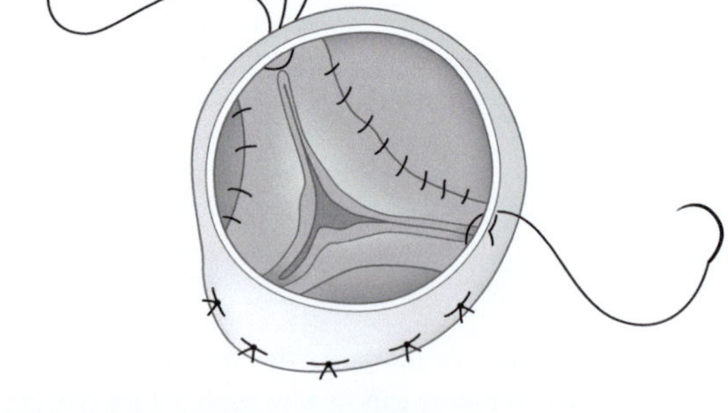

Fig. 15.5 The second-row suture

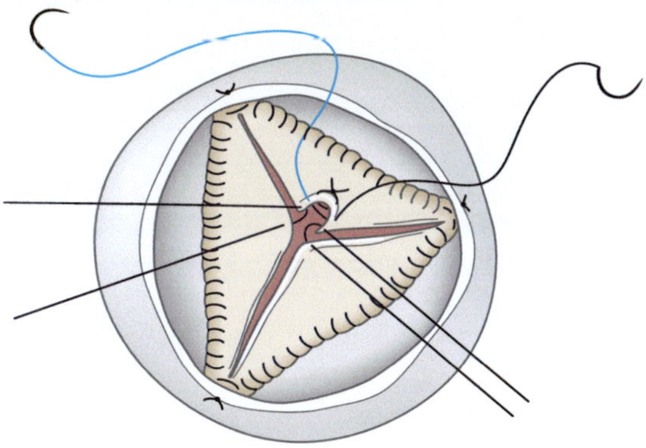

Fig. 15.6 Plication of the body of Arantius. Apply the marking stitch so that the distances from the commissures of the opposing valves are aligned and sew the excess portion of the leaflet edge at the center

and left ventricular outflow tract and confirm that there is no significant valvular regurgitation. At the same time, confirm the absence of hemorrhage at the suture lines. It is also important to correct the effective height of each leaflet to keep it above 8 mm. Particularly in a congenital bicuspid valve, it is essential to plicate the free edge of the non-fused cusp, which is the reference for the fused cusp, to keep the effective height sufficiently high.

Both coronary arteries are then anastomosed to the graft with 5-0 polypropylene suture by the button technique. The right coronary artery is sufficiently pulled cranially and anastomosed to the graft at a high level to avoid torsion after cardiac rhythm is resumed.

15.5 My Tips

In recent years, after the second-row sutures are placed, a fiberoptic endoscope is inserted from the upper right pulmonary vein, and the aortic valve is observed from the left ventricular side to evaluate the presence or absence of residual regurgitation [15, 16]. At this point, if leaflet prolapse is recognized, the bodies of Arantius in the center of the leaflets are gradually sutured with several 6-0 polypropylene sutures to correct the prolapse (Fig. 15.6).

15.6 Outcomes

In 1992, David et al. reported the results of ten consecutive reimplantation operations. The patient group included five patients with Marfan syndrome, five with severe aortic insufficiency, and four with acute aortic dissection, one of whom required reoperation for severe aortic regurgitation immediately after surgery. Other patients gained favorable results with an average follow-up period of 9 months [4]. From the beginning when this procedure was first announced, there were already discussions on the surgical indications for patients with Marfan syndrome and a congenital bicuspid valve. Thereafter, many reports on this procedure were published discussing the impact of various patients' backgrounds and an additional cusp maneuver. According to a study by Kallenbach et al., Marfan syndrome has emerged as a risk factor leading to reoperation. However, they considered the failures to be due to technical error during the early stage of their learning curve, so they concluded that this surgery is basically suitable for Marfan syndrome [17]. Regarding the adaptation of this procedure for congenital bicuspid valves, de Kerchove et al. reported the superiority of the reimplantation method over isolated aortic cusp repair at least in terms of fixation of the AVJ [18].

The results of reimplantation reported in a relatively large number of cases are shown in Table 15.1 [12, 17, 19–24]. The presence or absence of acute dissection and the severity of aortic regurgitation differ slightly depending on the series, but in all reports, the freedom from reoperation at 10 years is more or less 90%, which seems acceptable. Many facilities apply the Bentall operation as the standard for AAE cases with complex cusp pathologies. Although the proportion of valve-sparing root replacements for all AAE cases at each facility has not always been disclosed, the high rate of additional cusp repair might suggest that the surgical indications for valve-sparing root replacement have slightly expanded.

Table 15.1 Long-term clinical outcomes of reimplantation

First author	Published year	Reference number	Number of cases	Severe AR	BAV	MFS	AADA	Cusp repair	Freedom from reoperation	Freedom from moderate or severe AR
Reimplantation										
Kallenbach	2005	[17]	284	18 (6%)	17 (6%)	54 (19%)	53 (19%)	18 (6%)	87.1@10y	
Leontyev	2012	[19]	179	2 (1%)	16 (9%)	31 (17%)	28 (16%)	32 (18%)	96%@5y	94%@5y
Liebrich	2013	[20]	236	6 (3%)	35 (15%)	26 (11%)	14 (6%)	54 (23%)	87@10y	
Kvitting	2013	[21]	233	28 (12%)	63 (27%)	102 (44%)	0	105 (45%)	92.2@10y	
Miyahara	2015	[22]	183	89 (49%)	37 (20%)	45 (25%)	21 (12%)	111 (61%)	92.2@5y	
De Paulis	2016	[12]	124	20 (16%) (>IV)	15 (12%)	21 (17%)	7 (6%)	8 (6%)	90%@13y	87%@13y
Esaki	2016	[24]	123	80 (65%)	32 (26%)	8 (7%)	16 (13%)	N.A.	97%@7y	
David	2017	[23]	333	66 (20%)	45 (14%)	128 (38%)	28 (8%)	213 (64%)	97%@20y	92%@20y

15.7 Conclusion

We provided a detailed account of the history, techniques, and contemporary results of valve-sparing aortic root replacement with the reimplantation method. We hope this technique will increase in sophistication, provide durable long-term outcomes, and benefit more patients by eliminating prosthesis-related complications.

References

1. Bentall H, De Bono A. A technique for complete replacement of the ascending aorta. Thorax. 1968;23:338–9.
2. Silverman DI, Burton KJ, Gray J, Bosner MS, Kouchoukos NT, Roman MJ, et al. Life expectancy in the Marfan syndrome. Am J Cardiol. 1995;75:157–60.
3. Sarsam MA, Yacoub M. Remodeling of the aortic valve anulus. J Thorac Cardiovasc Surg. 1993;105:435–8.
4. David TE, Feindel CM. An aortic-valve sparing operation for patients with aortic incompetence and aneurysm of the ascending aorta. J Thorac Cardiovasc Surg. 1992;103:617–22.
5. David TE. The aortic valve-sparing operation. J Thorac Cardiovasc Surg. 2011;141:613–5.
6. David TE. Aortic root aneurysms: remodeling or composite replacement? Ann Thorac Surg. 1997;64:1564–8.
7. David TE, Feindel CM, Webb GD, Colman JM, Armstrong S, Maganti M. Long-term results of aortic valve-sparing operations for aortic root aneurysm. J Thorac Cardiovasc Surg. 2006;132:347–54.
8. Demers P, Miller DC. Simple modification of "T. David-V" valve-sparing aortic root replacement to create graft pseudosinuses. Ann Thorac Surg. 2004;78:1479–81.
9. Miller DC. Reprint of: rationale and results of the Stanford modification of the David V reimplantation technique for valve-sparing aortic root replacement. J Thorac Cardiovasc Surg. 2015;149(2 Suppl):S18–20.
10. Takamoto S, Nawata K, Morota T. A simple modification of 'David-V' aortic root reimplantation. Eur J Cardiothorac Surg. 2006;30:560–2.
11. De Paulis R, De Matteis GM, Nardi P, Scaffa R, Colella DF, Bassano C, et al. One-year appraisal of a new aortic root conduit with sinuses of Valsalva. J Thorac Cardiovasc Surg. 2002;123:33–9.
12. De Paulis R, Chirichilli I, Scaffa R, Weltert L, Maselli D, Salica A, et al. Long-term results of the valve reimplantation technique using a graft with sinuses. J Thorac Cardiovasc Surg. 2016;151:112–9.
13. Leyh RG, Schmidtke C, Sievers HH, Yacoub MH. Opening and closing characteristics of the aortic valve after different types of valve-preserving surgery. Circulation. 1999;100:2153–60.
14. de Kerchove L, Boodhwani M, Glineur D, Noirhomme P, El Khoury G. A new simple and objective method for graft sizing in valve-sparing root replacement using the reimplantation technique. Ann Thorac Surg. 2011;92:749–51.
15. Okita Y, Oka T, Miyahara S, Okada K. Direct visualization of the aortic cusp from the left ventricle during aortic root reimplantation. J Thorac Cardiovasc Surg. 2012;144:981–2.
16. Miyahara S, Oka T, Takahashi H, Inoue T, Matsumori M, Tanaka H, et al. Feasibility of intraoperative water testing in aortic valve repair: direct visualization from left ventricle with a videoscope. J Thorac Cardiovasc Surg. 2017;54:24–9.
17. Kallenbach K, Karck M, Pak D, Salcher R, Khaladj N, Leyh R, et al. Decade of aortic valve sparing reimplantation: are we pushing the limits too far? Circulation. 2005;112(9 Suppl):I253–9.
18. de Kerchove L, Boodhwani M, Glineur D, Vandyck M, Vanoverschelde JL, Noirhomme P, et al. Valve sparing-root replacement with the reimplantation technique to increase the durability of bicuspid aortic valve repair. J Thorac Cardiovasc Surg. 2011;142:1430–8.
19. Leontyev S, Trommer C, Subramanian S, Lehmann S, Dmitrieva Y, Misfeld M, et al. The outcome after aortic valve-sparing (David) operation in 179 patients: a single-centre experience. Eur J Cardiothorac Surg. 2012;42:261–6.
20. Liebrich M, Kruszynski MK, Roser D, Meisner C, Doll KN, Hemmer WB, et al. The David procedure in different valve pathologies: a single-center experience in 236 patients. Ann Thorac Surg. 2013;95:71–6.
21. Kvitting JP, Kari FA, Fischbein MP, Liang DH, Beraud AS, Stephens EH, et al. David valve-sparing aortic root replacement: equivalent mid-term outcome for different valve types with or without connective tissue disorder. J Thorac Cardiovasc Surg. 2013;145:117–26.
22. Miyahara S, Matsueda T, Izawa N, Yamanaka K, Sakamoto T, Nomura Y, et al. Mid-term results of valve-sparing aortic root replacement in patients with expanded indications. Ann Thorac Surg. 2015;100:845–51.
23. David TE, David CM, Feindel CM, Manlhiot C. Reimplantation of the aortic valve at 20 years. J Thorac Cardiovasc Surg. 2017;153:232–8.
24. Esaki J, Leshnower BG, Binongo JN, Lasanajak Y, McPherson L, Halkos ME, et al. Clinical outcomes of the David V valve-sparing root replacement compared with bioprosthetic valve-conduits for aortic root aneurysms. Ann Thorac Surg. 2017;103:1824–32.

History, Techniques, and Outcomes of the Remodeling Method

16

Takashi Kunihara

16.1 Introduction

Since the two valve-sparing root replacement procedures of aortic root remodeling and aortic valve reimplantation were introduced, they have rapidly gained attention in recent years. Both types have their advantages and disadvantages, and it is difficult to say which one is superior in general. They are compared in the section "ONE-POINT ADVICE: Experimental Comparison Between the Reimplantation Method and Remodeling Method" (Chap. 17).

This section focuses on aortic root remodeling and introduces the details of the surgical method, its results, and characteristics.

16.2 Transition of the Operation

Surgery for a dilated aortic root was introduced for the first time by Wheat et al. in 1964 [1]. Then, in 1968, Bentall and De Bono reported a method to replace the entire root component with a valved conduit (composite graft), and for a long time, this technique was the standard of choice [2]. Although the Ross operation using an autologous pulmonary valve was expected to achieve excellent long-term results, concerns regarding surgical invasiveness and reoperation to correct pulmonary valve position have remained, and thus this technique has not spread widely [3]. Root replacement with a stentless biological valve [4] or a composite graft using a biological valve [5] are not recommended for young people, who comprise the majority of the cases of aortic root enlargement. Therefore, in 1992, David and Feindel advocated the so-called aortic valve reimplantation method (hereinafter referred to as reimplantation) [6], and in 1993, Sarsam and Yacoub proposed the so-called aortic root remodeling method (hereinafter referred to as remodeling) [7] one after another, and as a consequence, valve-sparing root replacement has attracted much attention.

Thereafter, no major changes were made in the remodeling procedure itself, and David himself performed the remodeling method as the David-II operation and applied partial annuloplasty on the fibrous portion alone as the David-III operation (Fig. 16.1) [8]. Later, the emphasis focused on how to support the annulus, and for these details, see the next section "Variations and Outcomes of Annuloplasty" (Chap. 18).

16.3 Indications and Contraindications

The favorable indications for valve-sparing root replacement include a maximum diameter of the sinus of Valsalva equal to or greater than 40 to

T. Kunihara (✉)
Department of Cardiac Surgery, The Jikei University School of Medicine, Tokyo, Japan
e-mail: kunihara@jikei.ac.jp

T. Kunihara, S. Takanashi (eds.), *Aortic Valve Preservation*,
https://doi.org/10.1007/978-981-13-2068-2_16

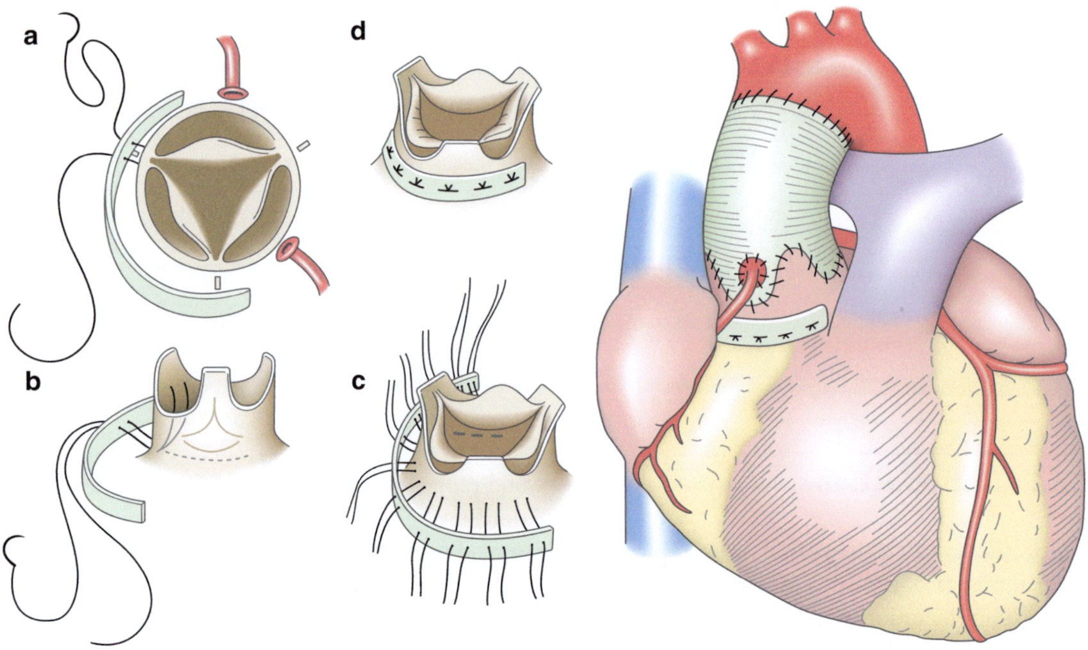

Fig. 16.1 Remodeling method with partial annuloplasty of the fibrous portion between the trigones alone (the so-called David-III operation)

45 mm and no obvious calcification or degenerative changes of the aortic cusps. The guidelines targeting Westerners state that a root with a diameter of at least 45 mm or more should be replaced at the time of surgery for the aortic valve [9, 10], but for smaller Japanese patients, 40 mm or more might be more appropriate. In addition, it is necessary to slightly lower this cut-off value for a bicuspid valve; for example, there are institutions in Europe and the United States where it is 43 mm [11, 12]. Strictly speaking, there are no contraindications, but in cases with advanced valvular calcification or retraction, it would be better to refrain from valve preservation unless the patient is very young. In terms of the physique of Westerners, it is recommended that valvuloplasty should be avoided in cases in which the length from the nadir of the cusp insertion to the tips of the cusp (geometric height) is 16 mm or less for a tricuspid valve and 19 mm or less for a bicuspid valve [13].

Next, when selecting between the two surgical procedures, it is common to select the reimplantation method when the aortic annulus diameter is large, and the remodeling method when the diameter is smaller. The cut-off value varies depending on the facility, but it seems to be around 28–30 mm in many cases [14] because long-term results after surgery worsened when this cut-off value was exceeded [11, 12]. Therefore, David, who advocated the reimplantation method in the first place, remarked that he performed the remodeling method for elderly patients with a normal annulus diameter [15]. There is also a strong tendency to select the reimplantation method for connective tissue disease represented by Marfan syndrome. Indeed, by 2010, the reimplantation method accounted for 259 (63%) of 413 valve-sparing root replacement surgeries for Marfan syndrome [16]. Also, in 239 cases registered in the international registry from 2005 to 2010, only one surgery (0.4%) was performed using the remodeling method [17].

For bicuspid valves, Svensson et al. recommends remodeling [18]. One reason is that with remodeling, it is easier to adjust the angle of the bicuspid configuration comparatively freely by way of cutting the tongue, and the second is due to the concern about contact between the cusp and the prosthesis with the reimplantation

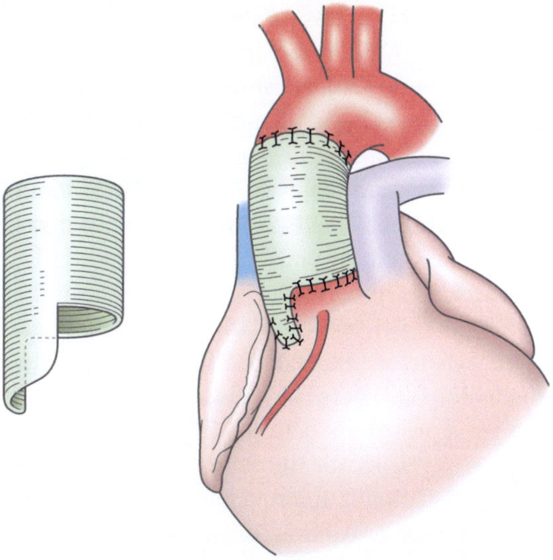

Fig. 16.2 Schema showing remodeling of only the non-coronary sinus

method. However, a graft with sinuses seems to eliminate the latter concern, and some groups have actually reported good outcomes from reimplantation in this subgroup [19].

Remodeling is an attractive option for acute type A aortic dissection because near-normal cusps and annulus diameter are seen in most of these cases, and the operation time should be shortened as much as possible according to the severity of the disease [18, 20, 21]. However, one group recommends the reimplantation method, advocating that if the aortic root is entirely covered with a prosthesis, although the operation time is slightly prolonged, the risk of bleeding is quite reduced [22]. However, there is still room for discussion in this area (see the section "Valve-Sparing Aortic Root Replacement to treat Acute Type A Aortic Dissection, Chap. 23). In addition, another alternative has been proposed: to repair only one or two Valsalva sinuses by the remodeling method [23, 24] (Fig. 16.2).

However, since annuloplasty has been added to the remodeling method as described later and grafts with sinuses have been used for the reimplantation method, the borders between both have clearly disappeared, and it seems that each institution should choose an appropriate surgical method according to their experience and the types of cases treated.

16.4 Advantages and Disadvantages

The greatest advantage of this procedure is that it provides more physiological hemodynamics. In the remodeling method, both the interleaflet triangles and the distensibility of the aortic root are maintained, and it has been shown both experimentally and clinically that valve opening and closing is more physiologic [25–27].

In comparison of up to 18–20% distensibility of the aorta at blood pressures of 100–120 mmHg, only about 3% distensibility is seen in a vascular graft [28]. In an in vitro study, remodeling without annuloplasty maintained approximately 9–10% annular distensibility, but it was only 5% with reimplantation with a tube graft [29]. However, as described above, if annuloplasty is added to remodeling and a graft with sinuses is used for reimplantation, the difference seems to be minimized. Reimplantation with a graft with sinuses improves distensibility at the Valsalva sinus level in comparison to a tube graft but not at the level of the annulus, where distensibility is only 4% and is similar to that of a tube graft [30]. Remodeling with an expansible external aortic ring maintained 4.8–9.1% annular expansibility during a median follow-up period of 19 months (maximum: 5 years) [31]. Although there are few studies comparing these two alternatives directly, some reports found that the stress on the cusps and Valsalva sinuses was the lowest in reimplantation performed by scalloping the prosthesis to create Valsalva sinuses, which seems interesting [32]. For these comparisons, see Chap. 17 ("ONE-POINT ADVICE: Experimental Comparison Between the Reimplantation Method and Remodeling Method").

The next advantage is that less dissection of the root is required than with reimplantation. This has important significance especially in patients in whom the discrepancy between the basal ring and the aorto-ventricular junction (AVJ) is very large, commonly found in the right coronary sinus (also referred to as a "paper-thin right coronary sinus wall") [33] (Fig. 16.3). In such cases, reimplantation requires surgical dissection up to the basal ring, with the associated risk of damaging the Valsalva sinus and the right ventricle. Another appealing aspect is that the

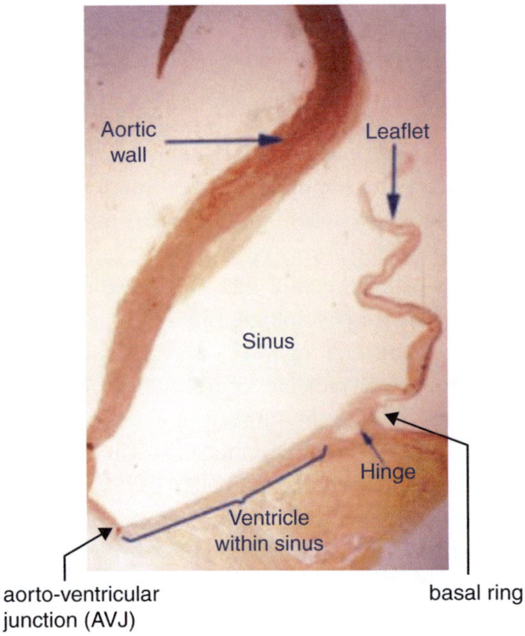

Fig. 16.3 Distinctive difference between the basal ring and aorto-ventricular junction. (Reproduced with permission from reference 33)

aortic cross-clamping time in remodeling can be considerably shortened as compared with that of reimplantation due to less surgical dissection, less suturing, and the possibility of always being able to suture from the outside [11].

Conversely, the disadvantage is that the risk of bleeding from suture lines is clearly higher than that with reimplantation. However, clinically this difference can be minimized by the ingenuity applied to the procedure as described later.

For further details with regard to this issue, please refer to the systematic review comparing the two alternatives [34].

16.5 Actual Practice

Selection of the Prosthesis

In the original method of Yacoub et al., the prosthesis size most frequently used was 30 mm, which seems quite large [35]. Currently in many institutions, the prosthesis used is one size smaller (or 10% less) than the AVJ diameter, unless the AVJ has significantly expanded (30 mm or less) [36], because the AVJ diameter is about 1.2 times larger than the sinotubular junction (STJ) diameter in normal adults [28]. In experienced facilities, it is empirically 24 mm if the body surface area is 1.8 m^2 or less, 26 mm if 1.9–2.2 m^2, and 28 mm if 2.3 m^2 or more [37]. However, it is important to select a prosthesis that is not too small because iatrogenic prolapse can occur when an expanded STJ is reduced too much [38, 39]. There is a highly interesting report that for a prosthesis between 26 and 34 mm, the long-term results for the reimplantation method show a remarkable improvement in performance with a larger prosthesis, whereas results of the remodeling method show that the smaller the better [14]. Recently, annuloplasty has been added routinely, so the annuloplasty size can be initially set according to the normal AVJ diameter based on the body surface area, and then a graft one size larger should be chosen [40]. Care must be taken when a graft with sinuses is used for both root replacement and external ring annuloplasty. The commissure height is set on the basis of the graft size, and the AVJ diameter becomes approximately 4 mm smaller than the ring diameter. Thus, a graft with sinuses with a diameter slightly larger than that for straight graft should be chosen [41]. Indeed, the reported mean size of grafts with sinuses used was 28.0 mm [41], whereas that of tube grafts was 25.4 mm [11]. For convenience, as the Brussels group has proposed, the height of the commissure between the left and non-coronary sinuses can indicate the graft size (or 1 mm larger when an odd number) because it is equal to or slightly smaller than the STJ diameter, and it is not greatly affected by root expansion [42].

Suturing

In the original method of Yacoub et al. for tricuspid cases, the tongue is cut into three equal parts of 1.5 times the native commissure height and sutured from the commissure to nadir, and

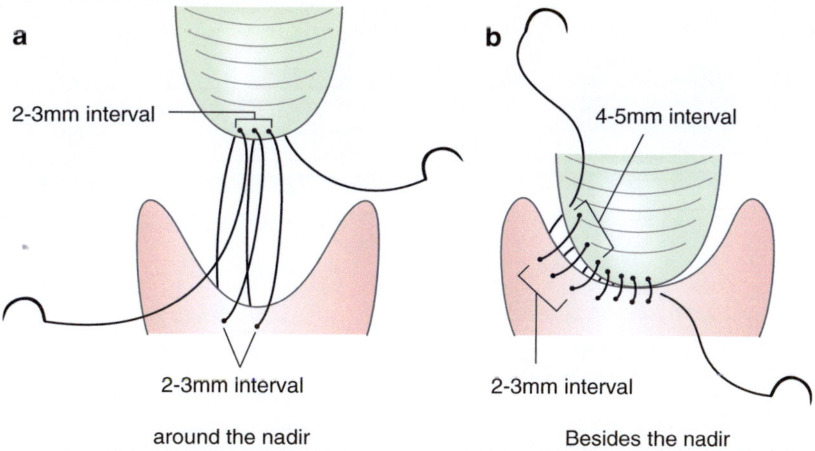

Fig. 16.4 How to create a Valsalva sinus by bulging the prosthesis. (**a**) At the nadir, each stich is of the same width on the native side and the prosthesis side. (**b**) As we move toward the commissure, however, we create bulging of the Valsalva sinus by widening the distance between each stitch from 2 to 3 mm on the native side to 4 to 5 mm on the prosthesis side

the remainder is cut off [35]. Conversely, another group stitched from the nadir to the commissure, and the prosthesis was further cut if necessary so that the commissure is lifted as much as possible [37]. The specific width of each stitch is the same between the native side and the prosthesis side at the nadir, but as we proceed to the commissure, we modify it from 2 to 3 mm on the native side to 4 to 5 mm on the prosthesis side to make bulge in the prosthesis to create a Valsalva sinus (Fig. 16.4). Continuous suturing using suture such as 4-0 polypropylene with a 17-mm 1/2 circle needle is recommended. When using a graft with sinuses, as described above, the commissure height is set on the basis of the graft size; thus, the tongue can be sutured from both the commissure and the nadir, and the sutures can be ligated in the middle [41].

For the bicuspid valve, it is recommended to cut the prosthesis with two equal tongues for three reasons: inferior long-term outcome with an angle of 160° or less between the two cusps [12], the best efficiency for cusp opening is at 180° [43], and procedural convenience in creating a symmetrical shape of the two cusps. If it is possible to improve the mobility of the fused cusp by excising the hardened part (raphe) towards the annulus as much as possible, in most cases, it will be unnecessary to add notches corresponding to this part in the prosthesis. In this way, when a cusp configuration with an angle of 180° or less is corrected to 180°, a bulge may always be produced in the fused cusp. If this is left untreated, the body of the cusp will bulge into the left ventricular side, which is considered a potential risk for recurrence of regurgitation over the long term [38, 44], so it is important to plicate the residual body of the cusps (Fig. 16.5).

Valve Evaluation

In cases requiring some annuloplasty, we perform it first and then move on to cusp evaluation. Three sutures ligated at each commissure should be retracted at the same angle, height, and tension in three directions to evaluate the cusp configuration exactly. The Arantius body is plicated with 5-0 or 6-0 polypropylene suture so that the longitudinal height from the nadir of cusp insertion to the tip of the cusp, the so-called effective height, becomes constant at all leaflets [45]. Its height for European and American patients is required to be 9 mm for tricuspid valves and 12 mm for bicuspid valves [46], but for smaller Japanese patients, it might

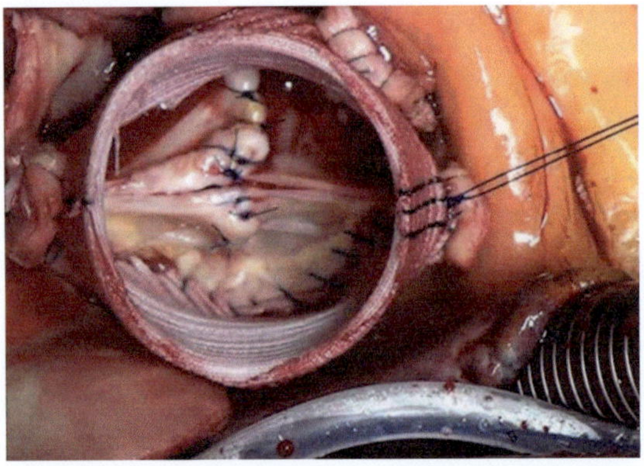

Fig. 16.5 Prevention of valvular bulging in a bicuspid valve. In a bicuspid valve, after plicating the cusp free margin, be sure to plicate the residual body of the cusp to prevent bulging of the cusp body into the left ventricular side

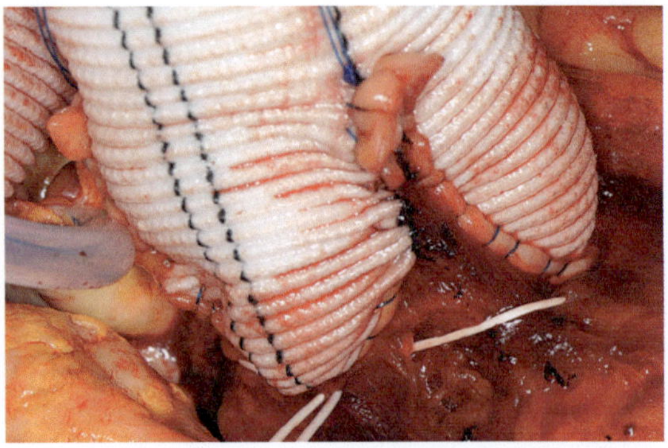

Fig. 16.6 Sewing of the prosthesis to the right coronary (right) and non-coronary (left) sides. It can clearly be seen that the prosthesis bulges to form a Valsalva sinus. To prevent postoperative bleeding, the prosthesis is inserted inside the remnant of the aortic wall

be at least 7 mm. In the case of a bicuspid valve, the non-fused cusp is plicated first until the effective height aimed for is reached, and then the fused cusp is adjusted accordingly by removing and suturing the raphe or simply plicating the Arantius body. For details of other information on valvuloplasty, please refer to the section "Tricuspid Aortic Valve" (Chap. 12).

16.6 My Tips

The key to success in the remodeling method is the control of bleeding. To create artificial Valsalva sinuses, the width of each stitch is wider on the prosthesis side, and thus the prosthesis should be positioned inside the remnant of the aortic wall to prevent bleeding (Fig. 16.6). For this purpose, it is therefore recommended to leave a height of the remnant aortic wall of approximately 4–5 mm. Our favorite prosthesis with regard to both handling and hemostasis is the InterGard™ (Intervascular SAS, La Ciotat, France) provided by the Getinge group in the elective setting and the J-graft™ (Japan Lifeline, Tokyo, Japan) in the emergent setting. Yacoub, who advocated the remodeling method in the first place, recommended using the slightly rigid Dacron tube graft for sufficient coaptation to the patient's tissues [35]. In addition, it is recommended to suture exactly along the firm cusp insertion line to prevent bleeding [35]. This maneuver is also believed to prevent late annular dilatation [47].

16.7 Results

To date, there have been only a few reports of long-term results of the remodeling method alone, and they are shown in Table 16.1 [15, 35, 37, 41, 48–50]. Reports with limited pathological conditions (bicuspid valve, Marfan syndrome, acute dissection, children, etc.), only one or two Valsalva sinuses replaced, or those with only a few cases were excluded. The report by Lansac et al. was a multicenter prospective registry from four institutions in France using an external ring annuloplasty in all cases [41]. Schäfers et al. reported the largest case volume at a single institution [37]. In reports in 2014 from the institution of Erasmi and his colleagues in Lübeck [51] and from the facility of David et al. in Toronto [52], the number of cases increased to 113 and 75 cases, respectively, but the long-term results of the remodeling method alone were not shown in detail and therefore are not described here. In the 2013 report from the institution of Jeanmart and his colleagues in Brussels, the number of cases had not increased at all [53].

Table 16.1 Long-term results of the remodeling method alone

First author	Published year	Reference number	Number of cases	Severe AR	Bicuspid aortic valve	Marfan syndrome	Acute aortic dissection	Cusp repair	Freedom from reoperation	Freedom from AR II or more	Comment
Yacoub	1998	[35]	158	28 (18%)	N.A.	68 (43%)	49 (31%)	13 (8%)[a]	85%@15y		[a]Cusp augmentation
Erasmi	2007	[48]	96	N.A.	13 (14%)	N.A.	21(22%)	22 (23%)	89%@54.7m		
Jeanmart	2007	[49]	48	9 (19%) (>IV)	11 (23%)	5 (10%)	0	23 (48%)	97%@5y	97%@5y	
David	2010	[15]	61	11 (21%)	2 (3%)	26 (42%)	7 (12%)	32 (52%)	90.4%@12y	82.6%@12y[a]	[a]Freedom from moderate or severe AR
Svensson	2011	[50]	72	7 (10%) (>IV)	17 (24%)	12 (17%)	19 (26%)[a]	N.A.	85%@10y		[a]Emergent: 14 (21%)
Schäfers	2015	[37]	747	405 (54%)	290 (39%)	29 (4%)	59 (8%)	690 (92%)	91%@15y		
Lansac	2017	[41]	177	32 (18%) (>IV)	59 (33%)	28 (16%)	2 (1%)	122 (69%)	89.5%@7y	77.4%@7y	

N.A. Not applicable; *AR* aortic regurgitation

Although there are variations in patient background among the facilities, the freedom from reoperation at 3 to 15 years is roughly 90% or more, excluding the report by Yacoub et al., which included many cases in the early series, and 43% with Marfan syndrome [35]. Freedom from the recurrence of aortic valve regurgitation ≥ grade II was as good as 80% or more. Comparisons with the reimplantation method were not significantly different in the reports from Lübeck and Brussels [48, 49] nor in previous reports from Homburg as well [11]. The only significant difference was found in the report from David et al. in Toronto that the reimplantation method provided superior freedom from recurrence of aortic valve regurgitation ($P = 0.035$) [15]. However, this difference had no statistical power in their recent series ($P = 0.52$) [52]. In their recent report, 31% of the cases in the remodeling group were of Marfan syndrome, and cusp repair was performed in 59% of the cases, yet they did not add annuloplasty or even partial reinforcement only, but these factors were considered to contribute to the inferiority of remodeling in their early series [8]. In fact, after the patients with Marfan syndrome were excluded, they reported that no patient in the remodeling group required reoperation or developed recurrent aortic valve regurgitation [52]. Indeed, a recent meta-analysis and multi-institutional analysis found that remodeling and reimplantation techniques provide comparable survival and valve durability results [54, 55].

The risks of long-term failure proved to be factors such as age [15], no cusp repair [56], large AVJ diameter, use of annuloplasty, use of a pericardial patch, low effective height, and myocardial ischemia time [37]. It seems that the use of annuloplasty is contradictory, but it is presumed that this is because annuloplasty used to be applied in complicated patients such as those with a large AVJ diameter or when using pericardial patches [37].

There were only a few reports of the long-term results of the remodeling method for bicuspid valves alone, and in the 2013 Homburg report, the 10-year freedom from reoperation was 89%, which was better than that for isolated valve repair (70%) [57], and aortic root replacement was identified as one of the favorable prognostic factors for long-term valve durability [12]. This result suggests that not the cusps alone but the entire aortic root complex should ideally be addressed in bicuspid valve repair. The same trend was also reported when performing reimplantation [19]. However, the same group later clarified that the cumulative incidence of reoperation increased up to 21.7% at 15 years, and cusp calcification and the use of a pericardial patch were associated with an increased risk of reoperation [58].

In a meta-analysis of 413 patients with Marfan syndrome, the reimplantation method resulted in a significantly lower re-intervention rate than the remodeling method (0.7%/year vs. 2.4%/year) [16]. Freedom from reoperation after the remodeling method was 86% at 8 years [59] and 67% at 15 years [60]. However, these are results from the era when effective annular support was not available. In the author's experience in Homburg with 21 cases of Marfan syndrome (including seven annuloplasties), the 5-year reoperation-free rate with the remodeling method was 100%, which seemed comparable with that of the reimplantation method [61]. Long-term valve durability after remodeling with annuloplasty in this cohort requires further evaluation.

The remodeling method for acute type A dissection was performed in eight patients by the Hannover University group in 2002, and half of them underwent reoperation during an average observation period of 23 months, which indicates a freedom from reoperation rate of 38% [62]. In recent years, as described above, repair of only one or two Valsalva sinuses by the remodeling method has resulted in favorable rates of freedom from reoperation of 90–100% at 5 years [23, 24]. In the author's experience in Homburg with 59 patients (with annuloplasty performed in 6 of them), freedom from proximal reoperation at 10 years after remodeling was 98%, which does not seem inferior to other alternatives [20] or remodeling for patients with stable chronic aneurysm [21].

16.8 Conclusion

Thanks to the addition of annuloplasty, the indications for remodeling are ever increasing. Hemodynamic differences from reimplantation have been minimized, and the greatest advantages are preservation of root distensibility along with less root dissection and shorter operation times. The largest concern is the lack of evidence, such as that from randomized trials, but presently, a large-scale registry is under way mainly in Europe, and a similar registry has just recently launched in Japan. Several meta-analyses and reviews have also been published, but it is hard to say that definitive conclusions have been obtained because there are too many variations in patient background and in the surgical procedures performed. Therefore, we currently recommend selecting the optimal procedure according to the aortic root pathology and the patient's background, as well as the experience of the surgeon.

References

1. Wheat MW Jr, Wilson JR, Bartley TD. Successful replacement of the entire ascending aorta and aortic valve. JAMA. 1964;188:717–9.
2. Bentall H, De Bono A. A technique for complete replacement of the ascending aorta. Thorax. 1968;23:338–9.
3. Davies H, Lessof MH, Roberts CI, Ross DN. Homograft replacement of the aortic valve: follow-up studies in twelve patients. Lancet. 1965;1:926–9.
4. Sievers HH, Lange PE, Bernhard A. Implantation of a xenogeneic stentless aortic bioprosthesis. First experience. Thorac Cardiovasc Surg. 1985;33:225–6.
5. De Paulis R, Scaffa R, Maselli D, Weltert L, Salica A, Bellisario A. Valsalva graft in the Bentall procedure: from mechanical valve to the BioValsalva, world's first biological aortic conduit. Surg Technol Int. 2008;17:216–21.
6. David TE, Feindel CM. An aortic-valve sparing operation for patients with aortic incompetence and aneurysm of the ascending aorta. J Thorac Cardiovasc Surg. 1992;103:617–22.
7. Sarsam MA, Yacoub M. Remodeling of the aortic anulus. J Thorac Cardiovasc Surg. 1993;105:435–8.
8. David TE. Aortic root aneurysms: remodeling or composite replacement? Ann Thorac Surg. 1997;64:1564–8.
9. Hiratzka LF, Bakris GL, Beckman JA, Bersin RM, Carr VF, Casey DE Jr, et al. ACCF/AHA/AATS/ACR/ASA/SCA/SCAI/SIR/STS/SVM guidelines for the diagnosis and management of patients with thoracic aortic disease. Circulation. 2010;121:e266–369.
10. Vahanian A, Alfieri O, Andreotti F, Antunes MJ, Baron-Esquivias G, Baumgartner H, et al. Guidelines on the management of valvular heart disease (version 2012): The Joint Task Force on the Management of valvular Heart Disease of the European Society of Cardiology (ESC) and the European Association for Cardio-Thoracic Surgery (EACTS). Eur Heart J. 2012;33:2451–96.
11. Kunihara T, Aicher D, Rodionycheva S, Groesdonk HV, Langer F, Sata F, et al. Preoperative aortic root geometry and postoperative cusp configuration primarily determine long-term outcome after valve-preserving aortic root repair. J Thorac Cardiovasc Surg. 2012;143:1389–95.
12. Aicher D, Kunihara T, Abou Issa O, Brittner B, Gräber S, Schäfers HJ. Valve configuration determines long-term results after repair of the bicuspid aortic valve. Circulation. 2011;123:178–85.
13. Schäfers HJ, Schmied W, Marom G, Aicher D. Cusp height in aortic valves. J Thorac Cardiovasc Surg. 2013;146:269–74.
14. Hanke T, Charitos EI, Stierle U, Robinson D, Gorski A, Sievers HH, et al. Factors associated with the development of aortic valve regurgitation over time after two different techniques of valve-sparing aortic root surgery. J Thorac Cardiovasc Surg. 2009;137:314–9.
15. David TE, Maganti M, Armstrong S. Aortic root aneurysm: principles of repair and long-term follow-up. J Thorac Cardiovasc Surg. 2010;140:S14–9.
16. Benedetto U, Melina G, Takkenberg JJ, Roscitano A, Angeloni E, Sinatra R. Surgical management of aortic root disease in Marfan syndrome: a systematic review and meta-analysis. Heart. 2011;97:955–8.
17. Coselli JS, Volguina IV, Lemaire SA, Sundt TM, Connolly HM, Stephens EH, et al. Aortic Valve Operative Outcomes in Marfan Patients Study Group. Early and 1-year outcomes of aortic root surgery in patients with Marfan syndrome: a prospective, multicenter, comparative study. J Thorac Cardiovasc Surg. 2014;147:1758–67.
18. Svensson LG, Pillai ST, Rajeswaran J, Desai MY, Griffin B, Grimm R, et al. Long-term survival, valve durability, and reoperation for 4 aortic root procedures combined with ascending aorta replacement. J Thorac Cardiovasc Surg. 2016;151:764–71.
19. de Kerchove L, Boodhwani M, Glineur D, Vandyck M, Vanoverschelde JL, Noirhomme P, et al. Valve sparing-root replacement with the reimplantation technique to increase the durability of bicuspid aortic valve repair. J Thorac Cardiovasc Surg. 2011;142:1430–8.
20. Kunihara T, Neumann N, Kriechbaum SD, Aicher D, Schäfers HJ. Aortic root remodeling leads to good

valve stability in acute aortic dissection and preexistent root dilatation. J Thorac Cardiovasc Surg. 2016;152:430–6.
21. Kunihara T, Neumann N, Kriechbaum SD, Nomura R, Schäfers HJ. Long-term outcome of aortic root remodeling for patients with and without acute aortic dissection. Circ J. 2017;81:1824–31.
22. Beckmann E, Martens A, Pertz J, Kaufeld T, Umminger J, Hanke JS, Schmitto JD, Cebotari S, Haverich A, Shrestha ML. Valve-sparing David I procedure in acute aortic type A dissection: a 20-year experience with more than 100 patients. Eur J Cardiothorac Surg. 2017;52:319–24.
23. Urbanski PP, Hijazi H, Dinstak W, Diegeler A. Valve-sparing aortic root repair in acute type A dissection: how many sinuses have to be repaired for curative surgery? Eur J Cardiothorac Surg. 2013;44: 439–44.
24. Subramanian S, Leontyev S, Borger MA, Trommer C, Misfeld M, Mohr FW. Valve-sparing root reconstruction does not compromise survival in acute type A aortic dissection. Ann Thorac Surg. 2012;94: 1230–4.
25. Graeter TP, Fries R, Aicher D, Reul H, Schmitz C, Schäfers HJ. In-vitro comparison of aortic valve hemodynamics between aortic root remodeling and aortic valve reimplantation. J Heart Valve Dis. 2006;15:329–35.
26. Fries R, Graeter T, Aicher D, Reul H, Schmitz C, Böhm M, et al. In vitro comparison of aortic valve movement after valve-preserving aortic replacement. J Thorac Cardiovasc Surg. 2006;132:32–7.
27. Leyh RG, Schmidtke C, Sievers HH, Yacoub MH. Opening and closing characteristics of the aortic valve after different types of valve-preserving surgery. Circulation. 1999;100:2153–60.
28. Kunzelman KS, Grande KJ, David TE, Cochran RP, Verrier ED. Aortic root and valve relationships. Impact on surgical repair. J Thorac Cardiovasc Surg. 1994;107:162–70.
29. Erasmi A, Sievers HH, Scharfschwerdt M, Eckel T, Misfeld M. In vitro hydrodynamics, cusp-bending deformation, and root distensibility for different types of aortic valve-sparing operations: remodeling, sinus prosthesis, and reimplantation. J Thorac Cardiovasc Surg. 2005;130:1044–9.
30. Matsumori M, Tanaka H, Kawanishi Y, Onishi T, Nakagiri K, Yamashita T, et al. Comparison of distensibility of the aortic root and cusp motion after aortic root replacement with two reimplantation techniques: Valsalva graft versus tube graft. Interact Cardiovasc Thorac Surg. 2007;6:177–81.
31. Wuliya M, Sleilaty G, Di Centa I, Khelil N, Berrebi A, Czitrom D, et al. An expansible aortic ring to preserve aortic root dynamics after aortic valve repair. Eur J Cardiothorac Surg. 2015;47:482–90.
32. Grande-Allen KJ, Cochran RP, Reinhall PG, Kunzelman KS. Re-creation of sinuses is important for sparing the aortic valve: a finite element study. J Thorac Cardiovasc Surg. 2000;119:753–63.
33. Anderson RH. Clinical anatomy of the aortic root. Heart. 2000;84:670–3.
34. Kunihara T. Valve-sparing aortic root surgery. CON: remodeling. Gen Thorac Cardiovasc Surg. 2017; https://doi.org/10.1007/s11748-017-0833-6.
35. Yacoub MH, Gehle P, Chandrasekaran V, Birks EJ, Child A, Radley-Smith R. Late results of a valve-preserving operation in patients with aneurysms of the ascending aorta and root. J Thorac Cardiovasc Surg. 1998;115:1080–90.
36. El Khoury GA, Underwood MJ, Glineur D, Derouck D, Dion RA. Reconstruction of the ascending aorta and aortic root: experience in 45 consecutive patients. Ann Thorac Surg. 2000;70:1246–50.
37. Schäfers HJ, Raddatz A, Schmied W, Takahashi H, Miura Y, Kunihara T, et al. Reexamining remodeling. J Thorac Cardiovasc Surg. 2015;149:S30–6.
38. Pethig K, Milz A, Hagl C, Harringer W, Haverich A. Aortic valve reimplantation in ascending aortic aneurysm: risk factors for early valve failure. Ann Thorac Surg. 2002;73:29–33.
39. Maselli D, De Paulis R, Scaffa R, Weltert L, Bellisario A, Salica A, et al. Sinotubular junction size affects aortic root geometry and aortic valve function in the aortic valve reimplantation procedure: an in vitro study using the valsalva graft. Ann Thorac Surg. 2007;84:1214–8.
40. Capps SB, Elkins RC, Fronk DM. Body surface area as a predictor of aortic and pulmonary valve diameter. J Thorac Cardiovasc Surg. 2000;119:975–82.
41. Lansac E, Di Centa I, Sleilaty G, Lejeune S, Berrebi A, Zacek P, et al. Remodeling root repair with an external aortic ring annuloplasty. J Thorac Cardiovasc Surg. 2017;153:1033–42.
42. de Kerchove L, Boodhwani M, Glineur D, Noirhomme P, El Khoury G. A new simple and objective method for graft sizing in valve-sparing root replacement using the reimplantation technique. Ann Thorac Surg. 2011;92:749–51.
43. Robicsek F, Thubrikar MJ, Cook JW, Fowler B. The congenitally bicuspid aortic valve: how does it function? Why does it fail? Ann Thorac Surg. 2004;77:177–85.
44. le Polain de Waroux JB, Pouleur AC, Robert A, Pasquet A, Gerber BL, Noirhomme P, et al. Mechanisms of recurrent aortic regurgitation after aortic valve repair: predictive value of intraoperative transesophageal echocardiography. JACC Cardiovasc Imaging. 2009;2:931–9.
45. Schäfers HJ, Bierbach B, Aicher D. A new approach to the assessment of aortic cusp geometry. J Thorac Cardiovasc Surg. 2006;132:436–8.
46. Bierbach BO, Aicher D, Issa OA, Bomberg H, Gräber S, Glombitza P, et al. Aortic root and cusp configuration determine aortic valve function. Eur J Cardiothorac Surg. 2010;38:400–6.
47. Furukawa K, Kamohara K, Yunoki J, Koga S, Itoh M, Morokuma H, Mukae Y, et al. Should the annulus be fixed in aortic valve-sparing root replacement with remodeling? Gen Thorac Cardiovasc Surg. 2017;65:200–5.

48. Erasmi AW, Sievers HH, Bechtel JF, Hanke T, Stierle U, Misfeld M. Remodeling or reimplantation for valve-sparing aortic root surgery? Ann Thorac Surg. 2007;83:S752–6.
49. Jeanmart H, de Kerchove L, Glineur D, Goffinet JM, Rougui I, Van Dyck M, et al. Aortic valve repair: the functional approach to leaflet prolapse and valve-sparing surgery. Ann Thorac Surg. 2007;83:S746–51.
50. Svensson LG, Batizy LH, Blackstone EH, Gillinov AM, Moon MC, D'Agostino RS, et al. Results of matching valve and root repair to aortic valve and root pathology. J Thorac Cardiovasc Surg. 2011;142:1491–8.e7.
51. Charitos EI, Stierle U, Tietze C, Hanke T, Karluss A, Misfeld M, et al. Clinical outcomes and lessons learned with aortic valve repair in 508 patients. J Heart Valve Dis. 2014;23:550–7.
52. David TE, Feindel CM, David CM, Manlhiot C. A quarter of a century of experience with aortic valve-sparing operations. J Thorac Cardiovasc Surg. 2014;148:872–9.
53. Price J, De Kerchove L, Glineur D, Vanoverschelde JL, Noirhomme P, El Khoury G. Risk of valve-related events after aortic valve repair. Ann Thorac Surg. 2013;95:606–12.
54. Arabkhani B, Mookhoek A, Di Centa I, Lansac E, Bekkers JA, De Lind Van Wijngaarden R, et al. Reported outcome after valve-sparing aortic root replacement for aortic root aneurysm: a systematic review and meta-analysis. Ann Thorac Surg. 2015;100:1126–31.
55. Kari FA, Doll KN, Hemmer W, Liebrich M, Sievers HH, Richardt D, et al. Residual and progressive aortic regurgitation after valve-sparing root replacement: a propensity-matched multi-institutional analysis in 764 patients. Ann Thorac Surg. 2016;101:1500–6.
56. Lansac E, Di Centa I, Sleilaty G, Bouchot O, Arnaud Crozat E, Blin D, et al. An aortic ring to standardise aortic valve repair: preliminary results of a prospective multicentric cohort of 144 patients. Eur J Cardiothorac Surg. 2010;38:147–54.
57. Aicher D, Schneider U, Schmied W, Kunihara T, Tochii M, Schäfers HJ. Early results with annular support in reconstruction of the bicuspid aortic valve. J Thorac Cardiovasc Surg. 2013;145:S30–4.
58. Schneider U, Feldner SK, Hofmann C, Schöpe J, Wagenpfeil S, Giebels C, et al. Two decades of experience with root remodeling and valve repair for bicuspid aortic valves. J Thorac Cardiovasc Surg. 2017;153:S65–71.
59. Patel ND, Weiss ES, Alejo DE, Nwakanma LU, Williams JA, Dietz HC, et al. Aortic root operations for Marfan syndrome: a comparison of the Bentall and valve-sparing procedures. Ann Thorac Surg. 2008;85:2003–10.
60. David TE, Armstrong S, Maganti M, Colman J, Bradley TJ. Long-term results of aortic valve-sparing operations in patients with Marfan syndrome. J Thorac Cardiovasc Surg. 2009;138:859–64.
61. Kunihara T, Aicher D, Rodionycheva S, Asano M, Tochii M, Sata F, et al. Outcomes after valve-preserving root surgery for patients with Marfan syndrome. J Heart Valve Dis. 2012;21:615–22.
62. Leyh RG, Fischer S, Kallenbach K, Kofidis T, Pethig K, Harringer W, et al. High failure rate after valve-sparing aortic root replacement using the "remodeling technique" in acute type A aortic dissection. Circulation. 2002;106:I229–33.

17 ONE-POINT ADVICE: Experimental Comparison Between the Reimplantation Method and Remodeling Method

Kenichi Sasaki and Kiyotaka Iwasaki

17.1 Introduction

The major difference between the aortic valve reimplantation method (hereinafter referred to as reimplantation) and aortic root remodeling methods (hereinafter referred to as remodeling) is the lack of annular support in the latter. Maselli et al. modified reimplantation into remodeling in the same aortic root and found that it significantly increased the Valsalva sinus diameter and aorto-ventricular junction diameter and, conversely, decreased the effective height and coaptation height [1]. This suggests the important effect of annular support on leaflet structure. However, at present, this drawback of the remodeling method can be overcome by adding annuloplasty (AP). In contrast, when a straight graft is used, a Valsalva sinus can be formed by the remodeling method but not by the reimplantation method, which is a disadvantage of the latter. As will be explained later, the Valsalva sinus has a significant influence on leaflet stress and smooth leaflet closure. However, even with the reimplantation method, Valsalva sinuses can be formed by using the currently available graft with sinuses. Therefore, clarification of the details of the features of both operation types on valve function will lead to ingenuity and improvement of both operations, and a clinical contribution is anticipated.

In this chapter, the effects of differences in root morphology with both operation types on valve function, valve durability, and hemodynamics are discussed. The first half discusses some of the studies reported up to the present, and the latter half discusses reports from our *in vitro* experiments.

17.2 History of the Research Evaluating Valve Durability with the Reimplantation and Remodeling Methods

Evaluation of the durability of the leaflets is roughly classified into the following two types of research introduced below.

Studies Evaluating Aortic Valve Behavior

One study evaluating aortic valve behavior focused on the responsiveness of the leaflets based on their opening and closing velocities.

K. Sasaki
Department of Cardiovascular Surgery, The Cardiovascular Institute, Tokyo, Japan

K. Iwasaki (✉)
Cooperative Major in Advanced Biomedical Sciences, Joint Graduate School of Tokyo Women's Medical University and Waseda University, Tokyo, Japan
e-mail: iwasaki@waseda.jp

T. Kunihara, S. Takanashi (eds.), *Aortic Valve Preservation*, https://doi.org/10.1007/978-981-13-2068-2_17

In 1990, Leyh et al. clinically observed and recorded the leaflet behavior from M-mode echocardiograms and reported that both the rapid valve opening and closing velocities increased and the ratio of slow systolic closure to total leaflet opening decreased with the reimplantation method. In the remodeling method, there was no difference in the rapid valve opening and closing velocities compared with those of the control group, and the ratio of slow systolic closure did not decrease. From these results, the reimplantation method was found to result in sudden opening and closing of the leaflets, and the authors concluded that the load applied to the leaflets was large [2]. Similar research was reported by Fries et al. and Graeter et al. in 2006 [3, 4]. They concluded that in comparison with the reimplantation method, the remodeling method maintains both normal valve movement and aortic root distensibility, leading to low leaflet stress. However, these experimental reimplantation models did not use a graft with sinuses, which is currently the mainstream graft used in clinical practice, but a straight graft. Thus, the clinical study of Matsumori et al. in 2007 showed that when using a graft with sinuses in the reimplantation method, the distensibility of the Valsalva sinus is almost equal to that of normal aorta [5].

Research Evaluating the Strength and Distribution of Leaflet Stress

The computer simulation analysis method of finite element analysis (FEA) enables calculation of the strength and distribution of stress and strain applied to the leaflets. In 2000, FEA performed by Grande-Allen et al. revealed the finding of increased leaflet stress with a straight graft rather than a graft with sinuses [6]. Similar studies were also reported by Beck et al. in 2001 and Katayama et al. in 2008 [7, 8]. Essentially, FEA revealed the occurrence of vortices in the Valsalva sinuses, and furthermore, these vortices were also involved in smooth closure of the leaflets.

17.3 Static Pressure Load Test

An experimental outline of the static pressure load test created by the authors is shown in Fig. 17.1. A tube was attached to the prepared model and the basal ring (BR) diameter, Valsalva sinus (VS) diameter, and sinotubular junction (STJ) diameter were measured under the condition of steady water pressures of 80 mmHg and 120 mmHg applied to the aortic side. Five of each of the following models were prepared for use in the experiments: remodeling model (RM) (22-mm J-graft, Japan Lifeline Co., Ltd., Tokyo, Japan); reimplantation-straight graft model (RI-S) (24-mm J-graft); remodeling-AP model (RM-AP) (22-mm J-graft + 20-mm annuloplasty); and reimplantation-graft with sinuses model (RI-V) (24-mm J-graft with a Valsalva sinus shape). Experiments 1–4 below were carried out, measurements were made by clinical echocardiography, and the results of each measurement are expressed as the mean value and standard deviation.

Experiment 1 (Table 17.1)

Method

In the static pressure load test circuit, the BR diameters of the RI-S group and the RM group were measured and compared. After measuring all of the BR diameters in the unloaded condition, an incision was made in the annulus, and the annular diameter was measured macroscopically.

Result

In the RI-S group, the expansion of the BR diameter was suppressed, whereas the annulus of the RM group was expanded by the static pressure load, suggesting that no annular support was provided by the remodeling method alone.

Experiment 2 (Table 17.2)

Method

We compared the BR, VS, and STJ diameters before and after the addition of a 20-mm AP by CV-0 suture to the RM model.

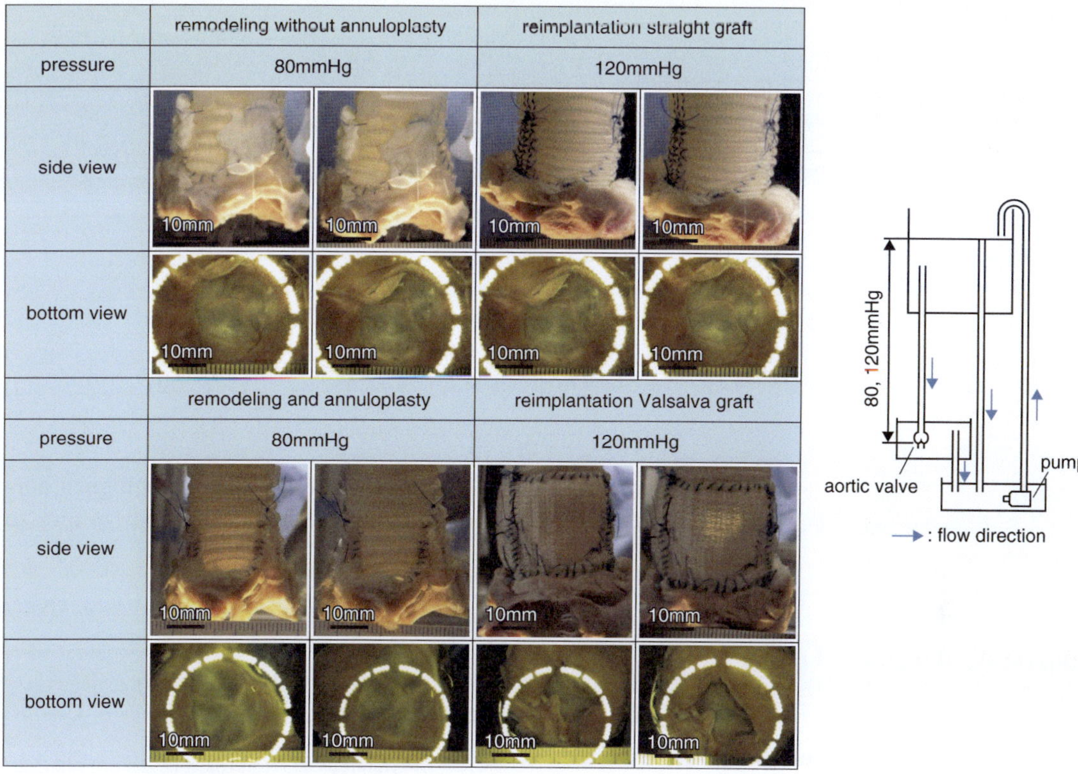

Fig. 17.1 Experimental outline of the static pressure load test

Table 17.1 Experiment 1

	Basal ring diameter				
	Unloading	80 mmHg	120 mmHg	P (Unloading vs. 120 mmHg)	P (80 vs. 120 mmHg)
RI-S (mm)	24.0 ± 1.3	20.5 ± 0.8	20.7 ± 1.3	< 0.01	0.71
RM (mm)	22.8 ± 1.1	24.4 ± 2.1	25.2 ± 1.6	0.02	0.52

Table 17.2 Experiment 2

	80 mmHg			120 mmHg		
RM	AP(−)	AP(+)	p	AP(−)	AP(+)	p
Basal ring	24.4 ± 12.1	20.9 ± 0.5	< 0.01	25.2 ± 11.6	21.4 ± 0.6	< 0.01
Valsalva sinus	27.8 ± 2.1	25.1 ± 2.0	0.06	28.5 ± 2.0	25.3 ± 2.1	0.03
STJ	25.8 ± 1.8	22.6 ± 1.0	0.01	25.4 ± 2.2	22.5 ± 1.2	0.04

Result

In the RM-AP group, the VS and STJ diameters were both significantly reduced by the addition of the AP.

Experiment 3 (Table 17.3)

Methed

The BR, VS, and STJ diameters were measured in the RI-S group and RI-V group.

Table 17.3 Experiment 3

	80 mmHg			120 mmHg		
	RI-S	RI-V	p	RI-S	RI-V	p
Basal ring	20.5 ± 0.8	21.3 ± 0.7	0.13	20.7 ± 1.3	21.8 ± 1.2	0.18
Valsalva sinus	23.8 ± 1.0	31.8 ± 1.9	< 0.01	23.9 ± 0.8	32.7 ± 1.9	< 0.01
STJ	24.4 ± 0.6	24.7 ± 1.3	0.68	24.7 ± 0.8	25.0 ± 1.8	0.84

Table 17.4 Experiment 4

	80 mmHg			120 mmHg		
	RI-V	RM-AP	p	RI-V	RM-AP	p
Valsalva sinus/basal ring	1.49 ± 0.07	1.22 ± 0.09	< 0.01	1.50 ± 0.05	1.21 ± 0.08	< 0.01
Valsalva sinus/STJ	1.29 ± 0.13	1.10 ± 0.07	0.03	1.32 ± 0.17	1.13 ± 0.08	0.05

Result
The VS diameter expanded significantly only in the RI-V group.

Experiment 4 (Table 17.4)

Methed
The VS/BR ratio and the VS/STJ ratio of the RI-V and RM-AP groups were compared, and the VS morphology was verified.

Result
Compared to the RM-AP group, the bulging of the VS could be reproduced in the RI-V group.

The results of the authors' research reconfirmed that the remodeling method provides poor annular stabilization and that AP compensates for it. It was further clarified that the improved graft with sinuses used in the reimplantation method has a sufficiently large VS.

17.4 Conclusion

The reimplantation method and the remodeling method are currently used clinically to compensate for the drawbacks of each other, but the research clearly showing their differences remains insufficient. The present study suggested that modifications to the two current methods functioned effectively. We plan to clarify the detailed hemodynamics of both types of operation under pulsatile flow using a mock circuit in the future. Further research is needed to reproduce a more physiological aortic root and to develop a technique to minimize leaflet stress.

References

1. Maselli D, Weltert L, Scaffa R, Nardella S, Guerrieri Wolf L, De Paulis R. Differences in aortic cusp coaptation between the reimplantation and the remodeling techniques of aortic valve-sparing surgery: an in vitro porcine model study. J Thorac Cardiovasc Surg. 2014;147(2):615–8.
2. Leyh RG, Schimidke C, Sievers H-H, Yacoub MH. Opening and closing characteristics of the aortic valve after different types of valve-preserving surgery. Circulation. 1999;100:2153–60.
3. Fries R, Graeter T, Aicher D, Reul H, Schmitz C, Böhm M, et al. In vitro comparison of aortic valve movement after valve-preserving aortic replacement. J Thorac Cardiovasc Surg. 2006;132(1):32–7.
4. Graeter TP, Fries R, Aicher D, Reul H, Schmitz C, Schäfers HJ. In-vitro comparison of aortic valve hemodynamics between aortic root remodeling and aortic valve reimplantation. J Heart Valve Dis. 2006;15(3):329–35.
5. Matsumori M, Tanaka H, Kawanishi Y, Onishi T, Nakagiri K, Yamashita T, et al. Comparison of distensibility of the aortic root and cusp motion after aortic root replacement with two reimplantation techniques: Valsalva graft versus tube graft. Interact Cardiovasc Thorac Surg. 2007;6(2):177–81.
6. Grande-Allen KJ, Cochran RP, Reinhall PG, Kunzelman KS. Re-creation of sinuses is important for sparing the aortic valve: a finite element study. J Thorac Cardiovasc Surg. 2000;119:753–63.
7. Beck A, Thubrikar MJ, Robicsek F. Stress analysis of the aortic valve with and without the sinuses of valsalva. J Heart Valve Dis. 2001;10:1–11.
8. Katayama S, Umetani N, Sugiura S, Hisada T. The sinus of Valsalva relieves abnormal stress on aortic valve leaflets by facilitating smooth closure. J Thorac Cardiovasc Surg. 2008;136:1528–35.

Variations and Outcomes of Annuloplasty

18

Takashi Kunihara

18.1 Introduction

Although annuloplasty for the aortic valve has been performed for quite a while, it has not been standardized for various reasons. However, in recent years, aortic valvuloplasty has aggressively been performed, and as it becomes clear that annular expansion is a risk factor for the recurrence of aortic regurgitation, annuloplasty is being recognized as an important option and various alternatives have been proposed. This section organizes and classifies the various types of annuloplasty, adds an overview, and clarifies their advantages and disadvantages.

18.2 History of the Operative Method

Aortic annuloplasty as performed so far can be classified as shown in Table 18.1, including those types in the experimental stage.

Suture Annuloplasty (Fig. 18.1)

External Annuloplasty

In 1958, Taylor et al. had already applied the "aortic circumclusion" method to 11 cases by suturing the aortic annulus from the outside in the beating heart [1]. However, this method was not retried for a while because of suboptimal outcomes, but it was spotlighted again half a century later after the Homburg group began to apply it to many cases (Fig. 18.1c) [2]. Originally, the intention was to compensate for annular stabilization, which was lacking in the aortic root remodeling method (remodeling), but due to its convenience, it has now also come to be used liberally for cases of isolated aortic valvuloplasty with annulus enlargement.

Internal Annuloplasty

The subcommissural annuloplasty advocated by Cabrol et al. in 1966 has spread widely due to its convenience [3], and Duran in 1988 [4] and Cosgrove et al. in 1991 [5] reported its usefulness (Fig. 18.1b). However, this method has not recently been in favor due to concerns such as the high risk of recurrence of aortic regurgitation due to partial reduction of the annulus, adverse effects of uneven plication on the movement of the leaflets, and inflammation caused by felt pledgets. In 2007, Kollar applied the same method from the outside of the aorta (Fig. 18.1d) [6], and in 2011, Mangini and his colleagues reduced 14% of annulus diameter by plicating the commissure at the level of half the height of the interleaflet triangle [7]; however, this procedure has also not been generalized.

T. Kunihara (✉)
Department of Cardiac Surgery, The Jikei University School of Medicine, Tokyo, Japan
e-mail: kunihara@jikei.ac.jp

T. Kunihara, S. Takanashi (eds.), *Aortic Valve Preservation*,
https://doi.org/10.1007/978-981-13-2068-2_18

Table 18.1 Classification of the various types of annuloplasty

	Suture				Ring	
	Full	Partial	Partial band		Rigid	Flexible
Internal	Carpentier Hydar Schöllhorn	Cabrol Mangini	(Haydar)	Hahm	Duran* Schomburg* Rankin Richardt*	Izumoto Fattouch Scharfschwerdt*
External	Taylor Schäfers	Kollar	David		Reimold*	Kawazoe Gogbashian* Scharfschwerdt* Lansac

*Animal study only

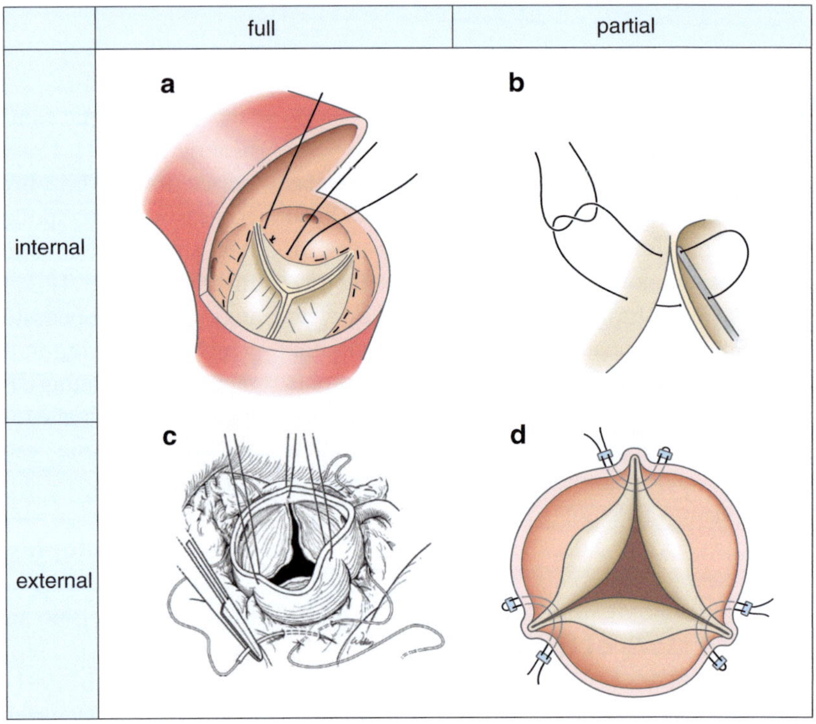

Fig. 18.1 The variations of suture annuloplasty. (**a**) Annular reduction using U-shaped continuous sutures at the cusp insertion line. (**b**) So-called subcommissural annuloplasty. (**c**) External circular suture annuloplasty (reproduced with permission from reference 2). (**d**) Subcommissural annuloplasty from the outside of the aorta

To compensate for these disadvantages, Carpentier in 1983 [8] and Haydar and his colleagues in 1997 [9] proposed another method of placing a U-shaped continuous suture along the aortic cusp insertion line to reduce the annulus size, and the long-term results were unknown in either case. However, in 2014, Schöllhorn and his colleagues modified this method and reported good results (Fig. 18.1a) [10].

Partial Band Annuloplasty (Fig. 18.2)

Haydar and his colleagues, as mentioned earlier, had reinforced the U-shaped continuous sutures using three autologous pericardial strips treated with glutaraldehyde in their early series [9] (Fig. 18.2a). David partially reinforced only the fibrous portion from the outside with a Dacron strip in 11 cases undergoing the remodeling method as the David-III operation [11] (Fig. 18.2b), and Hahm and his colleagues applied a method to reinforce the non-expansible strip from both the inside and the outside in 23 cases [12] (Fig. 18.2c). However, partial reinforcement is considered to have an insufficient effect on the prevention of annulus enlargement. The method of Hahm and his colleagues is called "comprehensive aortic root and valve repair (CARVAR)", and 397 cases were performed [13].

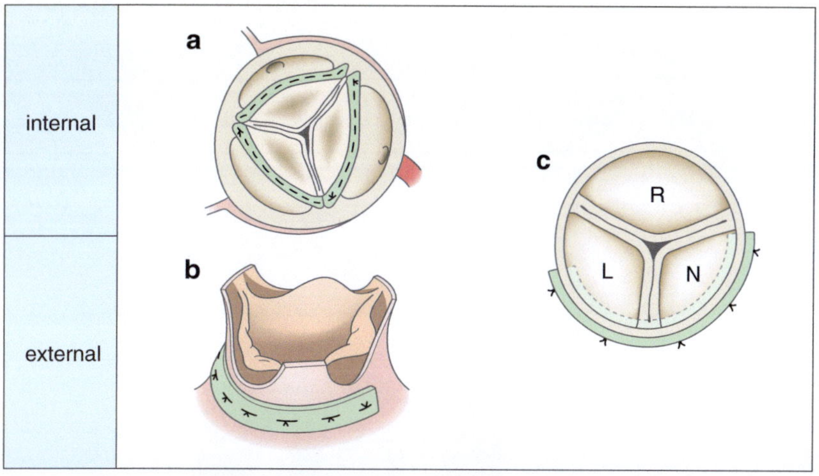

Fig. 18.2 The variations of partial band annuloplasty. (**a**) Annuloplasty using U-shaped continuous sutures reinforced with three autologous pericardial strips. (**b**) Partial reinforcement of the fibrous portion alone from the outside with a Dacron strip. (**c**) Partial reinforcement of the fibrous portion alone from both the inside and outside with a non-expansible strip. *R* right coronary cusp, *L* left coronary cusp, *N* non-coronary cusp

Ring Annuloplasty

Rigid Rings (Fig. 18.3)

In 1993, Duran et al. developed an internal ring (sigmoid ring) covered with Dacron that matched the shape of the aortic annulus, and they conducted animal experiments (Fig. 18.3a) [14]. A similar concept was later applied clinically by modifying the shape to form an elliptical ring after animal experiments were performed by Schomburg et al. [15] and Rankin et al. (HAART, Hemispherical Aortic Annuloplasty Ring Technology; BioStable Science and Engineering, Inc., Austin, TX, USA) (Fig. 18.3b) [16]. Currently, this ring is also available for bicuspid anatomy [17]. Contrastingly, Reimold and his colleagues applied external rings made of stainless steel or acrylic plastic in animal experiments in 1994, but they have not yet been applied clinically (Fig. 18.3d) [18].

Flexible Rings (Fig. 18.4)

Kawazoe et al. initially adapted glutaraldehyde-treated equine pericardium to cover the entire root from the outside (Fig. 18.4d) [19] and in 2002 applied an ePTFE (expanded polytetrafluoroethylene) strip placed directly under the aortic annulus using U-shaped sutures and reported acceptable long-term results (Fig. 18.4a) [20]. Fattouch et al. clinically applied a similar internal subvalvular annuloplasty method to 45 cases using a flexible band in combination with a coronal sinotubular junction (STJ) annuloplasty band with the legs fixed to the three commissures in 2011 and also reported good results (Fig. 18.4b) [21].

Meanwhile, in 2007, Gogbashian and his colleagues reported on animal experiments to tighten the aortic root from the outside with a size-adjustable loop-type nylon band for the control of aortic regurgitation, but it has not yet been applied clinically (Fig. 18.4e) [22]. Currently, the most widely applied ring in the clinic setting is the external expansible subvalvular aortic ring originally proposed by Lansac et al. in 2005 (Fig. 18.4g) [23]. They recently reported good long-term results of external ring annuloplasty combined with remodeling or isolated aortic valvuloplasty based on the aortic valve repair international registry (AVIATOR) [23, 24], and currently, the prospective CAVIAAR study to compare the effects of root replacement with or without valve preservation in the long-term phase is under way [25].

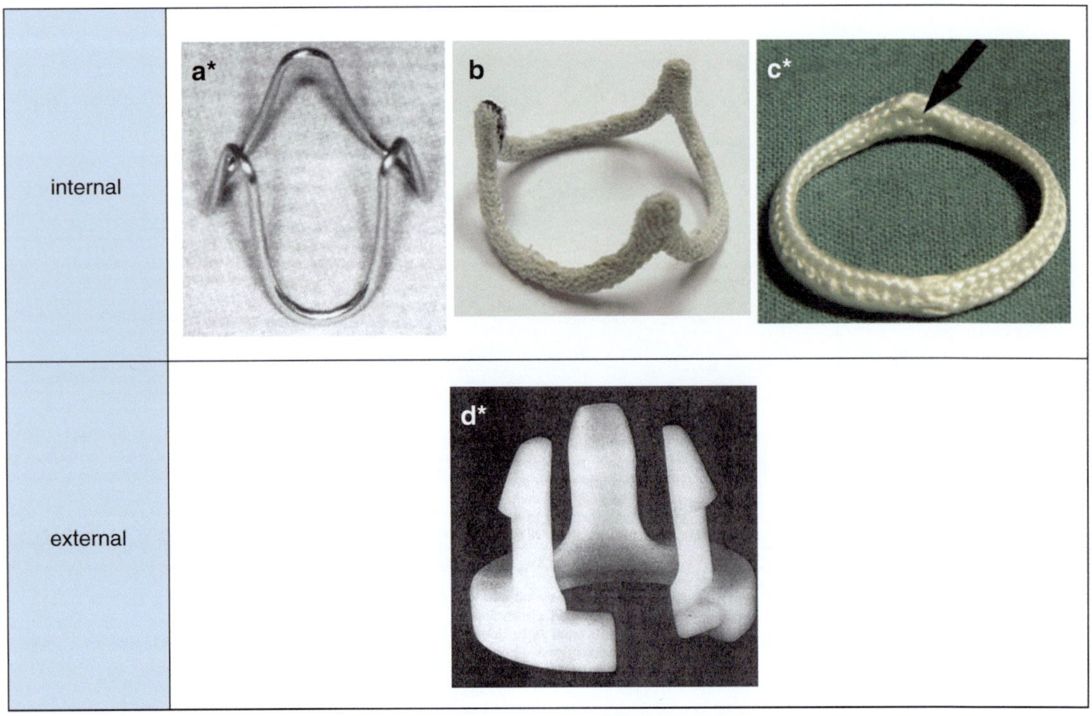

Fig. 18.3 The variations of rigid-ring annuloplasty. (**a**) Internal titanium ring covered with Dacron tailored to the annulus shape (sigmoid ring) (reproduced with permission from reference 14). (**b**) Elliptical HAART 300 internal rigid annuloplasty ring (reproduced with permission from Rankin JS, Beavan LA, Cohn WE. Technique for aortic valve annuloplasty using an intraannular "hemispherical" frame. J Thorac Cardiovasc Surg. 2011;142:933–6). (**c**) Rigid internal ring covered with soft Dacron. Atrioventricular block can possibly be prevented by positioning the part indicated by the arrow at the commissure between the right and non-coronary sinuses (reproduced with permission from reference 27). (**d**) External ring made of stainless steel or acrylic plastic (reproduced with permission from reference 18). *Animal study only

According to animal experiments performed by Scharfschwerdt and his colleagues to compare flexible external (Fig. 18.4f) and internal (Fig. 18.4c) rings, the latter was more advantageous in controlling aortic valve regurgitation [26]; therefore, this group is now investigating the rigid internal ring in animal experiments (Fig. 18.3c) [27].

18.3 Indications and Contraindications

Lansac et al. [28] and Schäfers et al. [29] added annuloplasty in patients with an annulus diameter of 25 mm or more and 27 mm or more, respectively, based on the fact that annulus enlargement is a risk factor for inferior performance after remodeling surgery [30, 31]. The addition of external suture annuloplasty to the remodeling method is very convenient, and it seems to have been performed in almost all cases in recent years to extend prevention of late annular expansion. Even in isolated aortic valvuloplasty cases, it appears to be frequently added to obtain better cusp coaptation.

A relative contraindication would be a unicuspid or a bicuspid valve with no marked annular dilation but at potential risk for causing aortic valve stenosis. Especially, subcommissural annuloplasty in these cases carries a high risk of aortic valve stenosis, and thus its application should carefully be discussed.

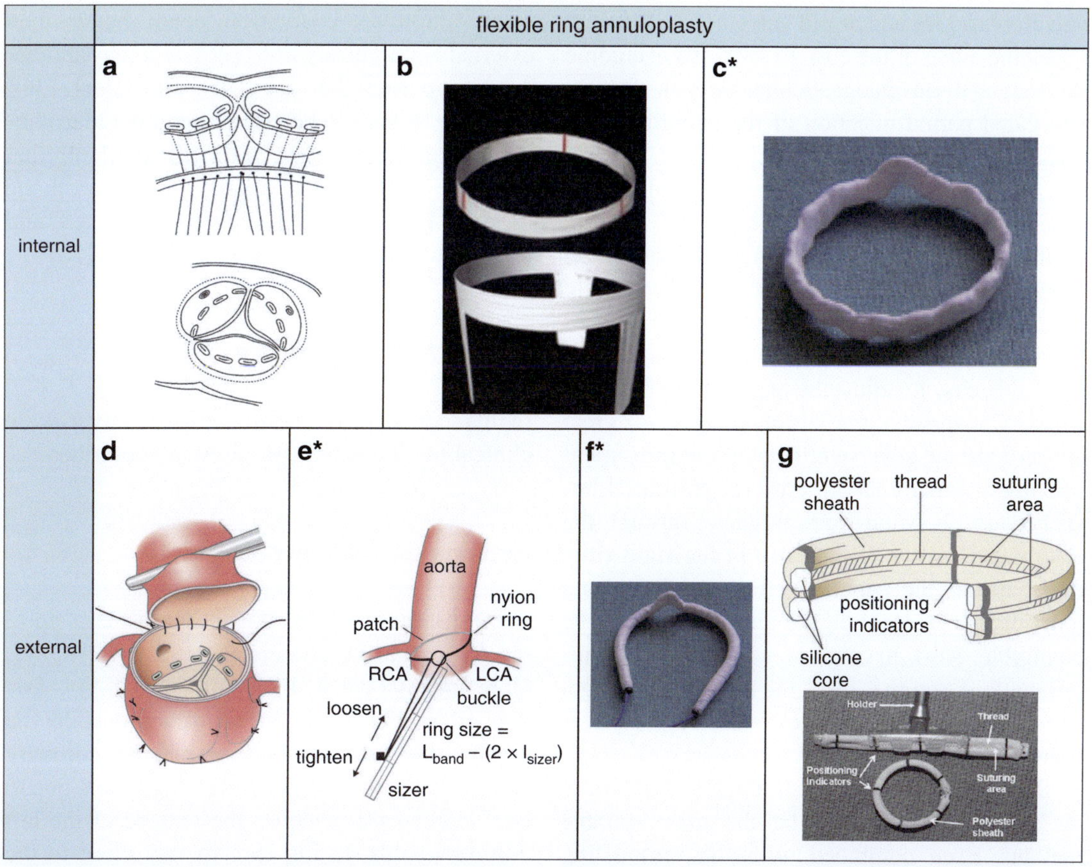

Fig. 18.4 The variations of flexible-ring annuloplasty. (**a**) Internal annuloplasty by fixing an ePTFE strip using U-shaped mattress sutures directly under the cusp insertion line (reproduced with permission from Mukaida M, Kawazoe K, Okabayashi H. Long-term results of aortic valve repair. Journal of JCS Cardiologists. 2012;20:65–70). (**b**) Combination of internal subvalvular annuloplasty and STJ annuloplasty band (reproduced with permission from reference 21). (**c**) A flexible internal ring to prevent atrioventricular block by positioning the convex upward part at the commissure between the right and non-coronary sinuses (reproduced with permission from reference 26). (**d**) External annuloplasty covering the entire root from the outside using glutaraldehyde-treated equine pericardium. (**e**) External annuloplasty in which the annulus is tightened from the outside with an adjustable loop-type nylon band. (**f**) Flexible external ring to prevent atrioventricular block by positioning the convex upward part at the commissure between the right and non-coronary sinuses. Sutures should be ligated at the commissure between the left and right coronary sinuses (reproduced with permission from reference 26). (**g**) External expansible subvalvular aortic ring (reproduced with permission from Lansac E, Di Centa I, Raoux F, Bulman-Fleming N, Ranga A, Abed A, et al. Expansible aortic ring for a physiological approach to conservative aortic valve surgery. J Thorac Cardiovasc Surg. 2009;138:718–24). *Animal study only

18.4 Advantages/Disadvantages

The advantages of external suture annuloplasty include its convenience, the requirement of less root dissection, and that it can also be evenly tightened. Therefore, it is easy to change the size, and it can also be removed easily when replacing the valve. Furthermore, the suture is tied around a Hegar dilator, resulting in a highly predictable postoperative annulus diameter. Conversely, there are two disadvantages. Especially in the right coronary sinus where the discrepancy between the basal ring and aorto-ventricular junction (AVJ) is particularly large (average 3.3–6.2 mm) [32, 33], it is uncertain whether the basal ring is exactly tightened or not. Moreover, in cases of isolated valvuloplasty for a bicuspid valve, it is difficult to adjust the angle of the cusp to 180°. To overcome this second disadvantage, Schneider et al. recently advocated partial plication of the annulus at the raphe in such a situation [34].

One advantage of internal annuloplasty, except for subcommissural annuloplasty, would be the certainty of reducing the basal ring size. The most attractive advantage is the complete elimination of root dissection, especially in cases of isolated valvuloplasty. Also, when a ring is used, it is easy to adjust the angle of the bicuspid valve. Conversely, the disadvantages of great concern are the adverse effects on the movement of leaflets, inflammation, erosion, and thrombosis because the sutures are threaded through the cusp insertion line. Especially in the rigid ring, the shape of the annulus differs subtly among individuals, so stress on the annulus will not be negligible. Also, in cases in which one continuous mattress suture is used, the resistance is large, and it is necessary to check whether the plications are even.

Because external ring annuloplasty stabilizes the basal ring, it might be the most reliable method. Even combined with the remodeling method, there is still the advantage that the distensibility of the root might be preserved. The disadvantage is that the root must be dissected up to the basal ring level, and in patients with a paper-thin right coronary sinus wall or those undergoing isolated valvuloplasty, the procedure becomes somewhat complicated and difficult. Care must be taken when dissection of the right ventricular myocardium is not adequate because the ring will be implanted in a tilted position, which might result in ineffective stabilization of the basal ring [35].

Regardless of whether internal or external, annuloplasty is known to increase the opening and closing velocity of the aortic valve [26, 36, 37]. Changes in hemodynamics caused by reduced compliance at the root and the decreased inner diameter are considered to be the underlying mechanism, but the clinical significance is still unknown. Morphologically, as mentioned above, one group reported that internal annuloplasty improves coaptation depth better than external annuloplasty does [26], whereas another group reported that they are equivalent [36]. However, at least in both cases, compared to subcommissural annuloplasty, there is no doubt that the valve orifice area is significantly reduced, the pressure gradient is significantly increased, and thus annular reduction is truly achieved. [36]

18.5 Actual Practice

In this section, three alternatives currently in wide clinical use in many institutions are described.

External Suture Annuloplasty

After dissection of the aortic root at least up to the AVJ, an ePTFE suture (Gore-Tex CV-0; WL Gore and Associates, Flagstaff, AZ, USA) is first applied to the septal myocardium outside the commissure between the left and right coronary sinuses at the level of the basal ring. Then, one to two stitches are made on the outside of the left coronary sinus, taking care to stay close to the annulus. The final stitch of the posterior arm is placed at the posterior half of the non-coronary sinus tangentially. Similarly, one to two stitches of the anterior arm are passed through the right ventricular myocardium outside of the right coronary sinus and one stitch at the counterpart of the non-coronary sinus. In the right coronary sinus and its adjacent commissure between the left coronary sinus, the suture should be passed deeply enough to reach the basal ring. Otherwise, it is sufficient to stitch shallowly so that the suture does not shift. Select a Hegar dilator one size smaller than the prosthesis used for the remodeling procedure and place it in the annulus and tie both arms of the suture at the center of the non-coronary sinus. In cases of isolated valvuloplasty, for example, the Hegar dilator size can be selected according to the normal annulus diameter per body surface area reported by Capps et al. [38] or according to the targeted annulus diameter to achieve a sufficient coaptation length of each cusp estimated by the actual measurement of geometric height.

External Expansible Subvalvular Aortic Ring

In this scenario, the root must be dissected up to the basal ring to place the aortic ring effectively. Next, six pledgeted 2/0 coated polyester sutures are passed inside out as U-stitches at the nadir of each cusp and at the base of each interleaflet triangle. However, a suture should be placed externally only at the commissure between the right and non-coronary sinuses to prevent atrioventricular block. The size of the ring is 1 mm less than that of the prosthesis, but conveniently, if there is no ring available, the prosthesis used for remodeling can be used by cutting it down into smaller pieces. Finally, these sutures are evenly passed through the ring and ligated. Sutures are not necessarily passed through the ring itself but are ligated looping the ring. If the commissure angle needs to be adjusted to 180° in the case of a bicuspid valve, sutures at two commissures should be passed in line with the bisection of the ring. A split ring is used, and both ends are finally joined in cases of isolated valvuloplasty.

Internal Rigid Hemispherical Ring

The greatest feature of this ring is that it is elliptical and mimics the physiological shape of the annulus. The sizes include 19, 21, 23, and 25 mm, and size is determined by the free margin length of the cusps, based on the smallest leaflet. The left ventricular side of the subcommissural annuloplasty is performed by passing pledgeted 4/0 polypropylene sutures through the ring. Next, two 4/0 polypropylene sutures placed between each commissure loop the ring and are passed through the cusp insertion line from the left ventricular side to the aortic side and ligated on the pledget. To avoid interference with the valve, the pledget should be small and thin, and the suture should be cut as short as possible.

18.6 My Tips

The major complications of external suture annuloplasty are obstruction or stenosis of the circumflex coronary artery, atrioventricular block, and ventricular septal perforation. Therefore, no suture is placed on the commissure between the right and non-coronary sinuses. In the case of isolated valvuloplasty, the aorta is transected immediately above the STJ, the aortic root is sufficiently dissected under both coronary arteries, and it is visually confirmed from the inside that the suture is passed through just outside the annulus. The commissure between the right and left coronary sinuses is sufficiently dissected off from the pulmonary artery trunk so as to place a suture at an adequate depth, and attention should be paid that the suture does not shift to the peripheral side. Also, a hemoclip is attached at the end of the knot to prevent slippage.

18.7 Results

The effects of annuloplasty alone are difficult to interpret because the procedure does not have a long history, the case volume is small, and the procedure types vary. Therefore, the clinical results of the major types of annuloplasty used at present are described according to the classification listed in Sect. 18.2.

External Suture Annuloplasty

Schneider and his colleagues added both external and internal suture annuloplasty to 95 and 69 patients, respectively, with a bicuspid valve who underwent isolated valvuloplasty, and the 5-year rate of freedom from reoperation improved to 92.6% compared with 73.2% in patients treated with no annuloplasty but with subcommissural annuloplasty in 60% of the cases [39]. They also concomitantly performed sinus plication to reduce the circumference of the fused sinus and to realign unfavorable commissural orientation in 32 patients, which improved the stability of the repair [34]. Internal annuloplasty with polyester sutures in their early series was frequently associated with postoperative morbidities: ventricular septal defect, atrioventricular block, and ischemia of the circumflex artery, and thus it has currently been abandoned.

Internal Suture Annuloplasty

Aicher and her colleagues performed subcommissural annuloplasty in 100 of 316 patients with a bicuspid valve, which proved to be a significant risk factor for reoperation by univariate analysis, and the results could not be improved even in cases of expanded annulus with an AVJ >28 mm alone [31].

de Kerchove and his colleagues also compared 53 patients with a bicuspid valve of whom 46 (87%) underwent subcommissural annuloplasty with 53 matched patients treated by the reimplantation method and disclosed that both freedom from reoperation (90 ± 8% vs. 100%) and aortic regurgitation greater than grade II (77 ± 14% vs. 100%) were significantly inferior in the former patient group [40]. In addition, subcommissural annuloplasty was frequently associated with an increased postoperative transvalvular gradient of 25 mmHg or more (30% vs. 13%), which is considered to have a negative effect on late valve stability [41].

In the following univariate analysis in patients with a bicuspid valve by this same Brussels group, subcommissural annuloplasty was identified as an independent predictor of reoperation and recurrence of aortic valve regurgitation of grade I or more [42]. Especially when the AVJ is 30 mm or more, freedom from the recurrence of aortic regurgitation of grade I or more after subcommissural annuloplasty is extremely poor, which suggests the limit of this method. A similar finding was obtained in cases with an AVJ of 28 mm or more by the Pennsylvania group [43]. In the subsequent verification by the Brussels group, similar results were also obtained with tricuspid valves, and the reimplantation method was recommended when the AVJ is 28 mm or more [44].

Schöllhorn and his colleagues applied internal suture annuloplasty in 22 cases and reported no reoperations although the degree of aortic regurgitation increased by one grade in 2 of 16 cases during a 1-year follow-up period [10].

Partial Band Annuloplasty

David reinforced the fibrous portion in 11 of 41 remodeling cases, but the results of the annuloplasty itself are not yet clear [11]. Hahm and his colleagues carried out similar sandwich reinforcement in 23 of 69 patients who underwent isolated valvuloplasty with or without ascending aortic replacement surgery [12]. This method was found to be undesirable as the one-year cumulative reoperation rate was 5.65%/year in the follow-up study of 397 cases over the subsequent 3 years [13].

Ring Annuloplasty

Rigid Rings

In a multicenter collaborative study, the HAART 300 internal rigid annuloplasty ring was implanted in 65 patients, and 7 patients (10.8%) underwent aortic valve replacement during a follow-up period of up to 3 years (mean 2 years) [45]. The cause of reoperation might have been related to surgical technique because most repair failures occurred in the early phase and results stabilized after 6 months. However, critics did note the possible alarming hazards of placing a rigid ring so close to the delicate aortic cusps [46].

Flexible Ring

Izumoto and his colleagues conducted subvalvular internal annuloplasty and leaflet suspension using an ePTFE strip in 19 cases and reported that the freedom from reoperation at 48 months was 88.9 ± 7.4% [47]. This same group combined this annuloplasty with remodeling in 60 patients, and the freedom from reoperation at 5 years was 82.5 ± 11.3% [48].

Fattouch et al. used an internal subvalvular annuloplasty and STJ annuloplasty band in 45 patients and found that no reoperations were necessary over an average follow-up period of 22 months [21].

A multicenter prospective registry (AVIATOR) from four institutions in France reported that an external ring annuloplasty combined with remodeling using a graft with sinuses in 177 patients provided freedom from reoperation of 89.5% at 7 years [24]. The rate was better for bicuspid valves (100%) than for tricuspid valves (88.8%), but the difference was not significant ($P = 0.15$). Annuloplasty and effective height assessment proved to be protective factors against reoperation, although the former was not a statistically significant factor ($P = 0.057$, 0.044, respectively). These two interventions might contribute their excellent outcomes to being performed together; thus, the solo effect of annuloplasty remains unclear [49]. This same registry showed even better freedom from reoperation at 7 years for isolated valvuloplasty with (100%) or without (97.5%) supracoronary aorta replacement [23]. Of interest, the authors insisted that double annuloplasty by adding an external ring at the STJ level improved the freedom from recurrence of aortic regurgitation of $\geq$ grade 2 or 3 ($P = 0.070$ and 0.099, respectively) compared with single subvalvular annuloplasty.

Importantly, an expansible external ring is thought to preserve root distensibility, which has emerged as a major advantage of remodeling over the reimplantation procedure. Annular distensibility after reimplantation with a graft with sinuses remains at only 4% and is similar to that of a tube graft. [50] In contrast, Wuliya and his colleagues reported that an expansible external aortic ring combined with remodeling maintained 4.8–9.1% annular expansibility during a median follow-up period of 19 months (maximum, 5 years) [51]. A similar finding was also reported by Basmadjian and his colleagues, i.e., that 10% systolic expansion was preserved up to 2 years after implantation of an expansible external ring [52].

18.8 Conclusion

As insights into aortic valvuloplasty have deepened, annuloplasty has emerged to play an important role, and various alternatives have been proposed as mentioned in this article. Despite their advantages and disadvantages, the clinical results reported to date are generally good. However, the case volume is still small, the observation period is short, and the procedure is only performed in limited facilities with highly experienced staff; therefore, it is still too early to judge its superiority or inferiority. Precise investigations are required to determine which method is reproducible and effective and can become the standard option.

References

1. Taylor WJ, Thrower WB, Black H, Harken DE. The surgical correction of aortic insufficiency by circumclusion. J Thorac Surg. 1958;35:192–205.
2. Schneider U, Aicher D, Miura Y, Schäfers HJ. Suture Annuloplasty in Aortic Valve Repair. Ann Thorac Surg. 2016;101:783–5.
3. Cabrol C, Cabrol A, Guiraudon G, Bertrand M. Treatment of aortic insufficiency by means of aortic annuloplasty. Arch Mal Coeur Vaiss. 1966;59:1305–12.
4. Duran CG. Reconstructive techniques for rheumatic aortic valve disease. J Card Surg. 1988;3:23–8.
5. Cosgrove DM, Rosenkranz ER, Hendren WG, Bartlett JC, Stewart WJ. Valvuloplasty for aortic insufficiency. J Thorac Cardiovasc Surg. 1991;102:571–6.
6. Kollar A. Valve-sparing reconstruction within the native aortic root: integrating the Yacoub and the David methods. Ann Thorac Surg. 2007;83:2241–3.
7. Mangini A, Lemma MG, Soncini M, Votta E, Contino M, Vismara R, et al. The aortic interleaflet triangles annuloplasty: a multidisciplinary appraisal. Eur J Cardiothorac Surg. 2011;40:851–7.
8. Carpentier A. Cardiac valve surgery—the "French correction". J Thorac Cardiovasc Surg. 1983;86:323–37.
9. Haydar HS, He GW, Hovaguimian H, McIrvin DM, King DH, Starr A. Valve repair for aortic insufficiency: surgical classification and techniques. Eur J Cardiothorac Surg. 1997;11:258–65.
10. Schöllhorn J, Rylski B, Beyersdorf F. Aortic valve annuloplasty: new single suture technique. Ann Thorac Surg. 2014;97:2211–3.
11. David TE. Aortic root aneurysms: remodeling or composite replacement? Ann Thorac Surg. 1997;64:1564–8.

12. Hahm SY, Choo SJ, Lee JW, Seo JB, Lim TH, Song JK. Novel technique of aortic valvuloplasty. Eur J Cardiothorac Surg. 2006;29:530–6.
13. Bae JM, Shin E, Heo DS. Safety of comprehensive aortic root and valve repair surgery: a retrospective outcomes research by national evidence-based health care collaborating agency, Korea. Korean Circ J. 2012;42:769–71.
14. Duran CM, Gallo R, Prabhakar G, Kumar N, Hainau B. New prosthetic ring for aortic valve annuloplasty. Cardiovasc Surg. 1993;1:166–71.
15. Schomburg JL, Lahti MT, Ruth GR, Bianco RW. Internal aortic annuloplasty: a novel technique. J Investig Surg. 2011;24:222–6.
16. Rankin JS, Conger JL, Tuzun E, Winkler JA, Harms KM, Beavan LA, et al. In vivo testing of an intra-annular aortic valve annuloplasty ring in a chronic calf model. Eur J Cardiothorac Surg. 2012;42:149–54.
17. Mazzitelli D, Pfeiffer S, Rankin JS, Fischlein T, Choi YH, Wahlers T, et al. A regulated trial of bicuspid aortic valve repair supported by geometric ring annuloplasty. Ann Thorac Surg. 2015;99:2010–6.
18. Reimold SC, Aranki SF, Caguioa ES, Solomon SD, Birjiniuk V, Cohn LH, et al. An external aortic root device for decreasing aortic regurgitation: in vitro and in vivo animal studies. J Card Surg. 1994;9:304–13.
19. Kawazoe K, Izumoto H, Satoh Y, Eishi K, Ishibashi K. Annuloaortic repair in the treatment of aortic regurgitation and aortic root pathology. Surg Today. 2001;31:27–31.
20. Izumoto H, Kawazoe K, Kawase T, Kim H. Subvalvular circular annuloplasty as a component of aortic valve repair. J Heart Valve Dis. 2002;11:383–5.
21. Fattouch K, Sampognaro R, Speziale G, Ruvolo G. New technique for aortic valve functional annulus reshaping using a handmade prosthetic ring. Ann Thorac Surg. 2011;91:1154–8.
22. Gogbashian A, Ghanta RK, Umakanthan R, Rangaraj AT, Laurence RG, Fox JA, et al. Correction of aortic insufficiency with an external adjustable prosthetic aortic ring. Ann Thorac Surg. 2007;84:1001–5.
23. Lansac E, Di Centa I, Sleilaty G, Lejeune S, Khelil N, Berrebi A, et al. Long-term results of external aortic ring annuloplasty for aortic valve repair. Eur J Cardiothorac Surg. 2016;50:350–60.
24. Lansac E, Di Centa I, Sleilaty G, Lejeune S, Berrebi A, Zacek P, et al. Remodeling root repair with an external aortic ring annuloplasty. J Thorac Cardiovasc Surg. 2017;153:1033–42.
25. Lansac E, Bouchot O, Arnaud Crozat E, Hacini R, Doguet F, Demaria R, et al. Standardized approach to valve repair using an expansible aortic ring versus mechanical Bentall: Early outcomes of the CAVIAAR multicentric prospective cohort study. J Thorac Cardiovasc Surg. 2015;149:S37–45.
26. Scharfschwerdt M, Pawlik M, Sievers HH, Charitos EI. In vitro investigation of aortic valve annuloplasty using prosthetic ring devices. Eur J Cardiothorac Surg. 2011;40:1127–30.
27. Richardt D, Bucsky B, Charitos EI, Sievers HH, Scharfschwerdt M. A novel rigid annuloplasty ring for aortic valve reconstruction: an in vitro investigation. Ann Thorac Surg. 2014;97:811–5.
28. Lansac E, Di Centa I, Bonnet N, Leprince P, Rama A, Acar C, et al. Aortic prosthetic ring annuloplasty: a useful adjunct to a standardized aortic valve-sparing procedure? Eur J Cardiothorac Surg. 2006;29:537–44.
29. Schäfers HJ, Raddatz A, Schmied W, Takahashi H, Miura Y, Kunihara T, et al. Reexamining remodeling. J Thorac Cardiovasc Surg. 2015;149:S30–6.
30. Kunihara T, Aicher D, Rodionycheva S, Groesdonk HV, Langer F, Sata F, et al. Preoperative aortic root geometry and postoperative cusp configuration primarily determine long-term outcome after valve-preserving aortic root repair. J Thorac Cardiovasc Surg. 2012;143:1389–95.
31. Aicher D, Kunihara T, Abou Issa O, Brittner B, Gräber S, Schäfers HJ. Valve configuration determines long-term results after repair of the bicuspid aortic valve. Circulation. 2011;123:178–85.
32. Khelil N, Sleilaty G, Palladino M, Fouda M, Escande R, Debauchez M, et al. Surgical anatomy of the aortic annulus: landmarks for external annuloplasty in aortic valve repair. Ann Thorac Surg. 2015;99:1220–6.
33. de Kerchove L, Jashari R, Boodhwani M, Duy KT, Lengelé B, Gianello P, et al. Surgical anatomy of the aortic root: implication for valve-sparing reimplantation and aortic valve annuloplasty. J Thorac Cardiovasc Surg. 2015;149:425–33.
34. Schneider U, Schmied W, Aicher D, Giebels C, Winter L, Schäfers HJ. Sinus plication to improve valve configuration in bicuspid aortic valve repair-early results. Ann Thorac Surg. 2017;103:580–5.
35. Holubec T, Higashigaito K, Belobradek Z, Dergel M, Harrer J, Alkadhi H, et al. An expansible aortic ring in aortic root Remodeling: exact position, pulsatility, effectiveness, and stability in three-dimensional CT study. Ann Thorac Surg. 2017;103:83–90.
36. de Kerchove L, Vismara R, Mangini A, Fiore GB, Price J, Noirhomme P, et al. In vitro comparison of three techniques for ventriculo-aortic junction annuloplasty. Eur J Cardiothorac Surg. 2012;41:1117–23.
37. Leyh RG, Schmidtke C, Sievers HH, Yacoub MH. Opening and closing characteristics of the aortic valve after different types of valve-preserving surgery. Circulation. 1999;100:2153–60.
38. Capps SB, Elkins RC, Fronk DM. Body surface area as a predictor of aortic and pulmonary valve diameter. J Thorac Cardiovasc Surg. 2000;119:975–82.
39. Schneider U, Hofmann C, Aicher D, Takahashi H, Miura Y, Schäfers HJ. Suture annuloplasty significantly improves the durability of bicuspid aortic valve repair. Ann Thorac Surg. 2017;103:504–10.
40. de Kerchove L, Boodhwani M, Glineur D, Vandyck M, Vanoverschelde JL, Noirhomme P, et al. Valve sparing-root replacement with the reimplantation technique to increase the durability of bicus-

pid aortic valve repair. J Thorac Cardiovasc Surg. 2011;142:1430–8.
41. Vohra HA, Whistance RN, de Kerchove L, Glineur D, Noirhomme P, El Khoury G. Influence of higher valve gradient on long-term outcome after aortic valve repair. Ann Cardiothorac Surg. 2013;2:30–9.
42. Navarra E, El Khoury G, Glineur D, Boodhwani M, Van Dyck M, Vanoverschelde JL, et al. Effect of annulus dimension and annuloplasty on bicuspid aortic valve repair. Eur J Cardiothorac Surg. 2013;44:316–22.
43. Vallabhajosyula P, Komlo CM, Szeto WY, Rhode T, Menon R, Desai ND, et al. Aortic annulus diameter affects durability of the repaired bicuspid aortic valve. J Heart Valve Dis. 2015;24:412–9.
44. de Kerchove L, Mastrobuoni S, Boodhwani M, Astarci P, Rubay J, Poncelet A, et al. The role of annular dimension and annuloplasty in tricuspid aortic valve repair. Eur J Cardiothorac Surg. 2016;49:428–37.
45. Mazzitelli D, Fischlein T, Rankin JS, Choi YH, Stamm C, Pfeiffer S, et al. Geometric ring annuloplasty as an adjunct to aortic valve repair: clinical investigation of the HAART 300 device. Eur J Cardiothorac Surg. 2016;49:987–93.
46. Cameron D. Why can't the aortic valve be more like the mitral? Eur J Cardiothorac Surg. 2016;49:994.
47. Izumoto H, Kawazoe K, Oka T, Ishibashi K, Yamamoto H, Yamamoto F. Leaflet suspension and subvalvular annuloplasty in aortic valve prolapse. Asian Cardiovasc Thorac Ann. 2009;17:278–81.
48. Kazui T, Tsuboi J, Izumoto H, Nakajima T, Ishihara K, Kawazoe K. Aortic root remodeling with aortic annuloplasty: mid-term results. Circ J. 2007;71:207–10.
49. Schäfers HJ. Aortic annuloplasty: the panacea of valve-preserving aortic replacement? J Thorac Cardiovasc Surg. 2017;153:1043–4.
50. Matsumori M, Tanaka H, Kawanishi Y, Onishi T, Nakagiri K, Yamashita T, et al. Comparison of distensibility of the aortic root and cusp motion after aortic root replacement with two reimplantation techniques: Valsalva graft versus tube graft. Interact Cardiovasc Thorac Surg. 2007;6:177–81.
51. Wuliya M, Sleilaty G, Di Centa I, Khelil N, Berrebi A, Czitrom D, et al. An expansible aortic ring to preserve aortic root dynamics after aortic valve repair. Eur J Cardiothorac Surg. 2015;47:482–90.
52. Basmadjian L, Basmadjian AJ, Stevens LM, Mongeon FP, Cartier R, Poirier N, et al. Early results of extra-aortic annuloplasty ring implantation on aortic annular dimensions. J Thorac Cardiovasc Surg. 2016;151:1280–5.

19 ONE-POINT ADVICE: Other Valve-Sparing Aortic Root Replacement Techniques

Masaru Sawazaki

19.1 Introduction

The standard techniques for valve-sparing aortic root replacement (VSARR) are the aortic root remodeling method (hereinafter referred to as remodeling) proposed by Yacoub et al. [1] and the aortic valve reimplantation method (hereinafter referred to as reimplantation) advocated by David et al. [2]. These techniques are usually employed because they are safe and the long-term outcomes are favorable. However, both techniques also have disadvantages, such as the long duration of cardiac arrest due to their complexity; for example, they are problematic when performing simultaneous mitral valve replacement (MVR) and aortic arch replacement surgery in patients with Marfan syndrome.

In 2005, Hess et al. from the University of Florida described an easy VSARR technique (the Florida sleeve) [3]. This technique entails covering the aortic root externally with a cylindrical vascular graft without resecting the enlarged sinus of Valsalva and then reducing the size of the sinotubular junction (STJ), sinus of Valsalva, and aortic annulus. This technique reduces the size of the aortic root and results in the reduction or elimination of concomitant aortic regurgitation (AR). However, it cannot be indicated in patients with leaflet prolapse causing type II AR, as described by Boodhwani et al. [4]. It is, however, indicated in patients with type I AR who have normal aortic valve leaflets and AR caused purely by aortic root dilatation.

19.2 Surgical Methods

The aorta is transected slightly superior to the STJ. Extensive external dissection from the area surrounding the left and right coronary arteries to the annulus is performed. At a position 2 to 3 mm below the annulus, four horizontal mattress sutures with pledgets are inserted below each commissure and the nadir of the non-coronary sinus.

A slit is made in the vascular graft sleeve to accommodate the right coronary artery, and the position of a slit to cover the left coronary artery is determined by covering the aortic root with the graft temporarily. The anchor sutures created in the preceding step are passed through the sleeve, and a Hegar dilator is inserted and ligated to avoid over-reduction of the annulus diameter (Fig. 19.1). The lower part of the openings that allow the coronary arteries to pass through the vascular graft are sutured. Care is taken to ensure that the three suture locations beneath the commissures are in the correct position, and running horizontal mattress sutures are used at the level of the sleeve and STJ. These are then sutured to the vascular graft used for the ascending aortic replacement (Fig. 19.2).

M. Sawazaki (✉)
Department of Thoracic Surgery and Valvular Disease Center, Komaki City Hospital, Komaki, Aichi, Japan
e-mail: sawamasa7007bb@nifty.com

T. Kunihara, S. Takanashi (eds.), *Aortic Valve Preservation*,
https://doi.org/10.1007/978-981-13-2068-2_19

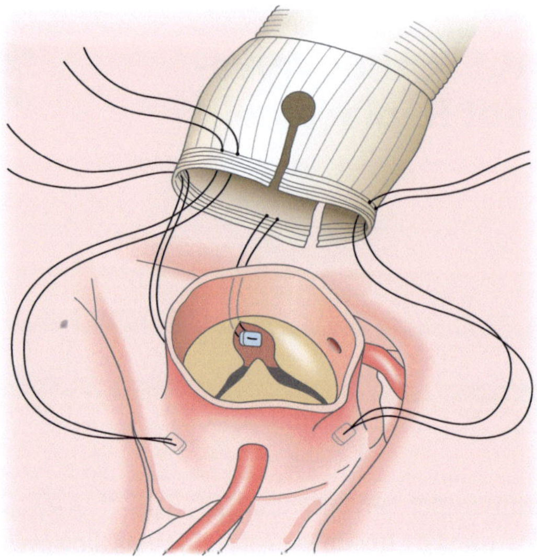

Fig. 19.1 Subannular sutures are inserted at three locations below each commissure and 2–3 mm below the nadir of the noncoronary cusp in the same horizontal plane, and horizontal mattress sutures are passed externally from the aortic root. A slit is made in the sleeve to accommodate the right coronary artery, and the sutures are passed through the lower end of the sleeve. Another slit is inserted to accommodate the left coronary artery to allow space for the two coronary arteries

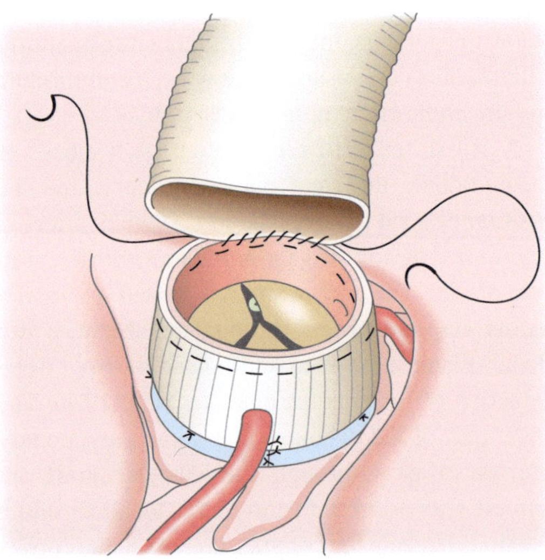

Fig. 19.2 Care is taken to ensure that the three suture locations beneath the commissures are in the correct position

19.3 Outcomes

Aalaei-Andabili et al. reported 3-year outcomes in 37 patients with Marfan syndrome [5]. The left ventricular end-diastolic diameter (LVEDD) decreased from 52.23 ± 5.29 mm preoperatively to 47.53 ± 8.89 mm at 1 week postoperatively ($n = 25$, $p = 0.086$). However, the left ventricular end systolic diameter (LVESD) did not improve from 35.53 ± 9.97 mm preoperatively to 36.58 ± 9.82 mm postoperatively ($p = 0.58$). The AR grade dropped from 1.76 ± 1.2 preoperatively to 0.48 ± 0.71 postoperatively ($p < 0.001$). The AR grade still improved to 0.85 ± 0.94 after 30 days ($n = 14$, $p = 0.002$). Nine patients had a postoperative follow-up echo at 5 years, and all were free from AR greater than grade 2 (mild).

19.4 Discussion

Seventeen years ago, the authors encountered a 40-year-old woman with Marfan syndrome who suffered from active infective endocarditis. Her aortic root dilatation measured 45 mm, and she suffered from mild AR. In addition to performing a mitral valve repair, a technique similar to the Florida sleeve procedure was performed. Using a method of so-called corset repair described by Kawazoe et al. [6], xenogeneic pericardium was used to reinforce the aortic root externally. During the 17 years postoperatively, the sinus of Valsalva did not enlarge to a size greater than 40 mm, and there was no further aortic dissection or AR. This same long-term outcome would be expected for patients treated with a Florida sleeve procedure. However, stenosis of the origin of both coronary arteries occurred 1 month postoperatively, and additional coronary artery bypass surgery was performed. Coronary artery stenosis may also occur after the Florida sleeve procedure, but it has not been observed in any of the 37 Marfan cases reported by Aalaei-Andabili et al. [5]. No patient experienced dissection or rupture throughout follow-up. During the follow-up period, only 1 patient (2.56%) required reoperation at the 112th month, secondary to ascending aortic pseudoaneurysm. This represented 100% freedom from reoperation at 8 years. The wall of the sinus of Valsalva may inadvertently become creased in the vascular graft sleeve when aortic root dilatation is severe, and a certain degree of residual AR may persist when the preoperative AR is severe; therefore, we believe this technique is better indicated for central AR in which the degree of root dilatation is mild or moderate.

References

1. Yacoub MH, Fagan A, Stassano P, Radley-Smith R. Results of valve conserving operations for aortic regurgitation. Circulation. 1983;68:311–21.
2. David TE, Armstrong S, Ivanov J, Feindel CM, Omuran A, Webb G. Results of aortic valve-sparing operations. J Thorac Cardiovasc Surg. 2001;122:39–46.
3. Hess PJ, Klodel CT, Beaver TM, Martin TD. The Florida sleeve: a new technique for aortic root remodeling with preservation of the aortic valve and sinuses. Ann Thorac Surg. 2005;80:748–50.
4. Boodhwani M, Kerchove L, Glineur D, Poncelet A, Ruby J, Astarci P, et al. Repair-oriented classification of aortic insufficiency: impact on surgical techniques and clinical outcomes. J Thorac Cardiovasc Surg. 2009;137:286–94.
5. Aalaei-Andabili SH, Martin T, Hess P, Klodell C, Karimi A, Arnaoutakis G, et al. Florida sleeve procedure is durable and improves aortic valve function in marfan syndrome patients. Ann Thorac Surg. 2017;104:834–9.
6. Kawazoe K, Izumoto H, Satoh Y, Eishi K, Ishibashi K. Annuloaortic repair in the treatment of aortic regurgitation and aortic root pathology. Surg Today. 2001;31:27–31.

ONE-POINT ADVICE: The Advantages and Disadvantages of Valsalva Grafts

20

Atsushi Shimizu

20.1 Introduction

The bulging shape characteristic of the sinuses of Valsalva plays an important role in opening and closing the aortic valve [1] and maintaining coronary perfusion. For this reason, various measures are attempted during valve-sparing aortic root reconstructions (VSARR) to recreate the sinuses of Valsalva. One of these measures involves the use of a Valsalva graft to perform VSARR during the reimplantation [2] or remodeling [3] procedure, and favorable outcomes have been reported.

We started to perform the reimplantation procedure using a Valsalva graft from 2006 onward and then began to perform a modified remodeling procedure from 2012 onwards. The modified remodeling procedure involves the use of a Valsalva graft during the remodeling procedure and securing a ring created from part of a vascular graft to the aortic annulus externally (Fig. 20.1).

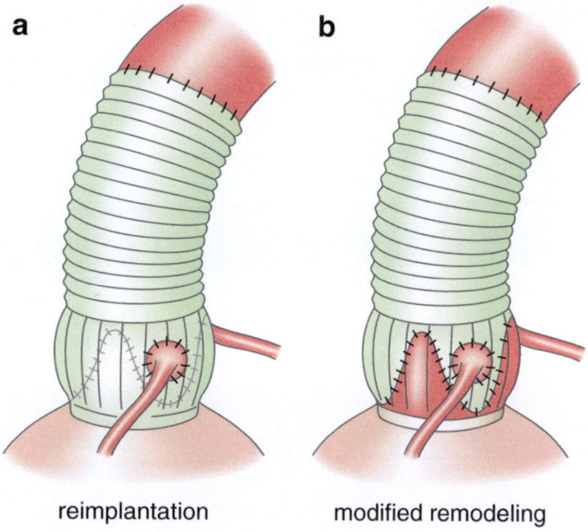

Fig. 20.1 (**a**) Reimplantation procedure using a Valsalva graft. (**b**) When performing the remodeling procedure using a Valsalva graft, a part of the vascular graft is used to create a ring, which in turn is used to secure the aortic annulus externally during a procedure known as modified remodeling

The Valsalva graft is designed to configure the height of the sinus of Valsalva portion to be equal to the diameter of the graft. In addition, the diameter of the sinus of Valsalva portion is equivalent to the vascular graft diameter plus an additional 8 mm (Fig. 20.2). Various reports have discussed how graft size should be determined, but we regard the following measurements as important: the annular diameter, which is also known as the aortoventricular junction (AVJ), the height of the leaflets (geometric height) [4], and the distance from the top of the noncoronary/left coronary commissure to a connecting line between the nadirs of the two adjacent cusps (Brussels height) [5]. The mean graft size at our hospital is 26.7 ± 1.6 mm, and 26 mm was the most frequently used size in a total of 58 patients.

A. Shimizu (✉)
Department of Cardiovascular Surgery, Sakakibara Heart Institute, Tokyo, Japan
e-mail: ashimizu@shi.heart.or.jp

T. Kunihara, S. Takanashi (eds.), *Aortic Valve Preservation*,
https://doi.org/10.1007/978-981-13-2068-2_20

We compared the aortic root morphology using 4D computed tomography after performing VSARR on 16 patients using the reimplantation procedure with a 26-mm Valsalva graft (reimplantation group) and on 11 patients using the modified remodeling method (remodeling group) (Fig. 20.3). The AVJ diameter was significantly smaller in the remodeling group (27.4 vs. 25.1 mm, $p < 0.01$).

The diameter of the sinus of Valsalva was significantly greater in the remodeling group (31.3 vs. 34.1 mm, $p < 0.01$), and there were no significant differences between the two groups in terms of the sinotubular junction (STJ) diameter (28.4 vs. 28.6 mm, $p = 0.066$).

Cautions and solutions in VSARR procedures with Valsalva grafts:

1. During VSARR by the reimplantation procedure using a Valsalva graft, if the first row of sutures is set at the sinus of Valsalva portion of the Valsalva graft, then depending on the circumstances, the AVJ diameter can sometimes be larger than the vascular graft diameter, and it may be possible to perform inadequate annular reduction (Fig. 20.4).

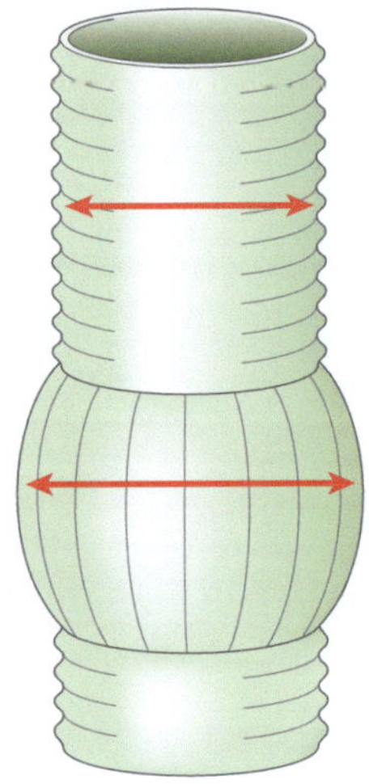

Fig. 20.2 The Valsalva graft is designed to configure the height of the sinus of Valsalva portion to be equal to the diameter of the graft, whereas the diameter of the sinus of Valsalva portion is equivalent to the vascular graft diameter plus an additional 8 mm

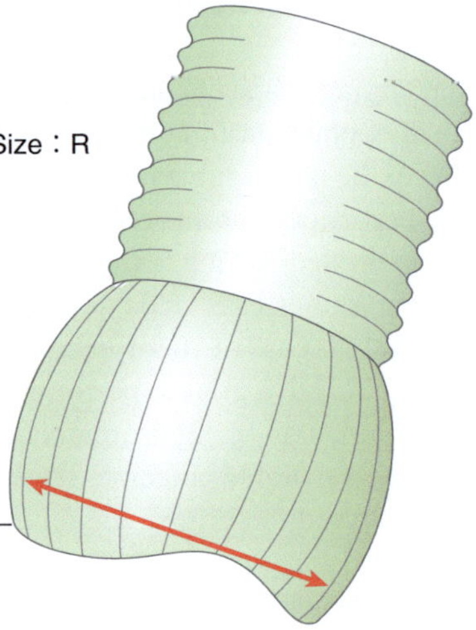

Fig. 20.4 During VSARR by the reimplantation procedure using a Valsalva graft, if the first-row sutures are set at the sinus of Valsalva portion of the graft, then depending on the circumstances, the AVJ diameter can sometimes be larger than the vascular graft diameter, which can lead to the possible performance of inadequate annular reduction

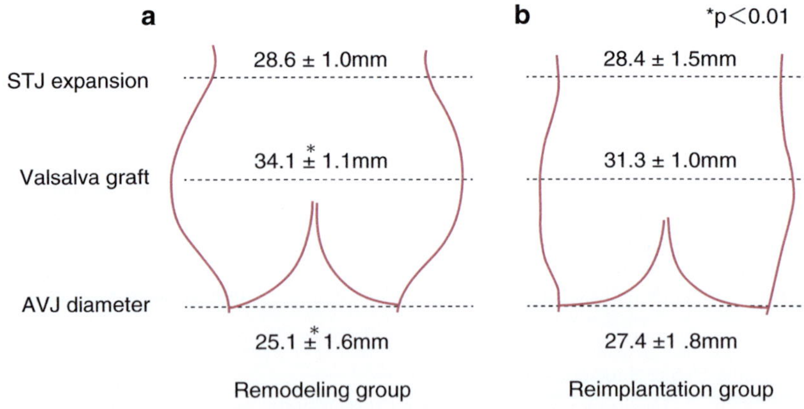

Fig. 20.3 (**a**) Remodeling group. (**b**) Reimplantation group. Compared to the reimplantation group, the AVJ diameter was significantly smaller in the remodeling group, and the sinus of Valsalva diameter was significantly greater

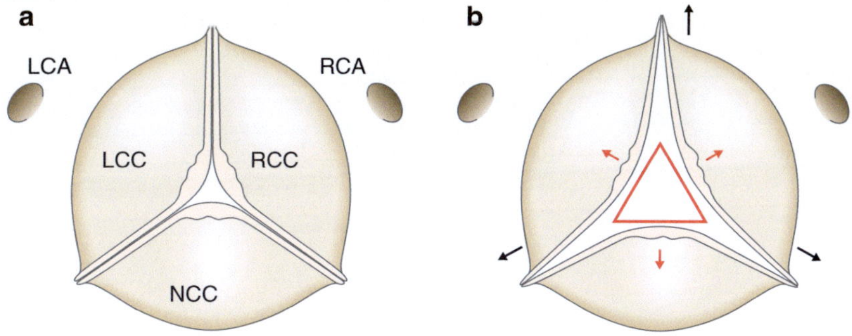

Fig. 20.5 (**a**) The STJ is not enlarged. (**b**) The STJ is enlarged. If the commissure is inadvertently included in the sinus of Valsalva portion and the STJ expands (black arrows), during diastole, tension will be applied to the free margins of the leaflets, which separate at the center (red arrows) and cause a gap to arise in the center of the leaflets

2. Each VSARR procedure can recreate the bulge of the sinus of Valsalva, although the remodeling procedure appears to be more advantageous in achieving it.
3. If the commissure is located within the sinus of Valsalva portion, then the STJ enlarges, and there is a risk of residual regurgitation from the center of the valve leaflets (Fig. 20.5).

The following measures have been devised to resolve these issues:

1. The remodeling procedure should be performed using a straight graft (when suturing, the suture pitch on the side of the graft is widened, which allows recreation of the bulge.
2. Short-type grafts can be used that are designed to set the height of the sinus of Valsalva portion to be lower than the graft diameter.
3. New types of grafts (e.g., the J Graft Shield Neo Valsalva produced by Japan Lifeline) have flat parts at the three commissure lines [6]. These allow us to prevent expansion of the interleaflet triangle during the reimplantation procedure or reduce bleeding in the remodeling procedure because of good coaptation of the suture line.

20.2 Conclusion

Valsalva grafts are favorably regarded because they exhibit high reproducibility and facilitate more physiological VSARR surgery. A novel elastic vascular prosthesis currently under development also appears promising to facilitate such surgery [7]. However, the potential risk of the late recurrence of regurgitation remains unless the graft structure is correctly understood and an appropriate graft size and design that match the patient are selected.

References

1. Pisani G, Scaffa R, Ieropoli O, Dell'Amico EM, Maselli D, Morbiducci U, et al. Role of the sinuses of valsalva on the opening of the aortic valve. J Thorac Cardiovasc Surg. 2013;145:999–1003.
2. De Paulis R, Scaffa R, Nardella S, Maselli D, Weltert L, Bertoldo F, et al. Use of the valsalva graft and long-term follow-up. J Thorac Cardiovasc Surg. 2010;140:S23–2.
3. Lansac E, Di Centa I, Sleilaty G, Crozat EA, Bouchot O, Hacini R, et al. An aortic ring: from physiologic reconstruction of the root to a standardized approach for aortic valve repair. J Thorac Cardiovasc Surg. 2010;140:S28–35.
4. Schäfers HJ, Schmied W, Marom G, Aicher D. Cusp height in aortic valves. J Thorac Cardiovasc Surg. 2013;146:269–74.
5. de Kerchove L, Boodhwani M, Glineur D, Noirhomme P, El Khoury G. A new simple and objective method for graft sizing in valve-sparing root replacement using the reimplantation technique. Ann Thorac Surg. 2011;92:749–51.
6. Richardt D, Karluss A, Schmidtke C, Sievers HH, Scharfschwerdt M. A new sinus prosthesis for aortic valve-sparing surgery maintaining the shape of the root at systemic pressure. Ann Thorac Surg. 2010;89:943–6.
7. Scharfschwerdt M, Leonhard M, Lehmann J, Richardt D, Goldmann H, Sievers HH. In vitro investigation of a novel elastic vascular prosthesis for valve-sparing aortic root and ascending aorta replacement. Eur J Cardiothorac Surg. 2016;49:1370–3.

21 Valve Surgery to Treat Connective Tissue Disease: Comparison Between Valve Replacement and Aortic Root Replacement

Tetsuro Morota and Minoru Ono

21.1 Introduction

Approximately a quarter of a century has passed since the David procedure for valve-sparing aortic root replacement (VSARR) (reimplantation method) was first published. We discuss some comparisons between this procedure and the Yacoub procedure (remodeling), another form of VSARR.

We also discuss whether it is possible to perform VSARR to treat annuloaortic ectasia (AAE) even when it is associated with connective tissue disease (CTD), and if it is possible, what long-term outcomes and, specifically, what kind of valve leaflet durability can be expected. To accomplish this, we have included outcomes from the literature and the authors' hospitals. In this chapter, CTD mainly refers to Marfan syndrome.

21.2 Changes in Surgical Technique

VSARR was first recognized in the 1990s to be an excellent technique for surgically treating AAE, and now there are two opposing procedures, namely remodeling, which reproduces the sinus of Valsalva morphology, results in less valve leaflet stress, and is advantageous for long-term outcomes, and reimplantation, which can prevent dilatation of the annulus. For this reason, there were also periods of time when reimplantation was selected for AAE associated with CTD and remodeling was selected for other conditions [1, 2].

Thereafter, the David-V procedure was published. This procedure involves performing the reimplantation procedure but also includes re-creation of the morphology of the sinuses of Valsalva, and a previous chapter has already described the course that elapsed from the time that the Valsalva graft designed for this purpose [3] first entered the market until it entered current mainstream use.

21.3 Indications and Contraindications for VSARR in Marfan Syndrome

If we consider the Bentall procedure to be the standard form of aortic root replacement, then the indications for selecting VSARR instead of the Bentall procedure vary depending on the hospital and the surgeon. The authors themselves have not made any modifications to the indications and contraindications for VSARR, even for Marfan syndrome. Even though there is marked valve

T. Morota (✉)
Department of Cardiovascular Surgery, Nippon Medical School, Tokyo, Japan
e-mail: morotat@nms.ac.jp

M. Ono
Department of Surgery, The University of Tokyo School of Medicine, Tokyo, Japan

T. Kunihara, S. Takanashi (eds.), *Aortic Valve Preservation*, https://doi.org/10.1007/978-981-13-2068-2_21

leaflet elongation in Marfan syndrome, this is unlikely to be a major obstacle due to the current advanced measures available for valve leaflet repair. Normally, the valve stiffness observed in patients with bicuspid valves is not seen in Marfan syndrome, and we believe that VSARR is indicated in all patients with advanced enlargement of the surgical annulus diameter (>30 mm).

21.4 Whether the Bentall Procedure or VSARR Should Be Indicated in Marfan Syndrome

The fundamental principle of a successful VSARR is that the "valves have normal morphology". Naturally, there are doubts regarding whether good short- and long-term outcomes can be obtained in patients with Marfan syndrome, who suffer from enlargement, elongation, and thinning of the valves, and are frequently noted to have fenestrations. "Although implicitly accepted by many that the durability of valve-sparing aortic root replacement in patients with bicuspid aortic valve disease and connective tissue disorders will be inferior", this excerpt taken from a paper from Stanford [4] shows that there are still many doubts in this regard (Fig. 21.1). There is no comparison to the Bentall procedure in this paper, which reported on long-term outcomes after the David procedure was performed on 233 patients (of whom 40% suffered from Marfan syndrome) over a mean observation period of 4.7 years. Respective 5- and 10-year survival rates were 98.7% and 93.5%, and at 10 years, freedom from reoperation on the aortic root was 92.2%, freedom from aortic insufficiency was 96.1%, and freedom from aortic regurgitation graded as moderate or greater was 95.3%. There were no statistically significant differences in terms of freedom from reoperation on the aortic root based on whether the underlying disease was CTD.

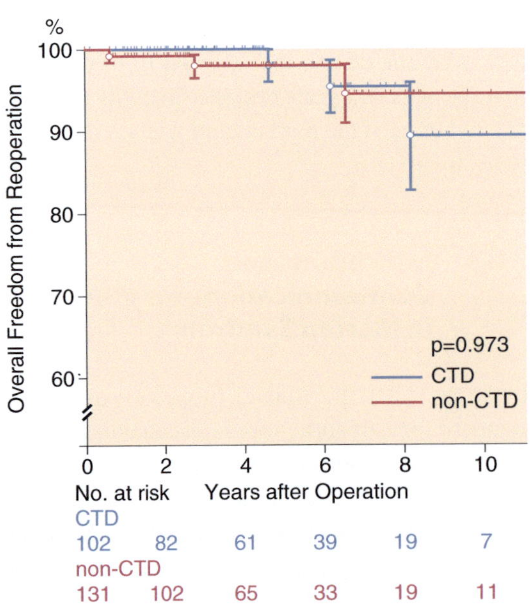

Fig. 21.1 Comparison of freedom from reoperation after VSARR for CTD and non-CTD patients (cited from Ref. [4] in modified form)

A report [5] on the outcomes of aortic root replacement in patients with Marfan syndrome from Hamburg, with a somewhat short mean observation period, stated that among 58 patients who underwent the David procedure, there were two mortalities, from cardiac failure and arrhythmia, during the observation period. This study reported that freedom from aortic regurgitation graded as moderate or greater was 80% at 10 years, and only two patients (3.4%) underwent repeat surgery of the aortic root, which was within the permissible range. A comparison was made to 30 patients who underwent the Bentall procedure, which showed that one benefit of the David procedure is a significantly lower rate of onset of endocarditis (Table 21.1), and although

Table 21.1 Comparison of complications in patients with Marfan syndrome who underwent the David procedure (AVS) or Bentall procedure (CVG)

	AVS ($n = 58$)	CVG ($n = 30$)	p value
Repeat sternotomy due to postoperative hemorrhage	2 (3.4%)	3 (10.0%)	0.333
Valve reoperation	2 (3.4%)	3 (10.0%)	0.333
Endocarditis	0	3 (10.0%)	0.037
Stroke	0	2 (6.7%)	0.114
Atrioventricular block	1 (1.7%)	3 (10.0%)	0.113
30-day mortality rate	0	0	
Mortality (>30 days)	2 (3.4%)	3 (10.0%)	0.333

Cited from Ref. [5]

no significant differences were observed in terms of freedom from cardiovascular events (death, endocarditis, stroke, repeat surgery to the aortic root) in patients with true aneurysms, the David procedure is superior (Fig. 21.2).

Kunihara et al. from Homburg compared 33 patients with Marfan syndrome who underwent VSARR (David procedure: 12, Yacoub procedure: 21) to 33 non-Marfan syndrome patients using propensity score matching [6]. The results showed that at 7 years, freedom from aortic regurgitation graded as moderate or greater was

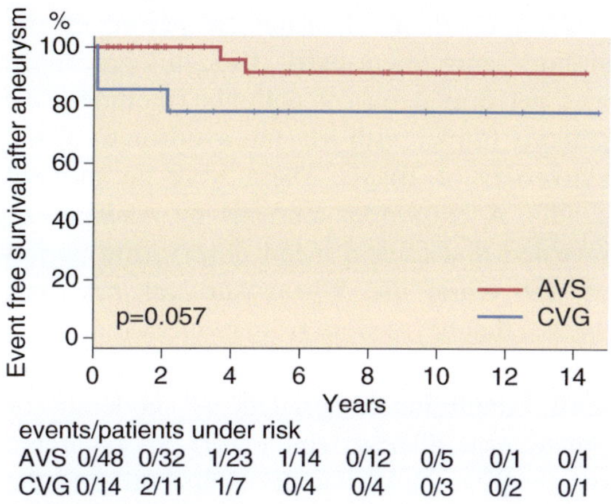

Fig. 21.2 Comparison of freedom from events in patients with Marfan syndrome who underwent the David procedure (AVS) or the Bentall procedure (CVG) (cited from Ref. [5] in modified form)

at 86% in the Marfan syndrome group versus 90% in the non-Marfan syndrome group, whereas freedom from reoperation on the aortic root was at 90 versus 100% in these respective groups, showing that no significant differences were observed (Fig. 21.3). There were also no differences based on whether the David or Yacoub procedure was performed. To summarize, the same long-term outcomes were achieved after VSARR in patients with and without Marfan syndrome.

Next, we refer to two excellent systematic reviews that performed a direct comparison between the Bentall procedure and VSARR to treat Marfan syndrome. Benedetto et al. [7] published a study documenting their analysis of 11 highly reliable articles from databases such as PubMed.

The long-term outcomes of 1385 patients with Marfan syndrome (Bentall procedure: 972 patients, VSARR: 413 patients) were investigated. The rate of reoperation on the aortic root was 0.3%/year after the Bentall procedure versus 1.3%/year after VSARR, with a lower rate observed after the Bentall procedure. The incidence of thromboembolism was 0.7%/year after the Bentall procedure versus 0.3%/year after VSARR, which was higher after the Bentall procedure. In addition, the rate of reoperation on the aortic root after VSARR was 0.7%/year after the David procedure versus 2.4%/year after the Yacoub procedure, indicating a significantly lower

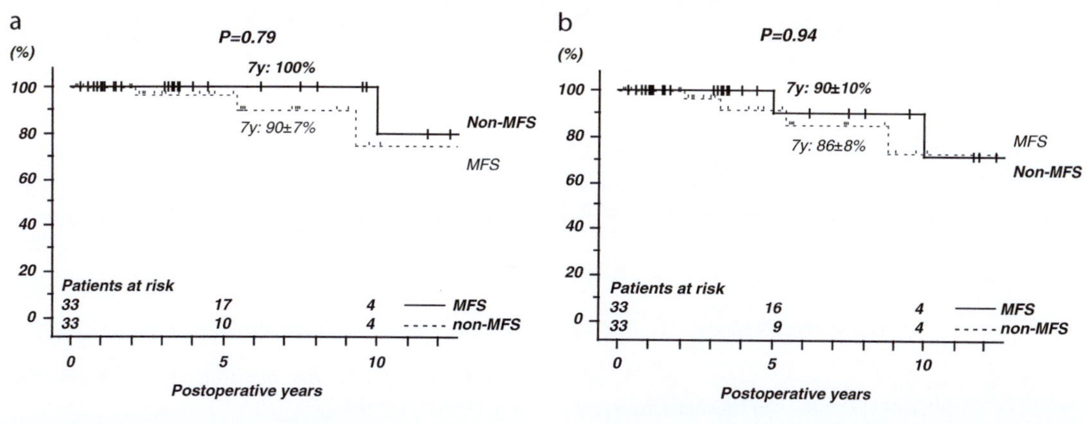

Fig. 21.3 Comparison of long-term outcomes after VSARR in Marfan syndrome (MFS) and non-Marfan syndrome patients. (**a**) Freedom from reoperation on the aortic root, (**b**) Freedom from aortic regurgitation graded as moderate or greater (From the presentation at the 6th Biennial Joint Meeting of the Society for Heart Valve Disease and Heart Valve Society of America held in Barcelona in 2011)

rate of reoperation after the David procedure. Six articles published by Hu et al. [8] were selected (including Ref. [5], which is from the same source as Ref. [6]). Subjects were 539 patients with Marfan syndrome; the risk ratio for complications (re-exploration for hemorrhage, early mortality, thromboembolism, endocarditis, repeat surgery on the aortic root, late mortality) of VSARR in comparison to the Bentall procedure was calculated using a 95% confidence interval. The incidence of regurgitation graded as moderate or greater was also investigated. The results verified the superiority of VSARR in terms of re-exploration for hemorrhage, thromboembolism, endocarditis, and late mortality. The incidence of regurgitation graded as moderate or greater occurred in 2–5% of patients who underwent the David procedure, in approximately 20% of those who underwent the Yacoub procedure, and in 0–8% of those in whom a Valsalva graft was used, and among the VSARR patients, those who underwent the Yacoub procedure had a higher incidence of regurgitation, which was the same as that noted in Ref. [6].

21.5 Authors' Experience and Outcomes

After conquering the learning curve associated with transitioning to the technique, the independently devised David-V University of Tokyo modification [9] has been consistently applied during all VSARR procedures from 2004 onwards. Characteristics of this method include the use of a straight vascular graft with a diameter of 32–34 mm, the placement of three pleats at the foot of the commissural posts that match the diameter of the left ventricular outflow tract, and the creation of longitudinal suture lines along three sections from the sinotubular junction to the tubular part. The advantages of the Valsalva graft are that the height of each valve leaflet commissure can be determined voluntarily, and the so-called second row of sutures can be made easily without causing overhang. During the period of the authors' enrollment until 2013, this procedure was performed on 59 patients (including 47 patients [80%] with Marfan syndrome) at the University of Tokyo. There were no surgical deaths. A classroom analysis by Ando et al. revealed that after a mean observation period of 4.9 years, the 5-year survival rate was 94.0%, that of freedom from reoperation on the aortic root was 95.7% and that of freedom from aortic regurgitation graded as moderate or greater was 88.9%, which were all favorable results (Fig. 21.4). Factors contributing to the incidence of adverse events were preoperative regurgitation graded as moderate or greater and the Z score for the surgical annulus diameter.

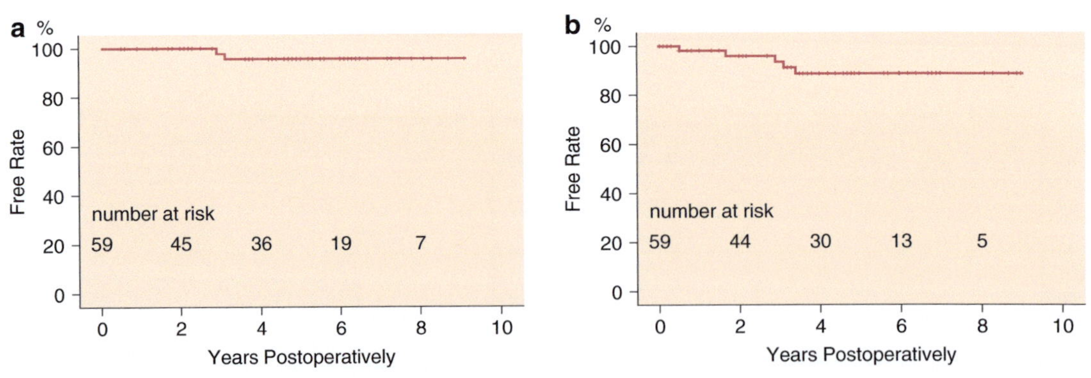

Fig. 21.4 Long-term outcomes after the David-V University of Tokyo modification. (**a**) Freedom from reoperation on the aortic root, (**b**) freedom from aortic regurgitation graded as moderate or greater (cited in modified form from Ref. [10])

21.6 Conclusion

VSARR should be proactively considered for young patients in particular as it offers the benefit of freedom from long-term events related to anticoagulation therapy and prosthetic valve infection, and it facilitates safer pregnancy and delivery in women. However, VSARR has not been established as a surgical technique with reliable reproducibility, and it must be borne in mind that this procedure involves advanced skills and includes valve leaflet repair, which requires experience.

On the basis of the above, cardiovascular surgeons should not hesitate to perform VSARR and particularly the David procedure, even in patients with CTD, as it is a surgical technique that is well indicated. The authors have been performing VSARR proactively since it was first introduced to Japan in 1993.

References

1. Miller DC. Valve-sparing aortic root replacement in patients with the Marfan syndrome. (Review). J Thorac Cardiovasc Surg. 2003;125:773–8.
2. Cameron DE, Alejo DE, Patel ND, Nwakanma LU, Weiss ES, Vricella LA, et al. Aortic root replacement in 372 Marfan patients: evolution of operative repair over 30 years. Ann Thorac Surg. 2009;87:1344–9.
3. Settepani F, Szeto WY, Pacini D, De Paulis R, Chiariello L, Di Bartolomeo R, et al. Reimplantation valve-sparing aortic root replacement in Marfan syndrome using the Valsalva conduit: an intercontinental multicenter study. Ann Thorac Surg. 2007;83:S769–73.
4. Kvitting JP, Kari FA, Fischbein MP, Liang DH, Beraud AS, Stephens EH, et al. David valve-sparing aortic root replacement: equivalent mid-term outcome for different valve types with or without connective tissue disorder. J Thorac Cardiovasc Surg. 2013;145:117–27.
5. Bernhardt AMJ, Treede H, Rybczynski M, Sheikzadeh S, Kersten JF, Meinertz T, et al. Comparison of aortic root replacement in patient with Marfan syndrome. Eur J Cardiothorac Surg. 2011;40:1052–7.
6. Kunihara T, Aicher D, Rodionycheva S, Asano M, Tochii M, Sata F. Outcomes after valve-preserving root surgery for patients with Marfan syndrome. J Heart Valve Dis. 2012;21:615–22.
7. Benedetto U, Melina G, Takkenberg JJ, Roscitano A, Angeloni E, Sinatra R. Surgical management of aortic root disease in Marfan syndrome: a systematic review and meta-analysis. Heart. 2011;97:955–8.
8. Hu R, Wang Z, Hu X, Wu H, Wu Z, Zhou Z. Surgical reconstruction of aortic root in Marfan syndrome patients: a systematic review. J Heart Valve Dis. 2014;23:473–83.
9. Takamoto S, Nawata K, Morota T. A simple modification of 'David-V' aortic root reimplantation. Eur J Cardiothorac Surg. 2006;30:560–2.
10. Ando M, Yamauchi H, Morota T, Taketani T, Shimada S, Nawata K, et al. Long-term outcome after the original and simple modified technique of valve-sparing aortic root reimplantation in Marfan-based population, David V University of Tokyo modification. J Cardiol. 2016;67:86–91.

22 ONE-POINT ADVICE: Significance of Aortic Valvuloplasty in the Elderly

Hirofumi Takemura

22.1 Bioprosthetic Valve Replacement in the Elderly

Bioprosthetic valves, such as porcine aortic valves and bovine pericardial valves, have provided favorable long-term outcomes thanks to the recent development of an anti-calcification treatment. The improvement in long-term outcomes for bioprosthetic valves has particularly been remarkable in the elderly, and thus it has emerged as an extremely reliable surgical technique in clinical practice except for patients on dialysis.

22.2 Comparison to Mitral Valve Replacement

Current guidelines recommend mitral valve repair rather than replacement according to the evidence of favorable early and long-term outcomes of the former. However, aortic valve repair has still not achieved a high grade of recommendation due to the lack of a high level of evidence because despite various endeavors to date, its long-term outcomes still have not surpassed the current outcomes of bioprosthetic valves. In addition, in contrast to the standardized valve replacement safely performed by both residents and attending surgeons, valvuloplasty is a procedure of craftsmanship performed by so-called top surgeons based on their abundant experience and decisions to use various surgical techniques according to each particular case. We also cannot deny that it is still too early for this skill-demanding and time-consuming surgical technique to become standard surgery for all patients, particularly the elderly.

22.3 Is this Technique Recommended in Young Patients?

We believe that valvuloplasty has great significance in the young. Although the details are dealt with in another section, as stated in the 2014 AHA guidelines, bioprosthetic valves are recommended for patients aged ≥70 years, whereas mechanical valves are strongly recommended for patients aged <60 years [1]. For patients between the ages of 60 and 70 years, the use of both alternatives is permitted considering various conditions. Mechanical valves, which are recommended for use in young patients, necessitate the life-long use of anticoagulants, and there are major concerns regarding their adverse effects, such as thromboembolism and hemorrhage. In contrast, valvuloplasty in young patients frees them from the use of anticoagu-

H. Takemura (✉)
Department of Thoracic, Cardiovascular and General Surgery, Kanazawa University, Kanazawa, Ishikawa, Japan
e-mail: takemura@med.kanazawa-u.ac.jp

T. Kunihara, S. Takanashi (eds.), *Aortic Valve Preservation*, https://doi.org/10.1007/978-981-13-2068-2_22

lants and is expected to provide better durability than bioprosthetic valves, so it is an attractive surgical option.

22.4 Is this Technique Recommended in Elderly Patients?

Bioprosthetic valves are recommended in elderly patients in favor of elimination of the use of anticoagulants and proven long-term durability. The indications for valvuloplasty cannot be clearly specified until long-term outcomes of valvuloplasty are proved to be equal to those of bioprosthetic valves. In addition, it will be acceptable to consider aortic valvuloplasty to avoid prosthesis-related complications including prosthetic valve endocarditis and thromboembolism. Currently, it is difficult to find implications to apply this skill-demanding and time-consuming surgical technique in open heart surgery for the elderly to obtain these benefits.

However, we think that this surgical technique may be preferable and should be indicated in unique situations. It is probably wise to proactively consider the indications for valvuloplasty in patients with a small aortic root at high risk for an increased transvalvular pressure gradient even with the smallest bioprosthetic valve or in hemodialysis patients in whom durable long-term outcomes of bioprosthetic valves are not expected.

22.5 What Are the Long-Term Outcomes of Bioprosthetic Valves?

The Cleveland Clinic recently reported on the outcomes of the use of the Carpentier-Edwards PERIMOUNT Aortic Heart Valve (Edwards Lifesciences, Irvine, CA), from the data of 12,569 cases covering 81,706 patient-years [2]. Among these subjects, 75% had stenosis and were different from the valvuloplasty subjects, who commonly suffered from insufficiency, but if we consider the real long-term outcomes of prosthetic valves, then these data can be used as reference. Figure 22.1 shows the relationship between patient age and the risk of reoperation over the 20 years after surgery, and we can see that the risk is extremely low once the patient is aged ≥70 years. In addition, Fig. 22.2 shows that the postoperative transvalvular pressure gradient is a risk factor for structural valve deterioration (SVD), although to a certain extent, the older the patients are, the lower these effects become. Also, 354 patients underwent reoperation, 41% because of infective endocarditis and 44% for SVD. If we consider these facts, avoiding infective endocarditis may be a reasonable background when selecting valvuloplasty.

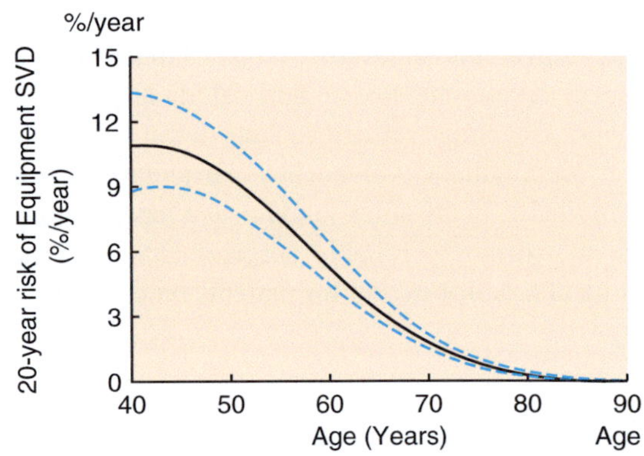

Fig. 22.1 The likelihood of bioprosthetic valve explant over 20 years stratified by age group (cited from Ref. [2] in modified form)

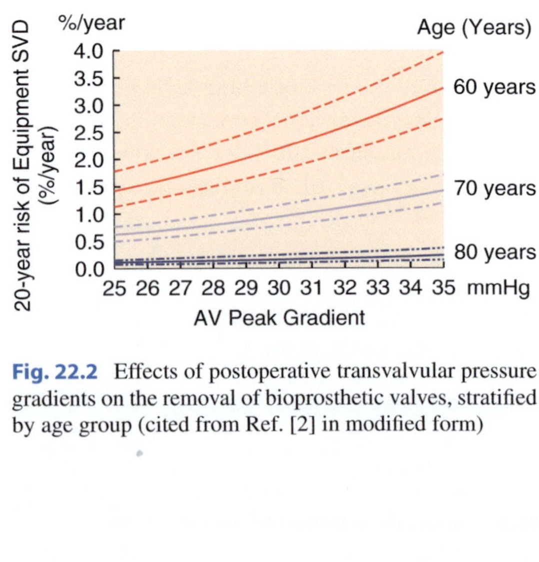

Fig. 22.2 Effects of postoperative transvalvular pressure gradients on the removal of bioprosthetic valves, stratified by age group (cited from Ref. [2] in modified form)

Borgiuinon et al. [3] also reported similar outcomes, and Fig. 22.3 shows a comparison of the freedom from SVD of bioprosthetic valves stratified by age group. Recent meta-regression analysis revealed the same trend regardless of the valve type and concluded that ages 60 to 65 years might comprise a gray area for considering a bioprosthesis [4] (Fig. 22.4). From Japan, Nishida et al. [5] also reported on long-term outcomes of the Carpentier-Edwards PERIMOUNT valve; they observed no cases of SVD during 20 years in patients aged ≥70 years, which indicates excellent outcomes.

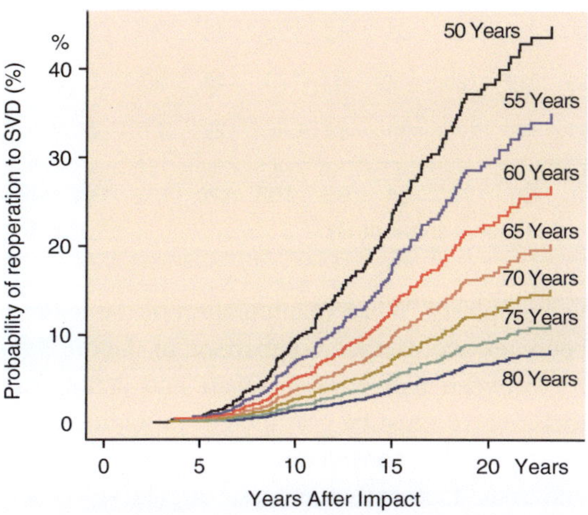

Fig. 22.3 Comparison of the onset of structural valve deterioration stratified by age group (cited from Ref. [3] in modified form)

22.6 What Are the Long-Term Outcomes After Aortic Valvuloplasty?

If we examine the patients reported by Schäfers and his colleagues [6], for whom stratification by age was not performed, patients with aortic insufficiency were in the majority, and their mean age was relatively young: 56 (1–86) years old. Accordingly, it is not possible to examine the long-term outcomes in the elderly alone. The freedom from reoperation at 10 years after valvuloplasty was 90% for bicuspid and 94% for tricuspid valves and was particularly favorable for tricuspid valves (Fig. 22.5).

It is not reasonable to consider these outcomes as those for elderly patients. However, since these results were obtained from the repair of native aortic valves regardless of patients' age, when these results are presumed to be similar to those for the elderly, then the outcomes cannot be said to be superior to those of bioprosthetic valves for the elderly.

Fig. 22.4 Mean structural valve deterioration (SVD)-free years (mean time to valve failure) versus mean patient age (cited from Ref. [4] in modified form)

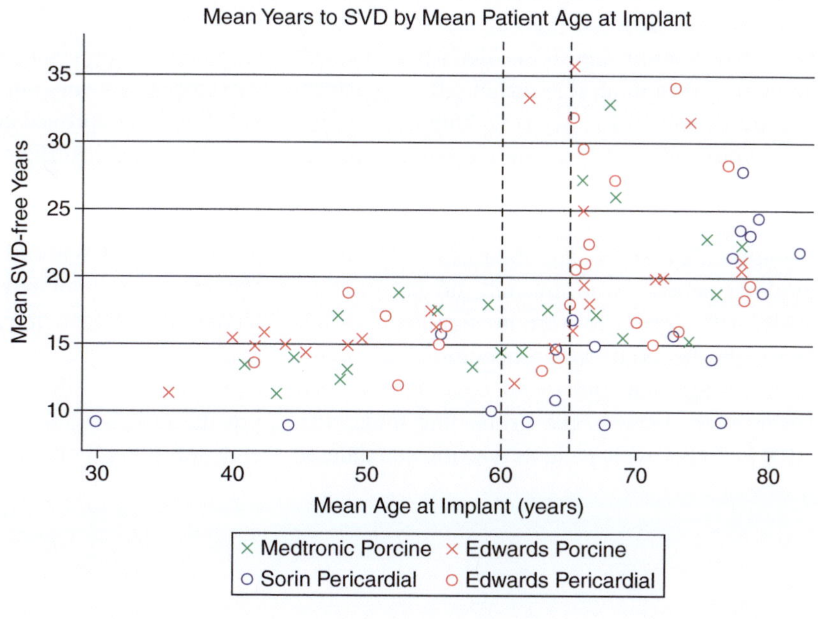

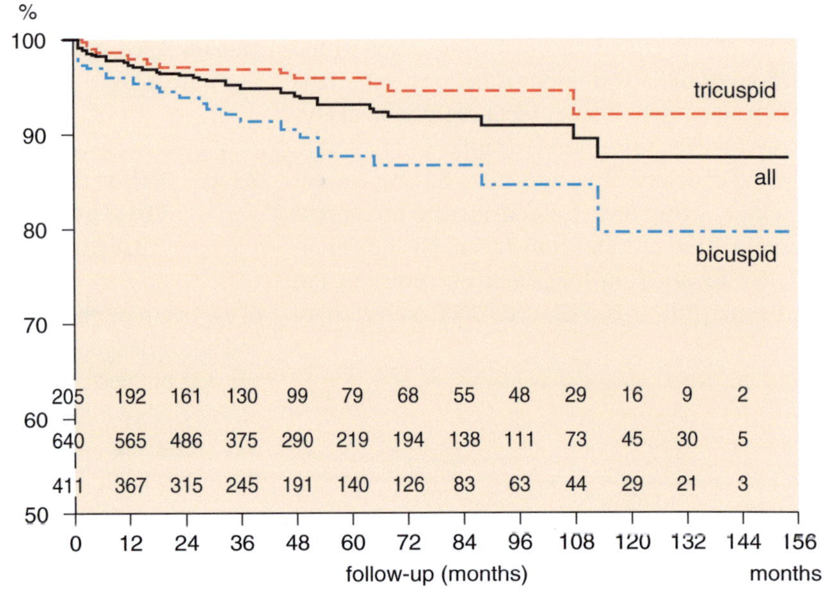

Fig. 22.5 Comparison of long-term outcomes for bicuspid and tricuspid valves (cited from Ref. [6] in modified form)

22.7 Discussion

The single word valvuloplasty encompasses a variety of surgical techniques. Conversely, an understanding of the structure of the aortic valve is essential. The history of aortic valvuloplasty started with aortic root reconstruction (ARR), i.e., the reimplantation and remodeling procedures, and was originally conducted for patients with normal leaflet morphology. Accordingly, the outcomes of ARR without leaflet repair were favorable. Naturally, even in elderly patients with aortic root dilatation, it is meaningful to perform already established surgical techniques, i.e., the reimplantation procedure or remodeling procedure, instead of performing valve replacement including a bio-Bentall procedure.

Figure 22.6 shows a comparison by Schäfers et al. of patients who did and did not undergo ARR. Although there were no significant differences, the freedom from reoperation was higher in the group that underwent concomitant ARR because, we believe, the group that underwent ARR included many patients who did not undergo valvuloplasty. When manipulation of the leaflets becomes necessary, a comparison of the durability between native valve repair and a bioprosthetic valve must be considered. In addition, we must give due consideration to the success rates and to the factors that increase surgical risk, such as the prolonged duration of surgery and cardiac arrest, in elderly patients.

22.8 Conclusion

Recently, several surgeons have begun to find valvuloplasty a very attractive option because we now have an improved understanding of the etiology of aortic insufficiency, the introduction of effective height as an indicator by Schäfers et al. [7], and a theoretical classification of aortic insufficiency by El Khoury and his colleagues [8]. Valvuloplasty is an extremely attractive surgical technique because it preserves the autologous leaflets, offers the benefit of eliminating anticoagulation, and reduces complications related to prosthetic valves, such as infective endocarditis and thrombembolism. However, bioprosthetic

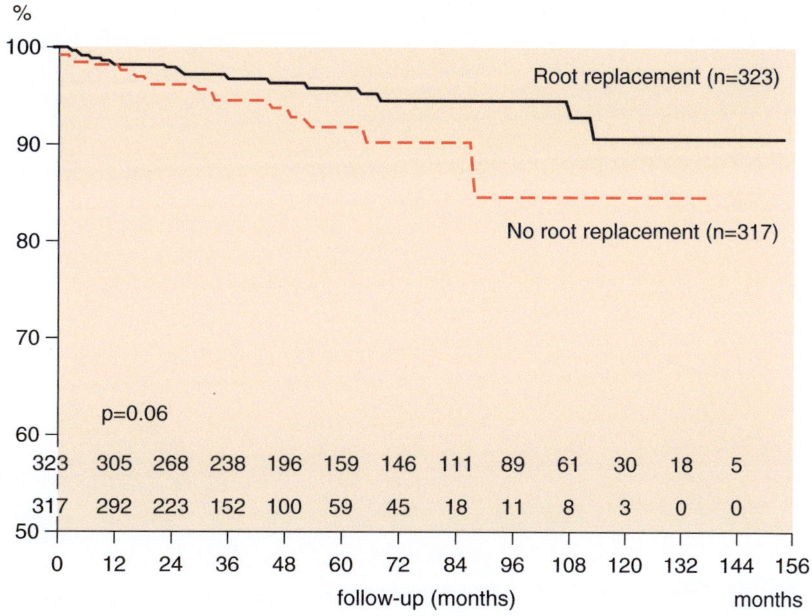

Fig. 22.6 Effects of aortic root replacement on long-term outcomes (cited from Ref. [6] in modified form)

valves have extremely superior long-term outcomes in the elderly, whereas depending on the technique, valvuloplasty may prolong the surgery due to complicated procedures or repair failure. Sufficient consideration must be given to these risks, and we believe the indications must carefully be selected.

References

1. Nishimura RA, Otto CM, Bonow RO, Carabello BA, Erwin JP 3rd, Guyton RA. et al, American College of Cardiology, American College of Cardiology/American Heart Association, American Heart Association. 2014 AHA/ACC guideline for the management of patients with valvular heart disease: a report of the American College of Cardiology/American Heart Association Task Force on Practice Guidelines. J Thorac Cardiovasc Surg. 2014;148:e1–e132.
2. Johnston DR, Soltesz EG, Vakil N, Rajeswaran J, Roselli EE, Sabik JF 3rd, et al. Long-term durability of bioprosthetic aortic valves: implications from 12,569 implants. Ann Thorac Surg. 2015;99:1239–47.
3. Bourguignon T, Bouquiaux-Stablo AL, Candolfi P, Mirza A, Loardi C, May MA, et al. Very long-term outcomes of the Carpentier-Edwards Perimount valve in aortic position. Ann Thorac Surg. 2015;99:831–7.
4. Wang M, Furnary AP, Li HF, Grunkemeier GL. Bioprosthetic aortic valve durability: a meta-regression of published studies. Ann Thorac Surg. 2017;104:1080–7.
5. Nishida T, Sonoda H, Oishi Y, Tatewaki H, Tanoue Y, Shiokawa Y, et al. Long-term results of aortic valve replacement with mechanical prosthesis or carpentier-edwards perimount bioprosthesis in Japanese patients according to age. Circ J. 2014;78:2688–95.
6. Aicher D, Fries R, Rodionycheva S, Schmidt K, Langer F, Schäfers HJ. Aortic valve repair leads to a low incidence of valve-related complications. Eur J Cardiothorac Surg. 2010;37:127–32.
7. Schäfers HJ, Schmied W, Marom G, Aicher D. Cusp height in aortic valves. J Thorac Cardiovasc Surg. 2013;146:269–74.
8. Boodhwani M, de Kerchove L, Glineur D, Poncelet A, Rubay J, Astarci P, et al. Repair-oriented classification of aortic insufficiency: impact on surgical techniques and clinical outcomes. J Thorac Cardiovasc Surg. 2009;137:286–94.

23 Valve-Sparing Aortic Root Replacement to Treat Acute Type A Aortic Dissection

Hiroyuki Kamiya

23.1 Introduction

The main forms of proximal operation to treat type A aortic dissection are (1) supracoronary aortic replacement, (2) aortic root replacement (ARR; Bentall procedure), (3) valve-sparing aortic root replacement (VSARR; David procedure, hereinafter referred to as reimplantation), and (4) VSARR (Yacoub procedure, hereinafter referred to as remodeling). If neither aortic root dilatation nor dissection in any of the sinuses of Valsalva is observed, and the patient does not suffer from aortic stenosis (AS) or regurgitation (AR), then supracoronary aortic replacement is considered to be the most appropriate form of surgery. In many cases, however, dissection has extended to the aortic root, and therefore, the surgical technique must be selected on the basis of the individual case.

This chapter focuses on my experience in Germany and mainly provides an explanation of the reimplantation method.

H. Kamiya (✉)
Department of Cardiac Surgery, Asahikawa Medical University, Asahikawa, Hokkaido, Japan
e-mail: hkamiya88@yahoo.co.jp

23.2 The Advantages and Disadvantages of Each Surgical Technique

Supracoronary Aortic Replacement

This is the most commonly used surgical technique. Gelatin-resorcin-formalin (GRF)-Glue (Cardial, Technopole, Sainte-Etienne, France) or Bio-Glue (CryoLife, Kennesaw, GA, USA) is injected into the false lumen in the aortic root to cause adhesion between the tunica intima and tunica adventitia. Next, felt is used to form the stump, which is then anastomosed to the vascular graft [1]. In this case, the commissure is automatically resuspended and secured, so any AR associated with the aortic dissection is usually well controlled. The benefits of this technique are its high reproducibility and short procedure time.

The disadvantage, although rare, is the reactive tissue damage caused by the glue, which might lead to coronary ostial stenosis or recurrent dissection of the aortic root over the long term. Patients might also sometimes present with AR associated with aneurysm formation of the sinus of Valsalva [2–4].

T. Kunihara, S. Takanashi (eds.), *Aortic Valve Preservation*,
https://doi.org/10.1007/978-981-13-2068-2_23

ARR (Bentall Procedure)

This technique is selected when the entry tear is present within the sinus of Valsalva or when the aortic root was originally dilated, i.e., the patient presented with annuloaortic ectasia (AAE) [5].

Although this technique offers excellent reproducibility, the aortic valve is also replaced even if it has no pathological lesions itself. This becomes problematic when selecting a prosthetic valve, particularly in young patients. Furthermore, the risk of bleeding is greater than that with supracoronary aortic replacement, and once bleeding occurs, it becomes extremely difficult to control it by additional sutures, so caution is required as the technique is challenging.

VSARR (Reimplantation)

As a rule, this procedure is indicated for cases of AAE that would have previously been treated surgically with the Bentall procedure and cases with advanced destruction of the aortic root due to dissection [6, 7]. The benefits of this technique are its excellent reproducibility and low risk of bleeding thanks to two suture lines. Also, no pathological aortic remnant remains, so favorable long-term outcomes can be expected. Furthermore, when performing the Bentall procedure, a certain pressure gradient will remain even if a large prosthetic valve is used. When performing the reimplantation procedure, however, virtually no pressure gradient is created, which makes the procedure superior to the Bentall procedure in this regard. One disadvantage is the longer procedure time than that of other surgical techniques.

VSARR (Remodeling)

The indications for this procedure are similar to those for the reimplantation method.

History of the VSARR Surgical Technique

Transition of the surgical techniques used to repair aortic root lesions are similar to those used for cases without aortic dissection and are discussed in detail in another chapter. Limited to VSARR, since the Hannover group stated that remodeling was an inferior technique [8], reimplantation has become the more mainstream technique. However, favorable outcomes have been reported for the so-called partial remodeling technique in recent years. This technique involves replacing only the sinuses of Valsalva that were damaged by the dissection [9]. Kunihara et al. also added annuloplasty to the remodeling procedure and reported that outcomes were the same as not only other standard techniques for dissection [10] but also the remodeling procedure for chronic aneurysm [11, 12].

23.3 Indications and Contraindications for the Reimplantation Technique

Comparing surgical techniques in Germany and Japan, ARR is more often performed in Germany than Japan whereas aortic arch replacement is more frequently performed in Germany than Japan. As a reflection of this surgical culture, we also proactively performed ARR to treat type A aortic dissection. Our personal surgical strategy is explained below.

1. As a rule, the sinuses of Valsalva that are damaged by the dissection are resected. Supracoronary ascending aorta replacement is performed when (a) the aortic root is not dissected at all or (b) the aortic root is dissected but the patient is in a severely compromised preoperative state and the surgery needs to be shortened as much as possible. In scenario (b), the dissected aortic root is repaired with glue.

2. If only the noncoronary cusp (NCC) sinus of Valsalva is affected by dissection, then the vascular graft is prepared in a lingular shape and the line of anastomosis lies immediately above the sinotubular junction (STJ) in the left and right coronary cusp (LCC, RCC, respectively) sinuses of Valsalva, whereas the line of anastomosis for the NCC sinus of Valsalva lies immediately above the annulus; in other words, partial (1/3) remodeling [9] is performed (Chap. 16, Fig. 16.2; Chap. 33, Fig. 33.1).
3. The Bentall procedure is only performed if organic changes to the aortic leaflets are observed.
4. If the dissection damages two or more sinuses of Valsalva, then the reimplantation procedure is performed.

23.4 Practical Surgical Techniques

The aortic valve is usually normal in cases of aortic dissection, and based on the valve characteristics, we believe that the patient with acute aortic dissection is a good candidate for the reimplantation procedure. Practically, these cases differ very little from normal AAE cases, but some cautionary notes are offered by the author.

Surgical Dissection of the Aortic Root

In some cases, the hematoma in type A aortic dissections extends to the tunica adventitia. Care must be taken not to detach the tunica adventitia by attempts to skeletonize the aortic root as is the case with reimplantation for chronic aneurysm. Close attention is also required to avoid separating the adventitia and intima. When the LCC and RCC sinuses of Valsalva are dissected up to the annulus over the coronary artery ostia, a comparatively normal aortic wall without dissection is usually seen, although the tunica adventitia of the NCC sinus of Valsalva is normally distended by hematoma. No attempt should be made to evacuate the hematoma because the operation can be performed safely when the distended adventitia is sutured together with the hematoma, despite the poor cosmetics. Caution is required not to dissect the root too deeply at the RCC sinus of Valsalva; otherwise, perforation of the right ventricle might occur. In the setting of acute dissection, the extent of dissection at the RCC sinus of Valsalva in particular should be limited. It is preferable to perform the first-row sutures somewhat from the inside at the subannular plane to the outside at the slightly upper plane.

Graft Sizing

In accordance with the rules used at the Hannover Medical School where the author used to be enrolled, the aortic root is examined macroscopically, and 28- to 30-mm straight grafts are selected for men, whereas 26- to 28-mm straight grafts are selected for women. However, a 24-mm graft is sometimes selected for Asian women with an extremely short stature. The same method of graft sizing is used at Ashikawa Medical School. When wavering on decisions regarding size, it is best to select a smaller size. Compared to a graft that is just the right size, implantation of an undersized graft will leave less space for the valve, possibly resulting in a poor final appearance, but it will not impair function. However, if the diameter of the aorta is extremely narrow in young patients, then we believe it is best to select a different surgical technique such as the remodeling procedure because selecting a graft $\leq$22 mm is likely to cause stenosis.

Adjusting the Intercommissural Distance and the Commissural Height

One of the advantages of the reimplantation procedure is that both the commissural height and intercommissural distance can freely be adjusted. However, as mentioned previously, the majority of patients with acute aortic dissection have a normal aortic valve, and therefore, the intercommissural distance is simply arranged equally in most cases. If the annulus of the NCC sinus of Valsalva is extremely larger than the others, then the intercommissural distance is sometimes also adjusted appropriately. When adjusting the commissural height, each commissure is maximally elevated without touching the graft (important!) when securing the graft to the annulus using the first-row sutures. An attempt is made to examine the overall balance in this position once the needles are passed into the graft.

Anastomosis of the Coronary Artery Ostia

The so-called Carrel patch is used for reconstruction of the coronary buttons, but in many cases, the coronary artery ostia themselves are affected by the dissection. Even if this is not the case, sometimes surgical manipulation results in detachment of the adventitia, so surgeons should perform meticulous manipulation. Glue is also not used to avoid long-term coronary artery complications. Surgeons must remain aware when securing the dissected adventitia using 4/0 polypropylene sutures to take large bites and widen the pitch. After the anastomosis is completed, the ostia are examined from inside the graft, and if there is any concern, then additional preventive stitches should be placed at this time.

23.5 Personal Tips

1. When adjusting the commissural height, the LCC/RCC commissure comes into contact with the pulmonary artery. To prevent the commissure from becoming elevated beyond a certain level, this commissure is first fixed to the graft and used as a reference point. Next, the LCC/NCC commissure is fixed to the graft, followed by the NCC/RCC commissure.

   The LCC/RCC commissural height acts as a reference point that never changes. Sometimes, cusp coaptation will be shallow when the NCC/RCC and the LCC/NCC commissures are excessively elevated, and then they may need to be fixed again a few millimeters inferior to the previous level.
2. When performing anastomosis of the right coronary artery (RCA) ostium in a normal anatomical position, weaning from the cardiopulmonary bypass may cause kinking of the RCA due to right ventricular volume overload, and patients may sometimes present with right ventricular failure. To prevent kinking of the RCA, the RCA ostium should be placed at the level of the STJ and the course of proximal RCA should be arranged in a straight fashion with no curves. This results in the proximal region of the RCA being in a somewhat extended state, which facilitates the prevention of RCA ischemia. If myocardial ischemia is suspected, it is theoretically possible to repeat the anastomosis of the ostia, although performing a bypass using a vein is also acceptable [13].

23.6 Outcomes

The International Registry of Acute Dissection (IRAD), published in 2014, is an analysis of type A aortic dissection [14]. According to this analysis, from a total of 1995 patients, 35% underwent ARR, with hospital mortality rates that were not significantly different between the two groups: 21% in the ARR group and 18% in the non-ARR group. This paper did not provide details about the surgical procedure used to perform ARR (reimplantation, remodeling, or Bentall). With regard to the reimplantation procedure, Leshnower et al. performed reimplantation on 43 patients with acute type A aortic dissection. They reported favorable outcomes, with an early mortality rate of 4.7% and freedom from reoperation of 100% during a 40-month observation period [15]. Kunihara et al. performed the remodeling procedure on 59 patients with type A acute aortic dissection. They reported extremely favorable outcomes, with an early mortality rate of 6.8% and freedom from reoperation rate of 98% over a 10-year observation period, which seems comparable with the other standard techniques for dissection [10] or the remodeling procedure for chronic aneurysm [12]. Quite recently, the Hannover group published their 20-year experience with 109 patients with acute type A aortic dissection who underwent a reimplantation procedure (David-I). The in-hospital mortality rate was 11% and freedom from valve-related reoperation at 10 years was 85% [16].

The author's personal experience is described below.

Surgical Outcomes at the University of Düsseldorf

We operated on 53 patients with acute type A aortic dissection between September 2009 and March 2014 at the University of Düsseldorf and performed the reimplantation procedure on 30 of these 53 patients. A straight graft (the majority was Hemashield Platinum Plus graft (Intervascular SAS, La Ciotat, France) provided by the Getinge group) was used during the procedure on all patients. Furthermore, total arch replacement was performed on 11 patients. The mean duration of surgery was 384 min, that of cardiopulmonary bypass support was 245 min, and that of aortic cross-clamping was 169 min. An extensive postoperative cerebral infarction occurred in one patient, and mesenteric ischemia occurred in four patients. All of these patients died, bringing the 30-day mortality to 16%. This is a high operative mortality rate, but when we consider that the mean operative mortality rate for acute type A aortic dissection in Germany is 17% [17], then we believe that these outcomes are reasonable. We have currently experienced no proximal reoperations in this subgroup over the long-term.

Surgical Outcomes at Asahikawa Medical University

We operated on 22 patients with acute type A aortic dissection at Asahikawa Medical University between April 2014 and April 2015. Five of these patients underwent the reimplantation procedure, and a graft with sinuses was used in two patients. Three patients also underwent total arch replacement using 4-branched prosthesis (J-Graft, Japan Lifeline, Japan). The mean duration of surgery was 451 min, that of cardiopulmonary bypass support was 238 min, and that of aortic cross-clamping was 181 min. There were no surgical deaths, but one surgical death was observed in the patients who did not undergo the reimplantation procedure due to low cardiac output syndrome.

23.7 Conclusion

When dealing with acute type A aortic dissection, if the dissection extends to the aortic root, the reimplantation procedure is theoretically an ideal surgical technique that does not leave any dissected, pathological aortic wall. In addition, patients with advanced aortic root dilatation who would previously have been treated using the Bentall procedure are good candidates for the reimplantation procedure, even if there is only minor dissection of the aortic root. The drawback is that the surgical technique is complex and time-consuming, but a complex procedure does not necessarily mean technical difficulty. Going forward, we believe this surgical technique in this scenario will likely become increasingly popular.

References

1. Bachet J, Goudot B, Teodori G, Brodaty D, Dubois C, De Lentdecker P, et al. Surgery of type A acute aortic dissection with Gelatine-Resorcine-Formol biological glue: a twelve-year experience. J Cardiovasc Surg. 1990;31:263–73.
2. Casselman FP, Tan ES, Vermeulen FE, Kelder JC, Morshuis WJ, Schepens MA. Durability of aortic valve preservation and root reconstruction in acute type A aortic dissection. Ann Thorac Surg. 2000;70:1227–33.
3. Fukunaga S, Karck M, Harringer W, Cremer J, Rhein C, Haverich A. The use of gelatin-resorcin-formalin glue in acute aortic dissection type A. Eur J Cardiothorac Surg. 1999;15:564–9.
4. Modi A, Bull R, Tsang G, Kaarne M. Ostial left coronary stenosis following aortic root reconstruction with BioGlue. Interact Cardiovasc Thorac Surg. 2011;13:243–5.
5. Pacini D, Ranocchi F, Angeli E, Settepani F, Pagliaro M, Martin-Suarez S, et al. Aortic root replacement with composite valve graft. Ann Thorac Surg. 2003;76:90–8.
6. Subramanian S, Leontyev S, Borger MA, Trommer C, Misfeld M, Mohr FW. Valve-sparing root reconstruction does not compromise survival in acute type A aortic dissection. Ann Thorac Surg. 2012;94:1230–4.
7. Kallenbach K, Oelze T, Salcher R, Hagl C, Karck M, Leyh RG, et al. Evolving strategies for treatment of acute aortic dissection type A. Circulation. 2004;110(11 Suppl 1):II243–9.
8. Leyh RG, Fischer S, Kallenbach K, Kofidis T, Pethig K, Harringer W, et al. High failure rate after valve-sparing aortic root replacement using the "remod-

eling technique" in acute type A aortic dissection. Circulation. 2002;106:I229–33.
9. Urbanski PP, Hijazi H, Dinstak W, Diegeler A. Valve-sparing aortic root repair in acute type A dissection: how many sinuses have to be repaired for curative surgery? Eur J Cardiothorac Surg. 2013;44:439–44.
10. Kunihara T, Neumann N, Kriechbaum SD, Aicher D, Schäfers HJ. Aortic root remodeling leads to good valve stability in acute aortic dissection and pre-existent root dilatation. J Thorac Cardiovasc Surg. 2016;152:430–6.
11. Schäfers HJ, Raddatz A, Schmied W, Takahashi H, Miura Y, Kunihara T, et al. Reexamining remodeling. J Thorac Cardiovasc Surg. 2015;149(2 Suppl):S30–6.
12. Kunihara T, Neumann N, Kriechbaum SD, Nomura R, Schäfers HJ. Long-term outcome of aortic root remodeling for patients with and without acute aortic dissection. Circ J. 2017;81:1824–31.
13. Shahriari A, Eng M, Tranquilli M, Elefteriades JA. Rescue coronary artery bypass grafting (CABG) after aortic composite graft replacement. J Card Surg. 2009;24:392–6.
14. Di Eusanio M, Trimarchi S, Peterson MD, Myrmel T, Hughes GC, Korach A, et al. Root replacement surgery versus more conservative management during type A acute aortic dissection repair. Ann Thorac Surg. 2014;98:2078–84.
15. Leshnower BG, Myung RJ, McPherson L, Chen EP. Midterm results of David V valve-sparing aortic root replacement in acute type A aortic dissection. Ann Thorac Surg. 2015;99:795–800.
16. Beckmann E, Martens A, Pertz J, Kaufeld T, Umminger J, Hanke JS, et al. Valve-sparing David I procedure in acute aortic type A dissection: a 20-year experience with more than 100 patients. Eur J Cardiothorac Surg. 2017;52:319–24.
17. Conzelmann LO, Weigang E, Mehlhorn U, Abugameh A, Hoffmann I, Blettner M, et al. Mortality in patients with acute aortic dissection type A: analysis of pre- and intraoperative risk factors from the German Registry for Acute Aortic Dissection Type A (GERAADA). Eur J Cardiothorac Surg. 2016;49(2):e44–52.

Pediatric Valvuloplasty

24

Kisaburo Sakamoto and Masaya Murata

24.1 Introduction

It is true that the absolute number of patients who have undergone surgical treatment on an anatomical aortic valve in childhood is not as high as that in adults. However, in recent years, treatments for the aortic valve have certainly advanced, and their number has increased even in children. Furthermore, if we consider the issue from the perspective of surgical treatment on a "systemic outflow tract valve", the absolute number is dramatically increasing. In addition, most of the patients who require intervention for systemic outflow tract valves in childhood may become candidates for late re-operation. The re-operative procedures can be more complex than expected for common adult cardiac surgeries because they have not yet gained experience in the conventional treatment of acquired aortic valve disorders. Considering such factors, in the twenty-first century, it seems very important that both pediatric and adult cardiac surgeons learn treatment strategies for patients with congenital heart disease affecting systemic outflow tract valves.

K. Sakamoto (✉) · M. Murata
Department of Cardiovascular Surgery, Mt. Fuji Shizuoka Children's Hospital, Shizuoka, Japan
e-mail: sabusabuno8@yahoo.co.jp

In this chapter, we provide an outline of the treatment strategies for systemic outflow tract valves in congenital heart disease that are conducted in childhood, particularly focusing on aortic valvuloplasty.

24.2 Pediatric Patients Who Require Treatment on the Systemic Outflow Tract Valve in Childhood (Fig. 24.1)

The following is a broad classification of the patients who require treatment of the systemic outflow tract valve in childhood.

When the Systemic Outflow Tract Valve Is Only An Anatomical Aortic Valve

This subgroup is classified into the following two subcategories. One is congenital aortic stenosis (N2 group, N3 group with bicuspid valves), frequently accompanied by coarctation or interruption of the aorta. The other is aortic regurgitation associated with dilatation of the aortic annulus and ascending aorta including the Valsalva sinuses in patients with congenital heart disease accompanied by pulmonary stenosis or atresia (N4 and N5 groups such as tetralogy of Fallot or a ventricular septal defect (VSD) accompanying pulmonary

T. Kunihara, S. Takanashi (eds.), *Aortic Valve Preservation*,
https://doi.org/10.1007/978-981-13-2068-2_24

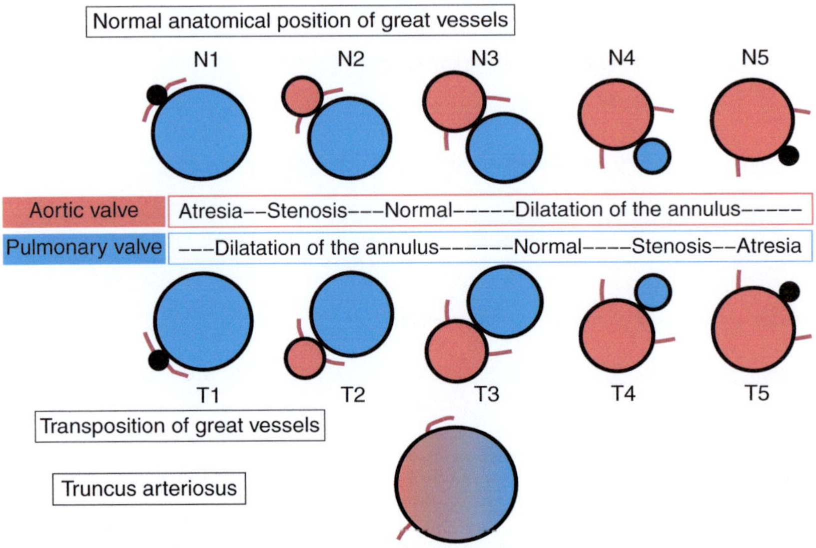

Fig. 24.1 Patients requiring treatment on a systemic outflow tract valve in childhood

atresia or T4 and T5 groups such as transposition of the great vessels with left ventricular outflow tract stenosis). Aortic regurgitation associated with dilatation of the aortic annulus and ascending aorta commonly does not appear in childhood because the dilatation progresses relatively slowly. Many patients have clinical features of adult annuloaortic ectasia (AAE).

Children with aortic regurgitation associated with collagen disorders such as Marfan syndrome or aortic regurgitation and/or stenosis associated with infectious diseases such as rheumatic fever are often symptomatic and occasionally indicated for surgical intervention during their childhood.

When the Systemic Outflow Tract Valve Is Only An Anatomical Pulmonary Valve

Neo-aortic valve deteriorations after either the arterial switch procedure for transposition of the great vessels (T3, T2, and part of T4) or Ross procedure (N2, T2, and part of N3) belong to this subgroup. In a number of cases, the anatomical pulmonary valve that maintains the systemic circulation as the neo-aorta may enlarge over time, and patients can present with clinical features similar to those in AAE. Dilatation of the neo-aortic valve also progresses relatively slowly; therefore, symptoms commonly occur in the mid or late postoperative period. In addition, aortic regurgitation may occur due to deformation of the neo-aorta associated with coronary translocation.

When the Systemic Outflow Tract Includes Both the Aortic and Pulmonary Valves

Systemic outflow tract valve deteriorations (mainly regurgitation) after either the Norwood procedure or Damus-Kaye Stansel (DKS) procedure (N1, T1, part of N2 and T2) are included in this subgroup because of deformation associated with the aorto-pulmonary anastomosis or enlargement of the anatomical pulmonary valve. Patients expected to undergo univentricular repair with the bi-directional Glenn or Fontan procedure are common.

Others

Valve problems (both regurgitation and stenosis) of the truncal valve.

24.3 Characteristics of Pediatric Aortic Valvuloplasty (Fig. 24.2, Table 24.1)

The major characteristics are that the indications for valvuloplasty and the techniques of valvuloplasty are different from those in adults. In adults, we make the decision to choose valve repair or valve replacement based on a comparison of superiority and inferiority between the two. However, we may sometimes have to choose valvuloplasty in small pediatric patients because valve replacement is not a choice. In practice, small or dysplastic valves in the neonatal period that have not yet reached a diameter of 5 mm may also become therapeutic targets, and it is not possible to choose valve replacement in these groups. Therefore, after it is resolved to perform palliative management, a life-saving valvuloplasty may be selected in a number of cases. In infants, the annulus diameter increases to around 10 mm in size, but common valve replacement is not possible even on them because the smallest available prosthetic valve is 16 mm in diameter. Under this background, valve replacement in small children has to be compared with procedures such as the Konno procedure or Ross procedure, which have a higher degree of difficulty. However, as it is actually not easy to achieve consistent outcomes with valvuloplasty on these small aortic valves, only a minority of institutions proactively select this option nowadays. However, each hospital determines their own indications for children and teenagers if their annulus will allow the selection of normal valve replacement. Nevertheless, even when these indications are determined to resemble those in adults, The additional consideration of whether "anticoagulation therapy can be selected for a highly active adolescent" is also required.

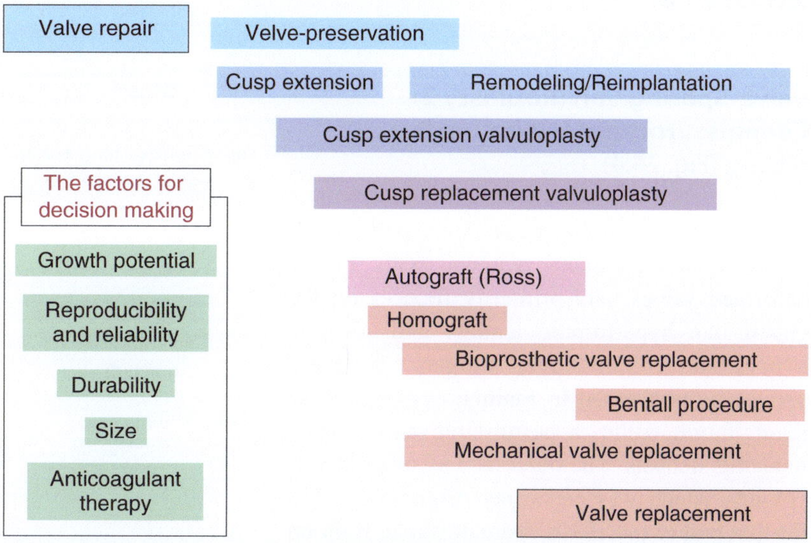

Fig. 24.2 Surgical treatment options for the aortic valve region

Table 24.1 Characteristics of treatment for pediatric aortic valves

– Small (absolute size and age)
– Growth (the body weight will treble from the neonatal period until 1 year of age!)
– No prosthetic valves with a diameter of <16 mm
– Early deterioration of graft materials (bioprosthetic valves)
– Difficult to manage anticoagulant therapy

24.4 Current State of Valvuloplasty in Pediatric Patients

Valve-Sparing Valvuloplasty 1: Peripheral Plication, Central Plication (Fig. 24.3)

These procedures have commonly been performed when a VSD is located just beneath both great vessels or at the outflow tract and is associated with regurgitation that causes a deformity linked to prolapse of the margins of the right- or non-coronary cusp. Due to recent advancements in echocardiographic diagnosis, it has become possible to close a VSD before the development of significant regurgitation, and thus the frequency of valvuloplasty in such cases has decreased.

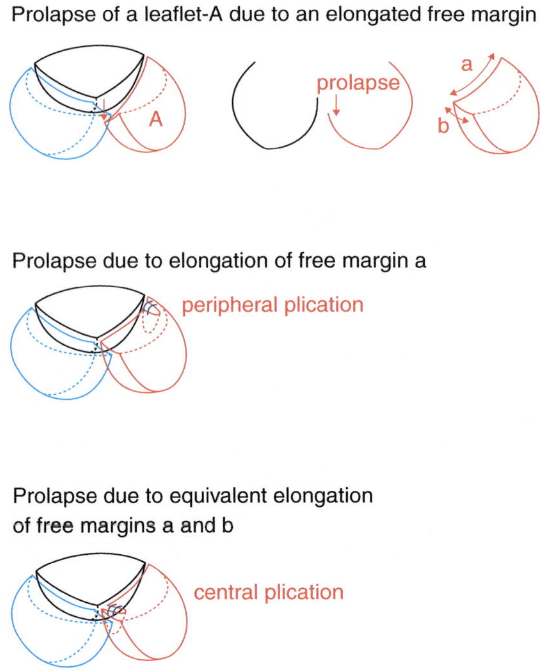

Fig. 24.3 Peripheral plication, central plication

Valve-Sparing Valvuloplasty 2: Commissurotomy and/or Leaflet Slicing (Fig. 24.4)

This is performed for aortic stenosis, particularly in neonatal or infant patients with highly deformed valves, and primarily focuses on the gelatin-like hypertrophic leaflets and severely hypoplastic commissures. Surgery in these patients is performed to maintain postoperative regurgitation within a permissible range while reducing stenosis. The outcomes of surgical valvotomy, which was performed from 1980 until the first half of the 1990s, were unstable. Balloon aortic valvotomy began to be performed in the 1990s, and reports indicated that it was effective and had less risk and better early outcomes than

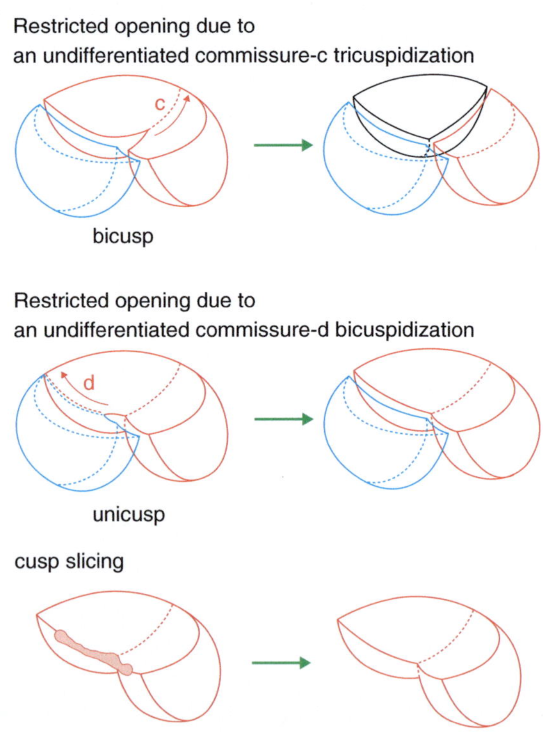

Fig. 24.4 Commissurotomy and leaflet slicing

those of surgery. However, in recent years, reports have also stated that when taking the long-term maintenance of adequate valve function into consideration, the prognosis following a highly accurate surgical valvotomy is superior to that of balloon valvotomy. Currently, different options are selected in each institution. Patients who can be discharged with mild stenosis or regurgitation after surgical valvotomy have a good mid-term prognosis, and this procedure is becoming the first choice of treatment for indicated cases. However, the prognosis for patients with highly deformed valves and regurgitation that is difficult to control is poor, and advanced valvuloplasty with cusp extension is being attempted to treat this group of patients.

Advanced Valvuloplasty Using Supplementary Materials 1: Commissuroplasty (Fig. 24.5a)

Usually, it is impossible to control regurgitation when commissurotomy is performed on a low-height raphe or fused commissure (as it is not possible to maintain the coaptation height after performing the procedure).

This is one of the effective surgical procedures making use of supplemental materials (such as autologous pericardium) to create reasonable valve function when treating severely hypoplastic commissures. However, advanced skills are required to increase the reproducibility of this procedure on small infants. It is effective for short- to mid-term control of regurgitation, but few reports have now shown reliability over the long term.

Advanced Valvuloplasty Using Supplemental Materials 2: Leaflet Extension (Fig. 24.5b)

When treating highly deformed leaflets that cannot be treated by means of a valve-sparing operation, this surgical technique uses supplemental materials to elongate the leaflet geometry (sometimes performed with partial resection) to maintain function and to handle the expected growth. There are numerous benefits such as the ability to freely determine the leaflet length and the coaptation height. Highly reproducible and reliable surgical techniques or procedures have not yet been established, so standardization or adjustment is difficult. At present, this technique

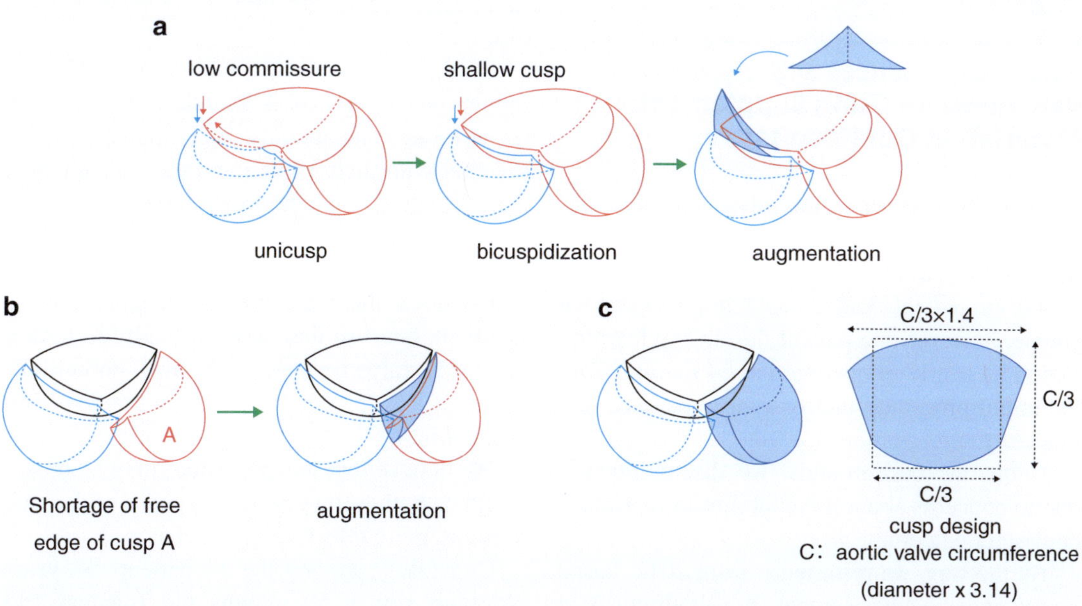

Fig. 24.5 Advanced valvuloplasty using supplementary materials. (**a**) Commissuroplasty, (**b**) leaflet extension, (**c**) leaflet replacement

is only performed at a limited number of experienced institutions. There are reports that a certain prognosis can be expected from late infancy onward, although there are few reports on young infants.

Advanced Valvuloplasty Using Supplemental Materials 3: Leaflet Replacement (Fig. 24.5c)

In performing this technique, the severely deformed leaflets are resected away from the attachment sites to the annulus, and supplemental materials are used to completely recreate the leaflets. It is now believed to be more easy and reliable than leaflet extension, and surgeons have started to choose this technique because all of the leaflets created in place have a reasonable coaptation height and the same pliability. Replacement is sometimes indicated for a single leaflet alone, although in some cases, two or three leaflets can be replaced. Although the annulus may grow, growth of the leaflets is not expected. This technique is now provisionally performed as a bridge to the next surgery in young children to maintain their general condition and cardiac function.

24.5 Experiences with Advanced Valvuloplasty Using Supplemental Materials at Our Hospital

We initially performed the advanced valuvuloplasty using supplemental Materials on 8 patients from 2008 to 2009.

All the patients had acceptable postoperative course, however one patient during my learning period had early re-operation at 24 months from his initial procedure and two other patients had moderate regurgitation at 2010.

Under the backgrounds, we discontinued it due to concerns about its reliability to reproduce consistent outcomes.

By the way, we restarted it from 2012, based on the positive advancements in valvuloplasty in adult field and the reasonable mid-term results of our initial experience without any re-operation except for the above-mentioned one.

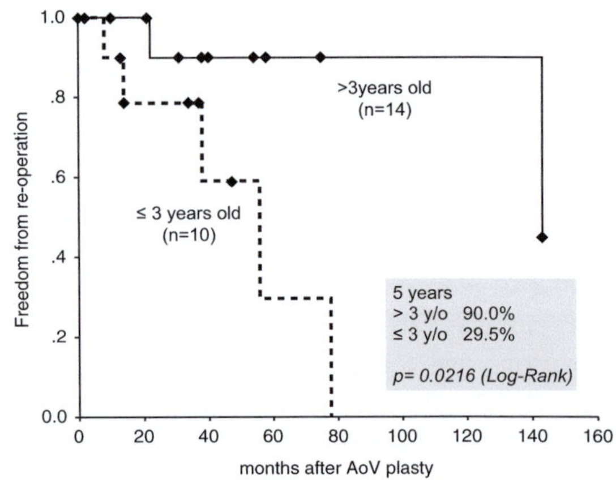

Fig. 24.6 Freedom from re-operation. (1) On the patients with 3 years old or less, mean age and body weight are 13±16 months old [median 3 months (0-43)], BW 6.7±4.3 kg. (2) On the patients with more than 3 years old, mean age and body weight are 140±50 months old [median 150 months (75-212)], BW 40.4±18.7 kg

We have experienced 24 patients up to 2017 and our result is shown in Fig. 24.6.

Freedom from re-operation rate is significantly different between the patients equal to or under 3 years old and those over 3 years old.

On the 10 patients ≤3 years old (age 13 ± 16 months old [median 3 months (0–43)], BW 6.7 ± 4.3 kg), the annulus surely increase in size together with their growth and the supplemental materials used may deteriorate rapidly.

For these reason, they have often required re-operation within 5 years or less.

However, there are little reasonable choices for them, because they have difficulty to have a prosthetic valve because of the size, poorer outcomes of Ross procedure in early infantile period and so on.

We believe that this procedure may be meaningful as both a life saving one and a bridge one to future more effective approaches.

Conversely, among the 14 patients >3 years old (age 140 ± 50 months old [median 150 months (75–212)], BW 40.4 ± 18.7 kg), only one patient, who had triple cusp plasty by means of one cusp replacement and two cusp extension, had re-operation at 143months postoperatively. Freedom from re-operation on them is 90% at 5 years so far.

On the basis of the experience, we believe that this procedure has potential to become an effective option for treating most of pediatric patients with aortic valve disease.

24.6 Conclusion

Treatment for pediatric systemic outflow valves including both the anatomical aortic valve and pulmonary valve is undoubtedly increasing now. Recently, valvuloplasty, including advanced procedures using supplemental materials, for systemic outflow valves has become a treatment option that cannot be ignored, and it is expected to be a reasonable and reliable choice in the near future.

25 ONE-POINT ADVICE: The Significance of Performing Aortic Valvuloplasty in Young Patients

Masafumi Yashima and Hirokuni Arai

25.1 Introduction

This chapter discusses the characteristics and problems of aortic valve replacement in young patients and the advantages and disadvantages of aortic valvuloplasty, focusing on young patients who have completed their physical growth.

25.2 Characteristics of Young Patients

High physical and metabolic activity are two characteristics of young patients. These patients are more likely to experience trauma, and they also like to participate in sports including contact play. The individuals most commonly injured during road-traffic accidents are in their 30s, followed by those in their 40s, and then by young individuals (16–24 years) [1]. For this reason, it is preferable to avoid medicines that promote hemorrhage. Furthermore, high cardiac output occurs during exercise, so it is desirable to perform surgical procedures that result in a lower transvalvular pressure gradient at the aortic position. Young patients are also frequently engaged in social activities and thus have little free time, so it is difficult for them to go to hospital regularly, and the cost of medication is an economic burden. Depending on the patients, they can also change their living environment, which may include dietary habits, as some may want to live alone. It is also possible for irregular lifestyle patterns caused by being busy with school or work to negatively affect their postoperative treatment, especially their adherence to oral medications. Physical activity may also include sexual activity as both boys and girls reach the reproductive age. The total blood volume in women during pregnancy increases by approximately 40% and places a burden on the heart, so reliable surgical treatment is preferred. The use of teratogenic agents such as warfarin is absolutely contraindicated during the period of fetal organogenesis, so women who wish to have children cannot undergo the implantation of a mechanical valve, which would necessitate the administration of warfarin as anticoagulant therapy. Meanwhile, the metabolic activity of calcium in young patients is high, so there is early progression of bioprosthetic valve calcification.

25.3 Problems of Prosthetic Valve Replacement

Structure

Mechanical valves have two leaflets and bioprosthetic valves three leaflets. The prosthetic valves are designed to obtain the maximum opening

M. Yashima · H. Arai (✉)
Department of Cardiovascular Surgery, Graduate School of Medicine, Tokyo Medical and Dental University, Tokyo, Japan
e-mail: hiro.cvsg@tmd.ac.jp

T. Kunihara, S. Takanashi (eds.), *Aortic Valve Preservation*,
https://doi.org/10.1007/978-981-13-2068-2_25

angle, but slight energy loss occurs when the leaflets open. A frame and sewing cuff must always be present around the leaflets, so the effective orifice area will always be smaller than the original physiologic orifice area. These functional and structural disadvantages increase the pressure gradient during exercise loads [2], which is unfavorable for highly active young patients.

Durability

Pyrolytic carbon is used for mechanical valves, and the durability of such material is not a problem. However, the greatest drawback of bioprosthetic valve is the structural valve deterioration (SVD) caused by calcification. The reported freedom from explantation at 15 years for SVD of a Mosaic valve (Medtronic Co., Ltd. Minneapolis, MN), which is a typical porcine valve, was 49.3% in patients aged ≤60 years, 80.8% for patients aged >60 to ≤70 years, and 98.6% for patients aged >70 years [3]. Similarly, freedom from reoperation at 15 years due to SVD of the Carpentier-Edwards pericardial (CEP) valve (Edwards Lifesciences Irvine, CA), which is a typical bovine pericardial valve, was 47.2% in patients aged <65 years and 94.4% in patients aged ≥65 years [4]. These results would all be unfavorable in younger patients. Bioprosthetic valve durability is poor in young patients because they have highly active calcium metabolism, which causes early and progressive calcification of the bioprosthesis. Therefore, the use of bioprosthetic valves in young patients is not recommended, except in exceptional cases, such as when a patient wishes to have children. Decellularized valves [5], which may possibly eliminate calcification, are the ideal material, but such valves have not become popular yet.

Valve Function Failure

Mechanical valves may fail due to thrombosis or tissue proliferation, which may result in either a restricted valve opening or insufficiency or a combination of the two. In addition to the above-mentioned causes, bioprosthetic valves may also fail as a result of SVD due to calcification, which causes stenosis or insufficiency.

Paravalvular Leakage

Paravalvular leakage can occur with both mechanical and biological prosthetic valves. It tends to occur particularly in cases of severe aortic stenosis with annular calcification. Nowadays, with the use of intraoperative transesophageal echocardiography, residual regurgitation is rarely overlooked.

Prosthetic Valve Infection

The incidence of early prosthetic valve infection (occurring within 1 year) is 5%, and subsequently, the risk is 0.91%/patient-year for bioprosthetic valves and 0.27%/patient-year for mechanical valves [6]. When it occurs in practice, the probability of repeat surgery is high at 48.9%, and the in-hospital mortality is also high at 22.8% [7]. Some patients may also require extensive surgery, such as aortic root replacement if this complication occurs.

Anticoagulant Therapy

Anticoagulant therapy is essential for patients with mechanical valves, and warfarin is the only reliable anticoagulant agent. The effect of warfarin is easily altered by diet and other drug intake, and it may sometimes cause life-threatening hemorrhagic events. The risk of hemorrhage increases with age. However, if the effect of warfarin is not sufficient, thromboembolism may occur. So, it is important to strictly monitor the effect of this anticoagulant medicine during treatment. Because self-measurement of PT-INR (prothrombin time calculated using the international normalized ratio) is not yet popular in Japan, patients usually need to visit their physician and undergo blood examinations periodically for the rest of their lives. Warfarin is teratogenic during the period of fetal organogenesis, so mechanical valves cannot be indicated for women who wish to bear children. Meanwhile, anticoagulant therapy is only administered for a few months after bioprosthetic valve implantation and is not required thereafter.

25.4 Ross Procedure

One of the options for treating aortic valve disease is the Ross procedure, which involves autologous transplantation of the patient's own pulmonary valve as an aortic valve graft. In addition to the excellent hemodynamic result, anticoagulant therapy can be avoided, so the indications for the Ross procedure should be considered in women who wish to bear children and patients at high risk of trauma due to sports or occupational reasons. However, the Ross procedure entails a moderately high risk (early mortality rate of 3.2%) [8], and this technique requires high surgical skills and should be performed at experienced institutions to obtain stable outcomes. The long-term outcomes show that the graft failure rates in patients aged >18 years are 1.14%/patient-year for aortic valves and 0.65%/patient year for pulmonary valves [8]. This means a total graft failure rate of 17.9% at 10 years postoperatively, which is certainly not low, and the Ross procedure can potentially convert single-valve disease into double-valve disease. The surgical indications should therefore be considered extremely carefully. However, excellent outcomes have been reported for the inclusion cylinder method [9], which so far has resulted in zero (0%) early mortality, and freedom from reoperation at 15 years on the aortic valves is 99%.

25.5 Advantages and Disadvantages of Aortic Valvuloplasty

Numerous drawbacks of prosthetic valves can be overcome by performing valvuloplasty, but it is necessary to know the actual results of both alternatives. Thirty-day mortality of mechanical aortic valve replacement in patients under 65 years old was 1.1%, and overall actual survival at 5 and 10 years was 95% and 87%, respectively [10]. Actual freedom from SVD was 95% and 91% at 5 and 10 years, respectively [10]. Meanwhile, hospital mortality for valvuloplasty was 3.4%. Freedom from reoperation at 5 and 10 years was 88% and 81% in bicuspid and 97% and 93% in tricuspid aortic valves [11]. In a report focusing on the quality of life of young patients (aged 18 to 45 years old), conspicuous differences were not observed between mechanical valve replacement and valvuloplasty [12].

For highly active young patients, valvuloplasty is an ideal treatment because it eliminates anticoagulation, frees patients from prosthesis-related complications, and avoids medications or frequent hospital visits. Valvuloplasty requires reliable lesion management and stable long-term outcomes similar to or better than prosthetic valve replacement; otherwise, reoperations may increase after aortic valvuloplasty. It seems reasonable to choose aortic valvuloplasty as the first choice in young patients when it is technically feasible, although the procedure still remains challenging.

25.6 Conclusions

Since prosthesis-related complications can be eliminated, aortic valvuloplasty has emerged as a novel alternative for young patients. On the other hand, durable repair by secure control of regurgitation is mandatory to overcome the long-term performance of prosthetic valve replacement. Thus indication for aortic valvuloplasty for young patients should be set critically according to the surgeons' experience.

References

1. National Police Agency. Traffic accidents situation in 2013 http://www.e-stat.go.jp/SG1/estat/List.do?lid=000001117549
2. Dumesnil JG, Yoganathan AP. Valve prosthesis hemodynamics and the problem of high transprosthetic pressure gradients. Eur J Cardiothorac Surg. 1992;6:S34–8.
3. Mosaic® aortic bioprosthesis 17-year Compendium. Medtronic Inc.

4. Minakata K, Tanaka S, Okawa Y, Shimamoto M, Kaneko T, Takahara Y, et al. Long-term outcome of the Carpentier-Edwards pericardial valve in the aortic position in Japanese patients. Circ J. 2014;78:882–9.
5. da Costa FD, Costa AC, Prestes R, Domanski AC, Balbi EM, Ferreira AD, et al. The early and midterm function of decellularized aortic valve allografts. Ann Thorac Surg. 2010;90:1854–60.
6. Piper C, Körfer R, Horstkotte D. Prosthetic valve endocarditis. Heart. 2001;85:590–3.
7. Wang A, Athan E, Pappas PA, Fowler VG Jr, Olaison L, Parè C, et al. Contemporary clinical profile and outcome of prosthetic valve endocarditis. JAMA. 2007;297:1354–61.
8. Takkenberg JJM, Klieverik LMA, Schoof PH, van Suylen RJ, van Herwerden LA, Zondervan PE, et al. The Ross procedure: a systematic review and meta-analysis. Circulation. 2009;119:222–8.
9. Skillington PD, Mokhles MM, Wilson W, Grigg L, Larobina M, O'Keefe M, et al. Inclusion cylinder method for aortic valve replacement utilising the Ross operation in adults with predominant aortic stenosis—99% freedom from re-operation on the aortic valve at 15 years. Glob Cardiol Sci Pract. 2013;46:383–94.
10. Bouhout I, Stevens LM, Mazine A, Poirier N, Cartier R, Demers P, et al. Long-term outcomes after elective isolated mechanical aortic valve replacement in young adults. J Thorac Cardiovasc Surg. 2014;148:1341–6.
11. Aicher D, Fries R, Rodionycheva S, Schmidt K, Langer F, Schäfers HJ. Aortic valve repair leads to a low incidence of valve-related complications. Eur J Cardiothorac Surg. 2010;37:127–32.
12. Aicher D, Holz A, Feldner S, Köllner V, Schäfers HJ. Quality of life after aortic valve surgery: replacement versus reconstruction. J Thorac Cardiovasc Surg. 2011;142:e19–24.

26 Aortic Valve Reconstruction to Treat Aortic Stenosis Using Autologous Pericardium: Ozaki Procedure

Shigeyuki Ozaki

26.1 Introduction

Tremendous advances have been made in the treatment of valvular disorders in recent years. Due to the development of new biological and mechanical valves and the evolution of valve-preserving surgical techniques, the search is on for surgical techniques that will not only improve curability but also lead to a higher quality of life. In recent years, the valvuloplasty techniques developed for mitral valves have also been used to treat aortic insufficiency (also known as aortic regurgitation or AR). However, there are still no established forms of valvuloplasty to treat aortic stenosis (AS). In our department, we perform aortic valve neo-cuspidization using autologous pericardium. This surgical technique was first used in April 2007, and by the end of December 2015, 850 patients had undergone the procedure at our hospital with extremely favorable outcomes [1–12].

S. Ozaki (✉)
Department of Cardiovascular Surgery, Toho University Ohashi Medical Center, Tokyo, Japan
e-mail: ozakis@oha.toho-u.ac.jp

26.2 Changes in Surgical Technique

An examination of the history of aortic valvuloplasty to treat AS shows that the Cavitron ultrasonic aspirator (CUSA) was used to remove calcifications from calcified cusps from the latter half of the 1980s until the 1990s. There was obvious improvement in cusp mobility, the pressure gradient across the aortic valve decreased, and the valve opening area was enlarged. However, AR worsened 2 years postoperatively, and CUSA was withdrawn from use. This device is no longer used to remove calcifications from valve cusps in patients with AS [13] unless the valve is replaced.

Aortic cusp extension is another technique that has increasingly been used to correct AR, and there have been several reports of favorable mid- and long-term outcomes. Although the technique had not been used to treat AS, Duran et al. began to use it to treat AS from the latter half of the 1980s [14]. This procedure involved the transplantation of a pericardial strip onto the leaflet after resection to achieve more complete coaptation. However, if this pericardial strip was too large, it could inadvertently occlude the coronary artery ostia, which in turn would potentially cause myocardial ischemia. For these reasons, Duran et al. withdrew the aortic cusp extension technique from use and began using a technique that involved replacing all valve leaflets with pericardium [15]. However, this technique

T. Kunihara, S. Takanashi (eds.), *Aortic Valve Preservation*,
https://doi.org/10.1007/978-981-13-2068-2_26

was only indicated for cases in which each commissure could be evenly located during the sizing stage because the size of all three leaflets created with pericardium had to be the same. This technique was therefore not indicated for bicuspid valves.

26.3 Advantages and Disadvantages

The biggest advantage of this technique is biocompatibility. No transplantation of a foreign body in the form of a prosthetic valve is required, so there are no rejection reactions, and the risk of cerebral infarction is also considered to be low.

1. No need to administer anticoagulants such as warfarin: The only oral postoperative antiplatelet agent used is aspirin, and there have been no actual cases of postoperative cerebral infarction.
2. Low pressure gradient across the aortic valve: Unlike with prosthetic valves, the effective valve opening area becomes equal to the aortic annulus; therefore, as mentioned previously, there is virtually no pressure gradient at all across the valve, even in patients with a narrow aortic annulus.
3. Saving medical resources: Autologous tissues are used during this procedure, so there are economic benefits associated with not using prosthetic valves.
4. Safety: No artificial materials are used, so there is a high level of resistance to infection.
5. Facilitation of redo surgery: There is no need to excise a firmly adherent prosthetic valve when repeat surgery is performed. Repeat surgery merely involves resection of the autologous pericardial valve.

26.4 Practical Surgical Techniques (Figs. 26.1, 26.2, 26.3, and 26.4)

The surgical technique that we use involves the resection of autologous pericardium, at least 7 × 8 cm in size, which is then processed with 0.6% glutaraldehyde for 10 min (Fig. 26.1). After resecting the calcified leaflets, calcified areas of the annulus are removed using a CUSA. Next, we use our original cusp sizer to measure the circumferential distance between each commissure (Fig. 26.1). Using our original template, glutaraldehyde-treated autologous pericardium is used to create cusps that correspond to these measured values (Fig. 26.2). During this process, 5-mm wing extensions are created at both edges of the leaflets (Fig. 26.2).

The leaflets are sutured directly to the annulus using a 4-0 polypropylene suture with 13-mm 1/2 circle needle as shown in Fig. 26.3. Finally, the wing extensions are fixed to 5 × 10-mm pledgets on the external aorta using a 4-0 polypropylene suture with 17-mm 1/2 circle needle (Fig. 26.4).

26.5 Personal Tips

Cusps of the same size will always be created when following the approach of Duran et al. He estimated the cusp free-edge length from the annulus diameter during valvuloplasty using pericardium [15, 16]. However, based on personal experience [4], the intercommissural distance was the same for all three cusps in 13% of cases, for two leaflets alone in 57% of cases, and every distance was different in 30% of cases. Based on this knowledge, it is doubtful that three cusps of identical size can be sutured to three native cusp insertion lines of different lengths. In addition, as shown in Fig. 26.5, the cusp contact point is lower than the vertical position of the commissure, and there are individual differences in height. Thus, if the cusp contact point is low, then the cusp free-edge length will increase, and when the cusp contact point is high, then the cusp free-edge length will shorten. It is quite difficult to derive the cusp free-edge length when taking everything from the annulus diameter to these factors into consideration.

Our method includes two essential points:

1. It is possible to derive the cusp free-edge length from each intercommissural distance.
2. The new pericardial cusp contact point is elevated to the height of a line connecting the commissures.

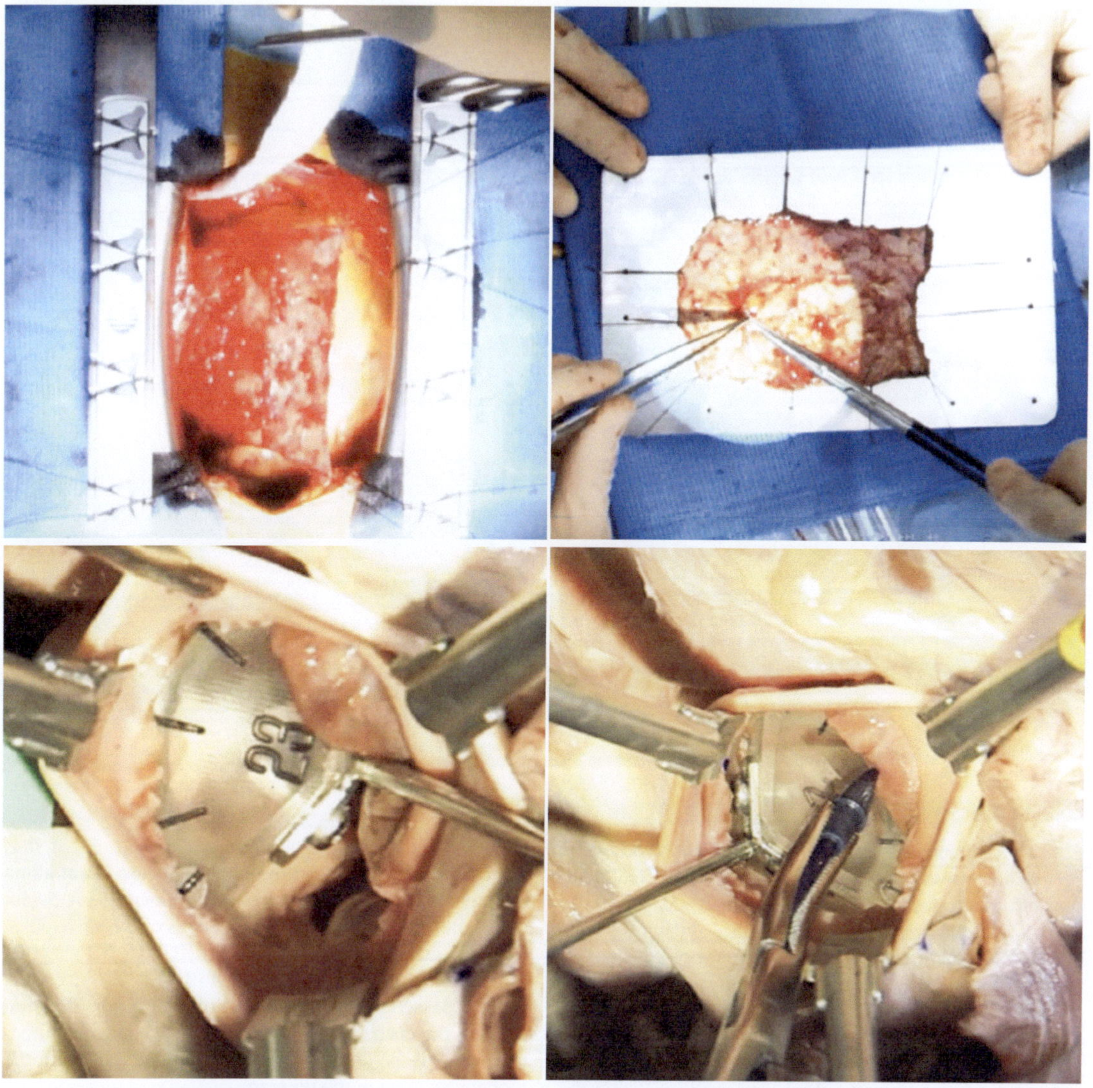

Fig. 26.1 Harvesting of the autologous pericardium and measurement of the intercommisural distance. Upper column: (1) The autologous pericardium is harvested at a size of at least 7 × 8 cm. (2) Before harvesting the pericardium, excess adipose tissue is removed using an ultrasound scalpel. (3) When harvesting the pericardium, gauze is placed between the pericardium and the heart to prevent myocardial injury. (4) The pericardium is fixed to a plate with sutures to prevent it from shrinking during the glutaraldehyde treatment. (5) The pericardium should always be fixed in such a way that the rough surface is facing upward during this process. (6) The shape of the pericardium is drawn onto a piece of paper, which is used at the end of surgery to cut a piece from a sheet of expanded polytetrafluoroethylene for repair of the pericardial defect. Lower column: (1) The intercommissural distance is measured, and at this time, the circumferential length connecting the commissures, and not the length of the annulus, is measured. (2) First, one part of the sizer is firmly attached to the commissures on one side, and another part of the sizer is used to confirm whether it will reach the contralateral commissure. (3) This is repeated until the appropriate size is measured. (4) If the measured value falls between two sizes, then we use the larger size. (5) Once the size has been determined, the midpoint of each annulus is marked

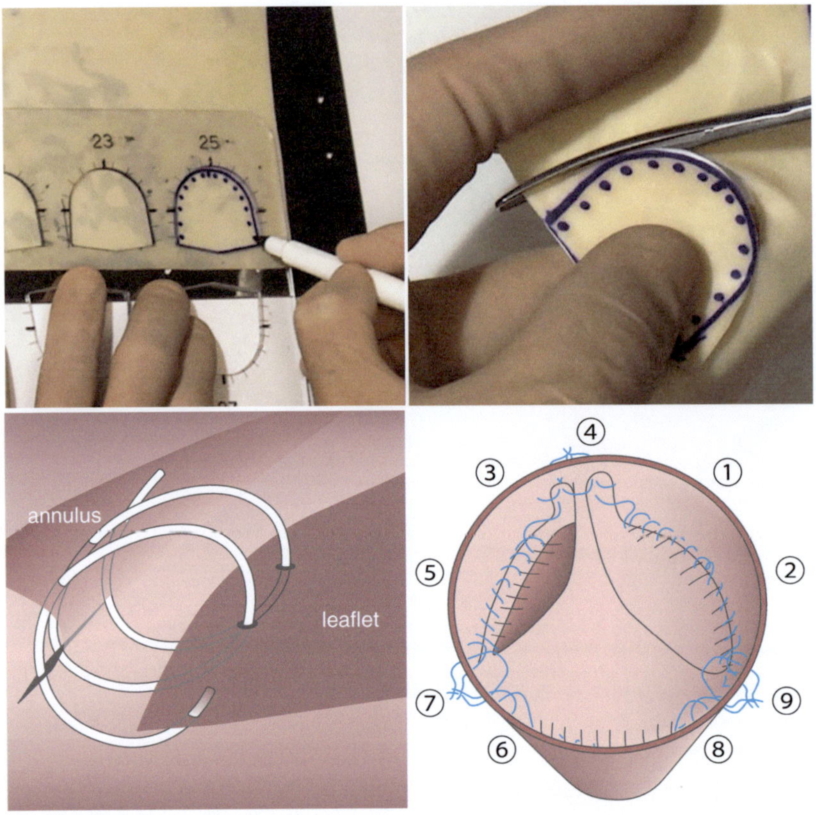

Fig. 26.2 Preparation and suturing of the autologous pericardial valve. Upper column: (1) After treatment, moisture is removed from the pericardium, and it is placed onto a plate with the smooth surface facing upward because it is not possible to draw on the rough surface. (2) A surgical skin marker is used to draw the leaflet along the window used for the template, and dots are also marked. (3) There are holes on both sides of the template for a 5-mm wing extension, which are also marked. (4) Large cusps are created from the thick pericardium facing the diaphragm. (5) The pericardium is easier to cut if it is glued to the paper protecting it. (6) The cusp is cut along the outside of the line that has been drawn. (7) A 5-mm wing extension is created on both edges of the valve cusp. Lower column: (1) The cusp is sutured in such a way that it is adherent to the annulus inferiorly. (2) The needle is usually passed from a superior to an inferior direction through the cusp, and from an inferior to superior direction through the annulus. (3) Each cusp is sutured in the sequence shown in the diagram

These points offer three advantages.

1. Enlargement of the coaptation zone.
2. The cusp contact point and each commissure will be in the same plane, there will be a 1:1 match between the intercommisural distance and the cusp free-edge length, and it is easy to derive the cusp free-edge length.
3. With the cusp contact point and each commissure in the same plane, when the leaflets are closed, they will support one another at the height of the commissure, which reduces the stress placed on the commissure.

Based on the above, the intercommissural distance is believed to define the cusp free-edge length, and a method was devised to create cusps based on the measured values [4].

26.6 Outcomes of Aortic Reconstruction to Date

Outcomes of aortic reconstruction to treat aortic valve disorders in our institution (Fig. 26.6).

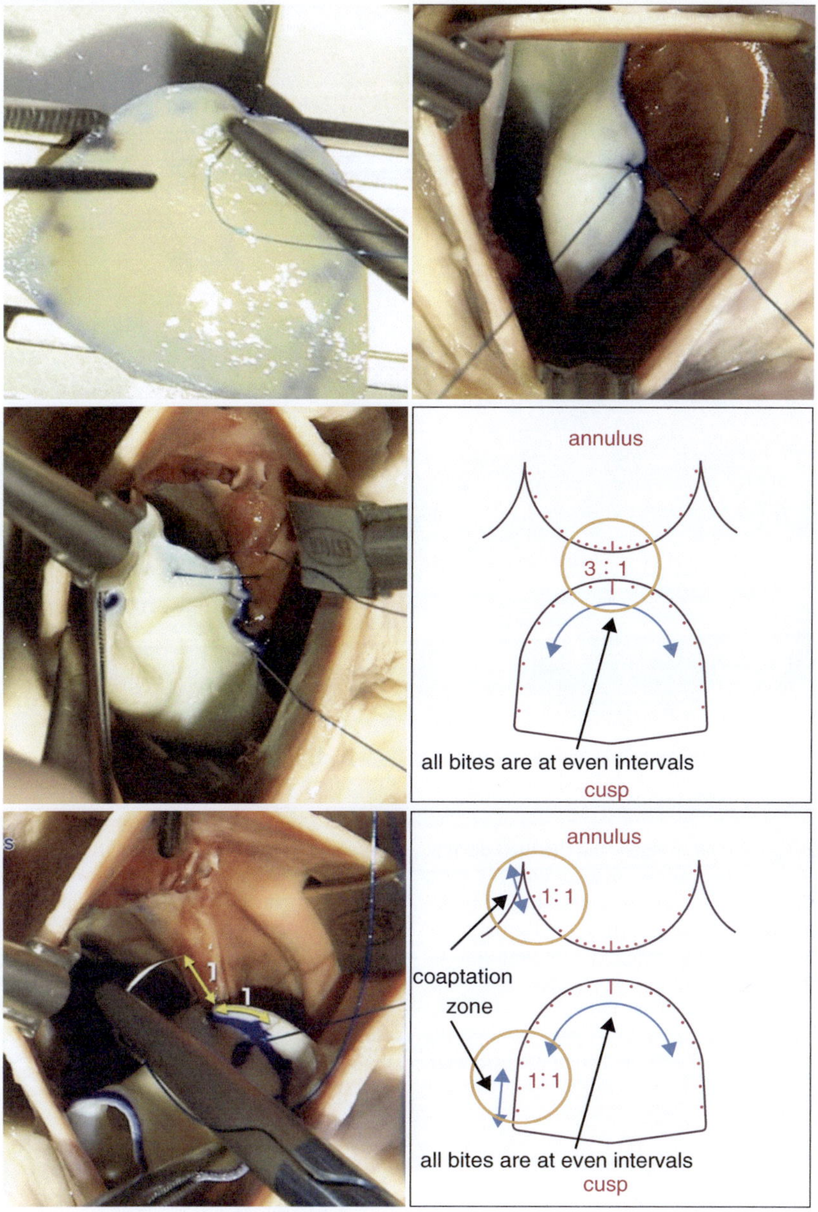

Fig. 26.3 Sequence of suturing the cusps. Upper column: (1) The cusps are sutured using a 4-0 polypropylene suture with a 13-mm 1/2 circle needle. (2) The smooth surface of the leaflet faces the left ventricle. The surface with the dots and lines drawn onto it will become part of the left ventricle. (3) First, the needle is passed through the center point of the cusp and the corresponding center point of the annulus. Then, after the cusp has descended into the left ventricle, three knots are created. Middle column: (1) The suturing continues as shown in the diagram. (2) Suturing is performed at equivalent intervals that correspond to the dotted line on the side facing the cusp. (3) The suture intervals on the side facing the cusp are created close to the base of the annulus and in such a way that they are 1/3 (1:3) of the intervals between the cusp sutures. (4) It is important to suture in such a way that the leaflet is firmly gathered close to the base of the annulus. Lower column: (1) The remaining cusp length is confirmed after some suturing has been performed at a ratio of 1:3. (2) During the part of the procedure when the remaining cusp length is either equal or slightly longer than the remaining annulus, the suture interval along the annulus is the same as that along the cusp. (3) The final point of suture insertion into the cusp is always 5 mm away from the margin. (4) If the dots have been marked within 5 mm of the margin, this should be ignored and the suture should be passed through the cusp at 5 mm from the margin. (5) After the final suture insertion point has been passed, the needle is straightened and used to pass through the aortic wall. The point at which the needle enters is 2–3 mm inferior to the commissure

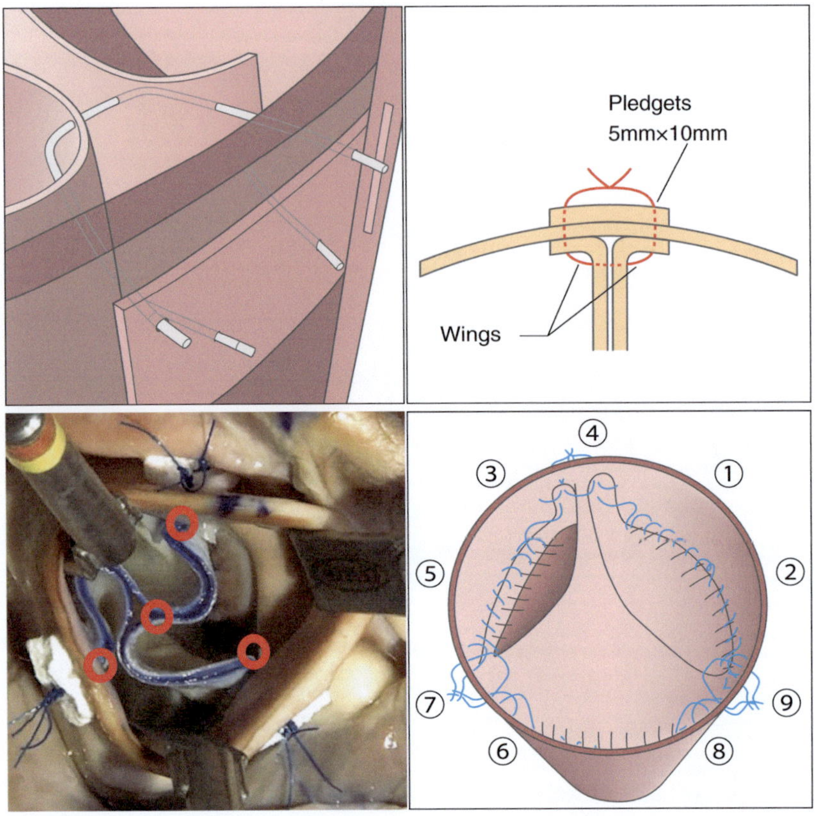

Fig. 26.4 Creating the commissures and the final design. Upper column: (1) A 4-0 polypropylene suture with a 17-mm 1/2 circle needle is used to create the commissures. (2) A new suture is passed as shown in the diagram. (3) This suture is passed at a middle height between the cusp margin and the final insertion point above the cusp. This is approximately 2.5 mm above the margin. (4) When the above-mentioned suture is used to pass through the aortic wall, four sutures will exit the external aortic wall. These four sutures are passed through 5 × 10 mm pledgets and ligated at the external aortic wall. Lower column: (1) The three commissures are created in the sequence shown in the diagram on the right (right coronary cusp—left coronary cusp—non-coronary cusp). (2) The three cusps are adjusted before closure of the aortic wall to form a windmill shape. (3) The three commissures and the middle contact point of the three leaflets are adjusted to lie in the same plane

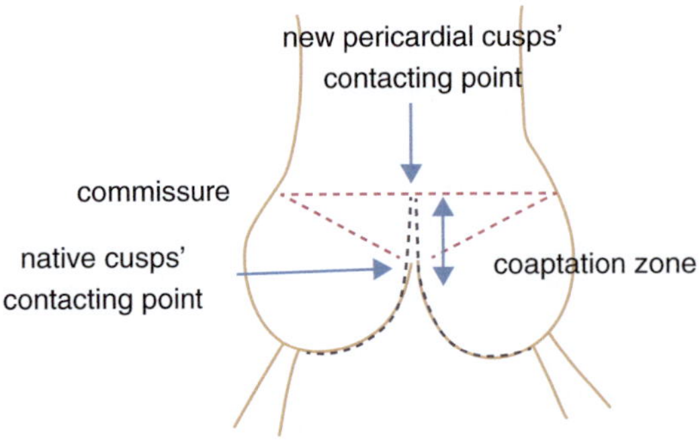

Fig. 26.5 Basic idea of aortic valve reconstruction

1. Period: From April 2007 to December 2015
2. There were 534 patients with aortic stenosis (AS), 254 with aortic regurgitation (AR), 61 with ASR, 19 with infective endocarditis, and five with a prior aortic valve procedure (including 444 men and 406 women). Among these patients, 224 valves were bicuspid, 28 were unicuspid, and two were quadricuspid.
3. Median patient age: 71 (range 13–90) years.
4. Mean preoperative annulus diameter: 20.9 ± 3.3 mm.

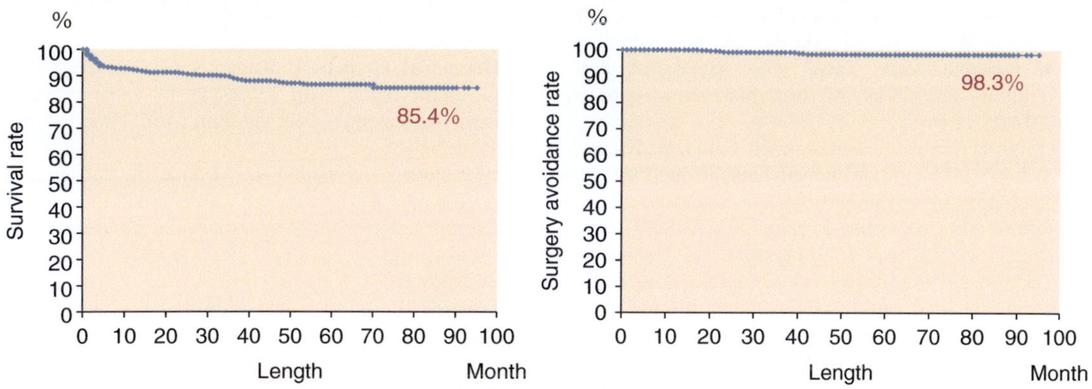

Fig. 26.6 Outcomes of aortic reconstruction to treat aortic valve disorders in our institution

5. Mean aortic cross-clamping time: 106.8 ± 27.5 min, mean cardiopulmonary bypass time: 150.4 ± 30.4 min.
6. Survival at 118 months: 85.9%, Freedom from reoperation at 118 months: 95.8%.

26.7 Conclusion

We have accumulated 10 years of experience with autologous pericardial aortic neo-cuspidization since April 2007. The freedom from reoperation rate is extremely favorable at 95.8%. There is no need for a prosthetic valve or for anticoagulants, which means infrequent onset of complications such as cerebral infarction. This surgical technique can also save medical resources. For these reasons, this surgery has been performed in all Asian countries (including China, Malaysia, Vietnam, South Korea, India, Thailand, and Turkey), Europe (UK, Germany, Italy, Belgium, Switzerland, Poland, Russia, and Ukraine), and the US (including at the Cleveland Clinic, Columbia University, the University of Pittsburgh, Boston Children's Hospital, UPMC, DeBakey VA Houston, etc.). It has received a high degree of interest from around the world, and there will be initiatives to develop more durable materials and continued communication from Japan to the rest of the world.

References

1. Ozaki S. Cardiac valvulopathy. In: Kusano E, Tabei K, editors. Cardiovascular complications and countermeasure in dialysis therapy. Tokyo: Nihon Medical Center; 2008. p. 161–74.
2. Ozaki S. Valvulopathy. Jpn J Clin Dial. 2008;24: 1643–52.
3. Ozaki, S. Aortic valvuloplasty using an original valve leaf former for aortic valve disease. In: Yamaguchi T, ed. Ann Rev (Circulatory Organ) . Tokyo: Chugai Igakusha; 2010. p.319–25.
4. Ozaki S, Kawase I, Yamashita H, Uchida S, Nozawa Y, Matsuyama T, et al. Aortic valve reconstruction using self-developed aortic valve plasty system in aortic valve disease. Interact Cardiovasc Thorac Surg. 2011;12:550–3.
5. Yamashita H, Ozaki S, Iwasaki K, Kawase I, Nozawa Y, Umezu M. Tensile strength of human pericardium treated with glutaraldehyde. Ann Thorac Cardiovasc Surg. 2012;18:434–7.
6. Kawase I, Ozaki S, Yamashita H, Uchida S, Nozawa Y, Matsuyama T, et al. Aortic valve reconstruction of unicuspid aortic valve by tricuspidization using autologous pericardium. Ann Thorac Surg. 2012;94:1180–4.
7. Kawase I, Ozaki S, Yamashita H, Uchida S, Nozawa Y, Matsuyama T, et al. Aortic valve reconstruction with autologous pericardium for dialysis patients. Interact Cardiovasc Thorac Surg. 2013;16:738–42.
8. Ozaki S, Kawase I, Yamashita H, Uchida S, Nozawa Y, Takatoh M, et al. A total of 404 cases of aortic valve reconstruction with glutaraldehyde-treated autologous pericardium. J Thorac Cardiovasc Surg. 2014;147:301–6.
9. Ozaki S, Kawase I, Yamashita H, Uchida S, Nozawa Y, Takatoh M, et al. Aortic valve reconstruction using autologous pericardium for patients aged less than 80 years. Asian Cardiovasc Thorac Ann. 2014;22:903–8.

10. Ozaki S, Kawase I, Yamashita H, Uchida S, Nozawa Y, Takatoh M, Hagiwara S, Kiyohara N. Reconstruction of bicuspid aortic valve with autologous pericardium—usefulness of tricuspidization. Circ J. 2014;78:1144–51.
11. Ozaki S, Kawase I, Yamashita H, Uchida S, Nozawa Y, Takatoh M, et al. Aortic valve reconstruction using autologous pericardium for patients aged less than 60 years. J Thorac Cardiovasc Surg. 2014;148:934–8.
12. Ozaki S, Kawase I, Yamashita H, Uchida S, Takatoh M, Hagiwara S, et al. Aortic valve reconstruction using autologous pericardium for aortic stenosis. Circ J. 2015;79:1504–10.
13. Kellner HJ, Pracki P, Hildebrandt A, Binner C, Eisele G, Struck E. Aortic valve debridement by ultrasonic surgical aspirator in degenerative, aortic valve stenosis: follow-up with Doppler echocardiography. Eur J Cardiothorac Surg. 1996;10:498–504.
14. Duran CM, Gometza B, Kumar N, Gallo R, Bjornstad K. From aortic cusp extension to valve replacement with stentless pericardium. Ann Thorac Surg. 1995;60:428–32.
15. Al Halees Z, Al Shahid M, Al Sanei A, Sallehuddin A, Duran C. Up to 16 years follow-up of aortic valve reconstruction with pericardium: a stentless readily available cheap valve? Eur J Cardiothorac Surg. 2005;28:200–5.
16. Chan KMJ, Rahman-Haley S, Mittal TK, Gavino JA, Dreyfus GD. Truly stentless autologous pericardial aortic valve replacement: an alternative to standard aortic valve replacement. J Thorac Cardiovasc Surg. 2011;141:276–83.

27 ONE-POINT ADVICE: Creating a Morphological Template for Autologous Pericardial Cusps

Masaru Sawazaki

27.1 Introduction

Many cardiovascular surgeons have by now attempted aortic valve replacement using autologous pericardium, although the only documented long-term outcomes involve the Duran method [1] described by Al Halees et al. [2] (Fig. 27.1). As shown in Fig. 27.1, the glutaraldehyde-treated autologous pericardium is trimmed and used to create the aortic valve. Their outcomes for 65 subjects with a mean follow-up period of 10.5 years and up to 16 years revealed that endocarditis had occurred in seven subjects (10.8%), which was relatively frequent. However, if we exclude endocarditis, then the freedom from structural valve deterioration (SVD) was 80 ± 5% at 10 years and 58 ± 9% at 15 years. These valves therefore do not compare favorably to prosthetic valves. However, when we consider that these outcomes are from 30 years ago, when echocardiography was in its infancy, we believe that surgical outcomes could further be enhanced by improving surgical precision.

Song's group [3] from Korea and Ozaki et al. [4] from Japan reported favorable short-term outcomes of the autologous pericardial valves. The incidence of endocarditis after the Ozaki procedure was low at 0.5%, so this surgical technique is considered to be beneficial because there are few factors, such as turbulent flows or regurgitant jets on the autologous pericardial valve, that would result in infection. A study of 404 subjects reported favorable short-term outcomes, with the maximum pressure gradient of 13.8 ± 10.2 mmHg at 3.5 years and the freedom from reoperation of 96.2% at 53 months [3]. However, the process of glutaraldehyde fixation was the same as previous reports when autologous pericardium was used, and the risk of the onset of SVD increases after 10 years, so at present, the procedure is believed to be well indicated in patients aged ≥70 years and particularly in patients with a small aortic root.

From a clinical perspective, the Ozaki method results in a large valvular area and favorable short-term outcomes, so there are no specific points of issue. However, when we examine the newly created aortic valve during echocardiogra-

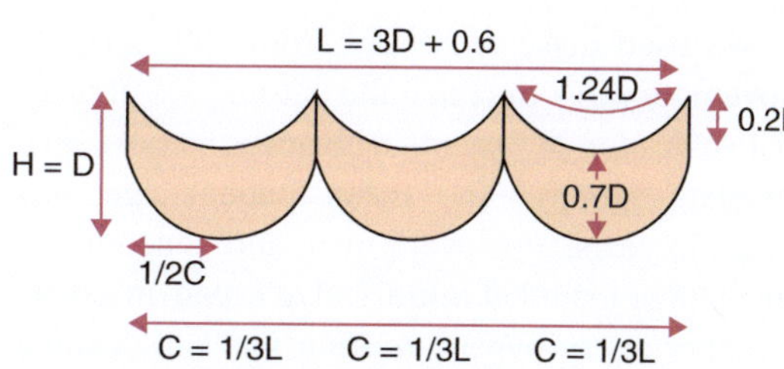

Fig. 27.1 Duran method template. *C* width of each leaflet, *D* annulus diameter, *H* patch height, *L* patch width

M. Sawazaki (✉)
Department of Cardiovascular Surgery,
Valvular Disease Centre, Komaki City Hospital,
Komaki, Aichi, Japan
e-mail: sawamasa7007bb@nifty.com

T. Kunihara, S. Takanashi (eds.), *Aortic Valve Preservation*,
https://doi.org/10.1007/978-981-13-2068-2_27

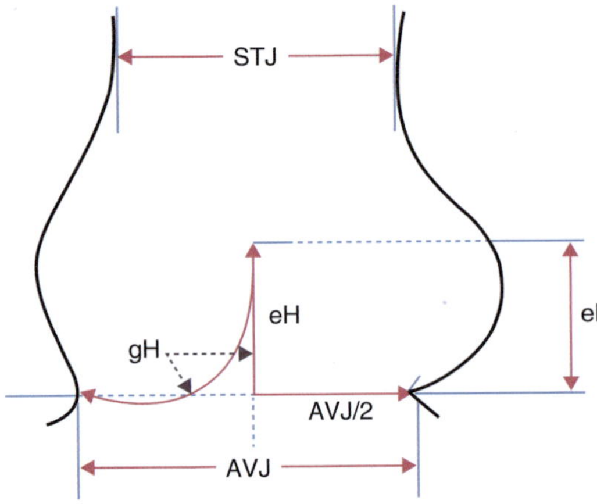

Fig. 27.2 gH = eH + AVJ/2. *AVJ* aorto-ventricular junction, *eH* effective height, *gH* geometric height, *STJ* sinotubular junction

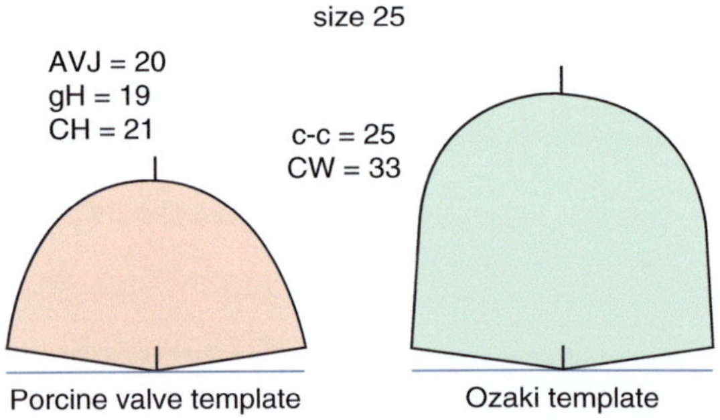

Fig. 27.3 Differences between the porcine valve template and Ozaki templates. *AVJ* aortoventricular junction, *c–c* intercommissural distance, *CH* height of the template cusps, *CW* width of the template cusps, *gH* geometric height

phy, we find that the cusp height is unnecessarily high. This is referred to as the safety margin, which is established to prevent aortic valve regurgitation, although the cusps are clearly larger than those that make up normal human or porcine aortic valves. For this reason, the author measured porcine cusps and derived the following formula for ideal leaflet height:

geometric height = effective height + annulus diameter/2 (Fig. 27.2).

The cusp height is then achieved by adding a 1-mm seam allowance, and a 1-mm wrinkle zone. The cusp width is approximately the same as that determined during the Ozaki procedure, but if we empirically designate the intercommissural distance as c–c, then the cusp width can be derived using the following formula: c–c/2 + 17.5 mm + seam allowance (1 mm × 2) (Fig. 27.2). A unique template was then created using this formula (Fig. 27.3).

We used these templates from July 2013 to November 2017 to create the autologous pericardial valves for 78 patients with aortic stenosis (the template group). The mean patient age was 78 ± 6.2 years, 36% were men, and concomitant procedures included mitral valve repair in seven, coronary artery bypass grafting in 11, ascending aorta replacement in 5, the maze procedure in one, and tricuspid annuloplasty in one patient. We designated nine patients who underwent the Ozaki procedure at our hospital as the control group.

27.2 Results

None of the patients had aortic regurgitation (AR) graded higher than mild, and all aortic valves were reconstructed. The mean postoperative pressure gradient was 5.9 ± 1.0 mmHg in the template group and 6.3 ± 0.6 mmHg in the control group ($p = 0.08$), with no significant difference between the two groups. The effective height assessed by echocardiography was 11.5 ± 0.5 mm in the template group and 16.6 ± 0.8 mm in the control group ($p < 0.001$), showing that the cusp height was lowered by approximately 5 mm. This is close to the values for normal human aortic valves.

27.3 Discussion

It goes without saying that the Ozaki method results in favorable clinical outcomes and is becoming an established form of autologous pericardial valve replacement surgery. However, autologous pericardial valves were indicated in 115 of 404 subjects to treat regurgitant lesions amenable to valvuloplasty using autologous pericardial patch. Meanwhile, patients treated using the template method have only been followed up for a short period of time, and long-term outcomes are still unknown. However, despite the fact that the height of the autologous pericardial cusps in the template group was already low, there has been no further restriction at 1 year postoperatively. By approximating the size of the normal human aortic valves, we believe that this technique offers new potential for aortic valvuloplasty, such as the option to perform valvuloplasty of a single cusp alone. Because the cusps are pericardium, they will eventually deteriorate. Also, the patients will be older. When selecting transcatheter aortic valve implantation, Ozaki's cusp is too high, and have the risk of coronary occlusion. On the contrary, our cusp never reaches the coronary orifice.

27.4 Conclusion

A morphological template for autologous pericardial valves was created by making reference to porcine valves. We created unique templates for clinical application and obtained favorable early outcomes. The long-term outcomes with sufficient case load remain to be confirmed.

References

1. Duran CM, Gallo R, Kumar N. Aortic valve replacement with autologous pericardium: surgical technique. J Card Surg. 1995;10:1–9.
2. AL Halees Z, AL Shahid M, AL Sanei A, Sallehuddin A, Duran C. Up to 16 years follow-up of aortic valve reconstruction with pericardium: a stentless readily available cheap valve? Eur J Cardiothorac Surg. 2005;28:200–5.
3. Liu X, Han L, Song Z, Tan M, Gong D, Xu Z. Aortic valve replacement with autologous pericardium: long-term follow-up of 15 patients and in vivo histopathological changes of autologous pericardium. Interact Cardiovasc Thorac Surg. 2013;16:123–8.
4. Ozaki S, Kawase I, Yamashita H, Uchida S, Nozawa Y, Takatoh M, et al. A total of 404 cases of aortic vakve reconstruction with glutaraldehyde-treated autologous pericardium. J Thorac Cardiovasc Surg. 2014;147:301–6.

Part III

Case Study: What to Do in Each Particular Case?

How to Manage Patients with Low Geometric Cusp Height

28

Atsushi Shimizu and Shuichiro Takanashi

Patient	44-year-old man, body height: 178.8 cm, body weight: 98.3 kg, body surface area: 2.17 m^2
Medical history	Hypertension, dyslipidemia
History of present illness	A heart murmur was indicated during a physical examination, and detailed investigations led to a diagnosis of mild aortic root dilatation, severe aortic regurgitation (AR), and left ventricular enlargement, so the patient was referred for surgical management.
Preoperative transthoracic and transesophageal echocardiogram (TTE, TEE) (Fig. 28.1)	Grade IV AR (left ventricular diastolic diameter during diastole: 61 mm, during systole: 40 mm), aortoventricular junction (AVJ): 27 mm, sinus of Valsalva diameter (SN): 40 mm, sinotubular junction (STJ): 31 mm, geometric height (gH) of the non-coronary cusp (NCC): 20 mm, left coronary cusp (LCC): 20 mm, right coronary cusp (RCC): 11 mm (19 mm during systole). There was bending at the center of the RCC, with prolapse and uneven regurgitation from the center of the valve to the anterior leaflet of the mitral valve.
Preoperative computed tomography (CT) scan (4D CT) (Fig. 28.2)	AVJ: 29 mm, SN: 44 mm, STJ: 36 mm, gH of the NCC: 21 mm, LCC: 20 mm, RCC: 16 mm, with bending at the center of the RCC also observed.

A. Shimizu (✉) · S. Takanashi
Department of Cardiovascular Surgery, Sakakibara Heart Institute, Fuchu, Tokyo, Japan
e-mail: ashimizu@shi.heart.or.jp

28.1 Surgical Technique

Replacement of the ascending aorta, aortic root remodeling, and external ring annuloplasty.

28.2 Surgical Method

We performed a median sternotomy and initiated cardiopulmonary bypass with aortic cannulation in the aortic arch and bicaval venous drainage. After cross-clamping the aorta, we dissected the aortic root and took intraoperative measurements (AVJ: 29 mm, gH of the NCC: 22 mm, LCC: 19 mm, RCC: 23 mm, the height of the NCC-LCC commissure [Brussels height]: 27 mm).

The free margin of the RCC near the LCC-RCC commissure was elongated. The fibrous band and a pouch were seen at the middle portion of the cusp and at the free margin, respectively. We performed the aortic root remodeling procedure using a 26-mm graft with sinuses. We measured the effective height (eH) and

T. Kunihara, S. Takanashi (eds.), *Aortic Valve Preservation*, https://doi.org/10.1007/978-981-13-2068-2_28

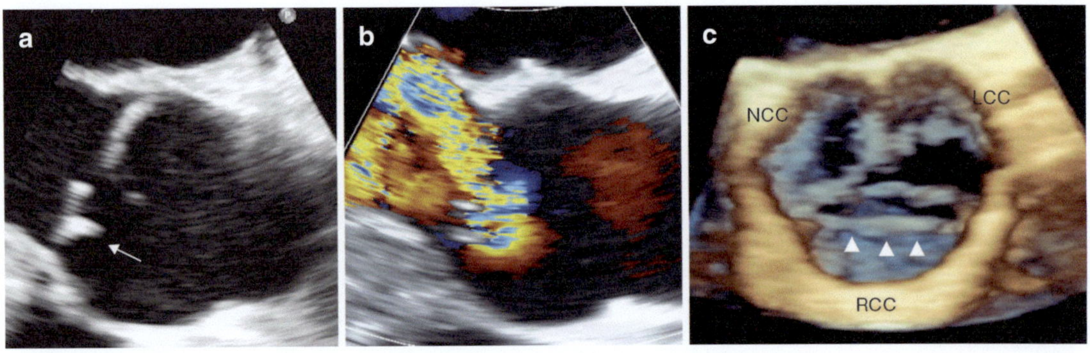

Fig. 28.1 Preoperative TEE. (**a**) Long-axis view. RCC prolapse with bending at the center of the valve (white arrow). (**b**) Color long-axis view. Uneven, severe AR from the center of the valve to the anterior leaflet of the mitral valve. (**c**) 3D view of the aortic valve, bending of the center of the RCC (three white arrowheads)

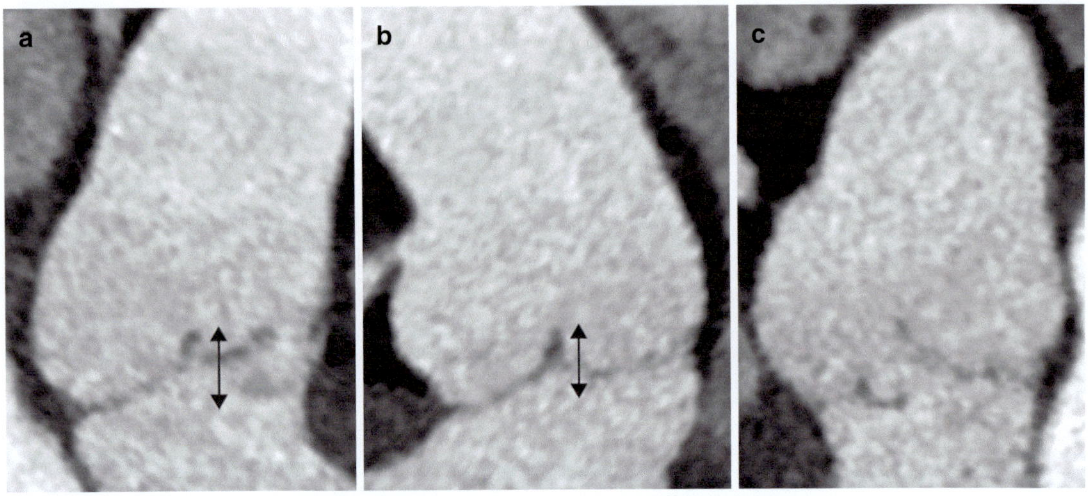

Fig. 28.2 Preoperative 4D CT. (**a**) NCC. gH: 21 mm, effective height (eH): 10 mm. (**b**) LCC. gH: 20 mm, eH: 10 mm. (**c**) RCC. gH: 16 mm, eH: Unable to measure due to prolapse

performed central plication of the LCC and RCC, but the eH of the RCC was still not elevated adequately and there was residual prolapse of the RCC on the LCC side. We then used an autologous pericardial patch treated with 0.6% glutaraldehyde to reinforce approximately one-half of the terminal edge of the RCC closest to the LCC. We performed additional central plication of the RCC, which resulted in an eH of 8 mm (Fig. 28.3). We used a ring created from the same 26-mm graft for external ring annuloplasty. After reattachment of the left and right coronary arteries and distal anastomosis, the aorta was unclamped. The patient was weaned from cardiopulmonary bypass uneventfully, and the intraoperative echocardiogram showed no residual AR.

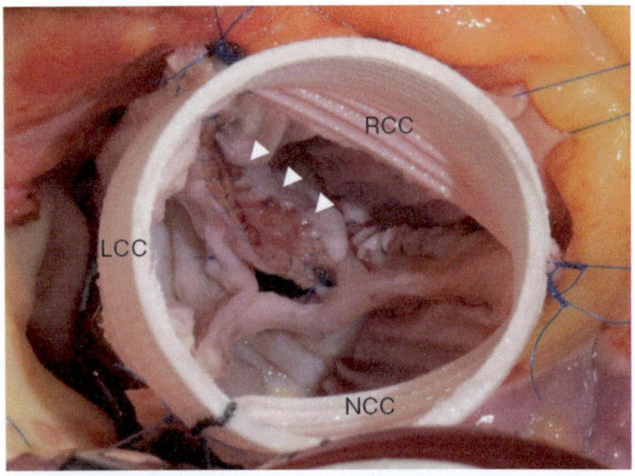

Fig. 28.3 Intraoperative photograph. Prolapse of the RCC was managed by sewing a concave lens-shaped pericardial patch to the RCC on the side facing the LCC (arrowheads). Additional central plication of the LCC and RCC was performed, resulting in an eH of 8 mm

28.3 Personal Tips

When using patches to recreate leaflets, there is a danger of suture dehiscence when you try to suture to a thin, healthy leaflet and avoid the diseased leaflet. Therefore, the bending fibrous band can be used for suturing. If the suture line extends to the thin leaflet, then use a fine suture, e.g., 7–0. Interlocking sutures should be used as well as multiple sutures, which will prevent scarring and contraction of the suture line.

28.4 Postoperative Course

The patient was extubated on the day of surgery and discharged from the intensive care unit on the next day after surgery. The patient was discharged ambulatory from the hospital on postoperative day 9.

28.5 Postoperative Echocardiogram

AR: trivial, AVJ: 22 mm, SN: 32 mm, STJ: 26 mm, eH: 9 mm (Fig. 28.4).

28.6 Postoperative 4D CT

AVJ: 25 mm, SN: 35 mm, STJ: 31 mm, eH: 8 mm (Fig. 28.5).

28.7 Key Points

An objective assessment of leaflet size is important to perform aortic valvuloplasty successfully. Although leaflet size can be evaluated using gH, the free margin length, and eH, we believe that gH is the most reliable parameter due to the ease of intraoperative measurement and good reproducibility. Schäfers et al. reported that patients with intraoperative gH measurements of ≤16 mm for tricuspid valves and ≤19 mm for bicuspid valves required aortic valve replacement in the early postoperative period, thus they proposed these values as gH cut-off values for aortic valvuloplasty.

In our case, preoperative measurement of the gH of the RCC, which was subject to bending, was 11–16 mm and was expected to be short. Although intraoperative measurement showed an adequate size of 23 mm, we were unable to obtain favorable leaflet morphology by means of central plication

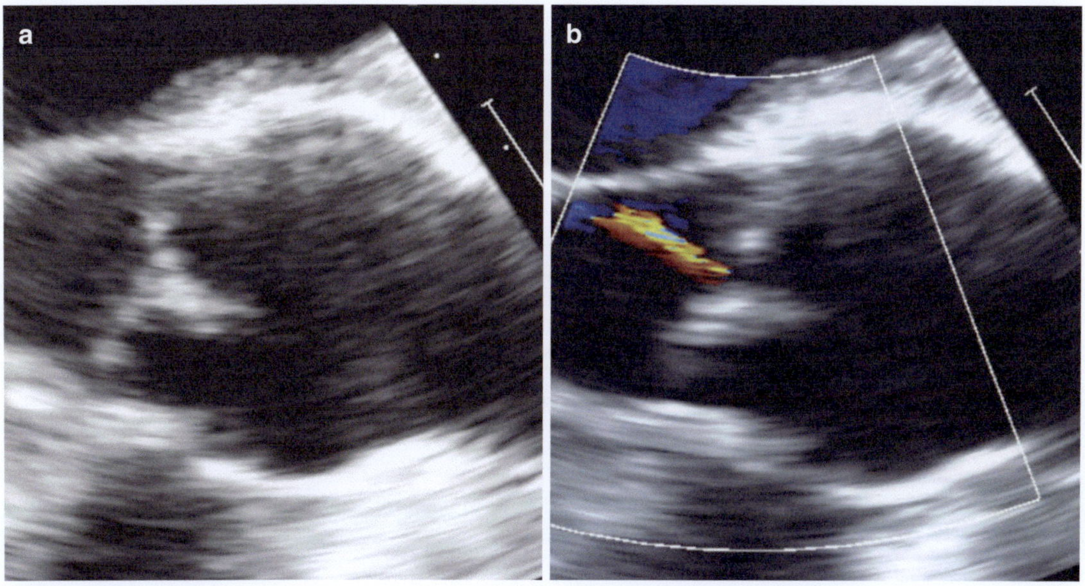

Fig. 28.4 Postoperative TEE. (**a**) Long-axis view. RCC prolapse has disappeared, and favorable coaptation has been achieved. (**b**) Color long-axis view. A trivial regurgitation jet straight from the center of the valve is present

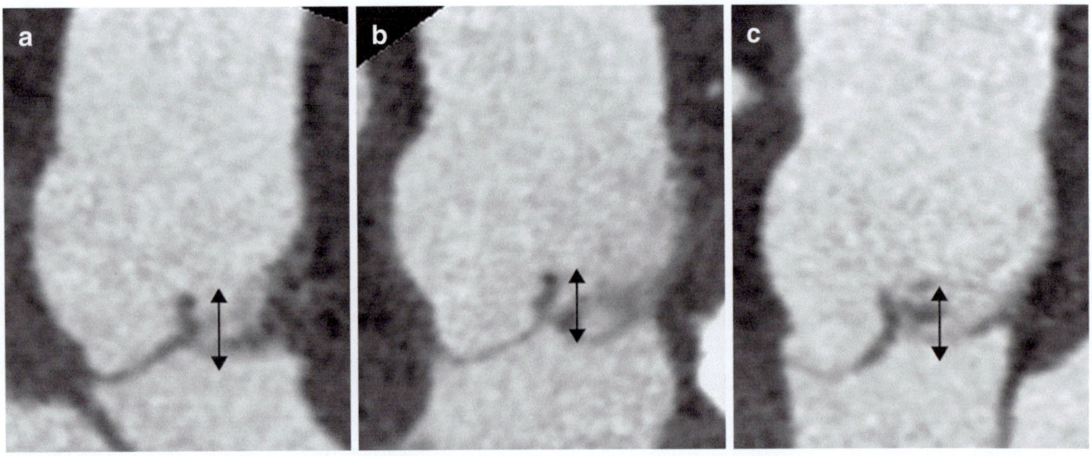

Fig. 28.5 Postoperative 4D CT. (**a**) NCC. gH: 19 mm, eH: 8 mm. (**b**) LCC. gH: 20 mm, eH: 8 mm. (**c**) RCC. gH: 20 mm, eH: 8 mm

alone. This suggests that when the leaflets are subject to deformities such as bending, the functional gH is shorter than the intraoperative gH measurement. It may be possible to predict gH from the preoperative, off-pump measurement. In addition, errors may occur during intraoperative gH measurement due to the leaflets being in an expanded or extended state. We believe it is important to make decisions by taking preoperative echocardiographic or CT measurement together into account.

If the gH is found to be low, and it is difficult to select an appropriate graft size for root replacement, then a smaller size should be selected, and the eH value should be targeted at 6–8 mm. The target eH value of 9 mm proposed by Schäfers et al. is focused on patients with a gH of 20–22 mm. If the gH is low, excessive adjustment will not result in an increased eH but in the curling of the free margin laterally, which is associated with increased central regurgitation. This is disadvantageous when the aim is to control regurgitation.

If it is not possible to control regurgitation despite this, consider extending the leaflet with the smallest possible autologous pericardium. However, when using autologous pericardium, it is important to examine the leaflets carefully, use the possibly smallest amount, pay attention to the patch design and suturing method, and prevent contraction of the suture line.

Finally, it should always be borne in mind that it is difficult to perform valvuloplasty in patients with a low gH, and it is important not to hesitate to switch to valve replacement while taking the patient's age into account.

How to Manage a Stenosed Bicuspid Valve

29

Kohei Abe and Kohei Kawazoe

29.1 Introduction

We believe that most patients with aortic valve stenosis are suitable candidates for valve replacement in the current era. However, valvuloplasty is indicated in some cases, such as young patients who will require reoperation for prosthetic valves over the long term and suffer from concomitant stenosis due to localized sclerotic lesions. The methods for valvuloplasty include decalcification and slicing of the sclerotic lesion, and partial cusp replacement using tissue such as the autologous pericardium. We present two applicable cases.

Patient 1	61-year-old woman, body height: 151 cm, body weight: 49 kg, body surface area (BSA): 1.44 m^2
Medical history	Rheumatic fever at the age of 16 years, hypertension from the age of 49 years, and hyperlipidemia from the age of 55 years.
History of present illness	The patient was admitted to our hospital when she was 16 years old for a high fever. She was diagnosed as having rheumatic fever and has been followed up on an outpatient basis since then. In 2006, an echocardiogram revealed a bicuspid aortic valve and moderate aortic regurgitation (AR). The AR became severe in 2011, and she fulfilled the indications for surgery as she was experiencing palpitations during exertion.
Preoperative echocardiogram	Severe AR, moderate aortic stenosis (AS), maximum aortic valve velocity (Vmax): 3.3 m/s, maximum/mean transvalvular gradient (AVG): 45/27 mmHg, aortoventricular junction (AVJ): 24 mm, sinus of Valsalva (SV): 36 mm, sino-tubular junction (STJ): 35 mm, left ventricular diastolic/systolic diameter (LVDd/LVDs): 51/34 mm, left ventricular ejection fraction (LVEF) 68%, bicuspid aortic valve with fusion of the right/left coronary cusp (RCC/LCC) and sclerosis of the raphe.
Preoperative computed tomography (CT) scan	No significant stenosis of the coronary arteries. Ascending aorta dilated with a maximum diameter of 52 mm.

K. Abe (✉)
Cardiovascular Center, St. Luke's International Hospital, Tokyo, Japan
e-mail: koabe@luke.ac.jp

K. Kawazoe
Cardiovascular Disease Center, Kansai Medical University Medical Center, Osaka, Japan

T. Kunihara, S. Takanashi (eds.), *Aortic Valve Preservation*,
https://doi.org/10.1007/978-981-13-2068-2_29

29.2 Surgical Technique

Replacement of the ascending aorta and aortic valvuloplasty (creation of a tricuspid valve and use of the autologous pericardium).

29.3 Surgical Method

We performed a median sternotomy, cannulated the ascending aorta, placed one drainage cannula in the right atrium and established cardiopulmonary bypass. We cross-clamped the aorta and then examined the aortic valve. The raphe between the RCC and LCC was sclerosed, and the intercommissural distances were equivalent, with the NCC measuring 35 mm, the RCC measuring 33 mm, and the NCC measuring 33 mm. The sclerotic portion, including the raphe, was resected, and we replaced this portion with the autologous pericardium, which was treated with 0.7% glutaraldehyde, as shown in Figs. 29.1 and 29.2. The new commissure was adjusted to lie at the same height as the other two commissures. The annulus measured 27 mm, so subcommissural annuloplasty was performed between the NCC/RCC and NCC/LCC. The height of each leaflet was confirmed, and central plication of the NCC was performed to yield an effective height of 8 mm. We then replaced the ascending aorta and concluded the procedure.

29.4 Personal Tips

If the autologous pericardium is used as a free margin, it is beneficial to use pericardium treated with glutaraldehyde as it does not shrink.

29.5 Postoperative Course

The patient was extubated on the day of surgery, discharged from the intensive care unit (ICU) on the postoperative day (POD) 2 and then discharged from hospital in an ambulatory state on the POD 11.

29.6 Postoperative Echocardiogram

AR: trivial (central), aortic valve area: 1.7 cm^2, Vmax: 2.0 m/s, maximum/mean AVG: 16/9 mmHg, AVJ: 30 mm, SV: 32 mm, STJ: 24 mm.

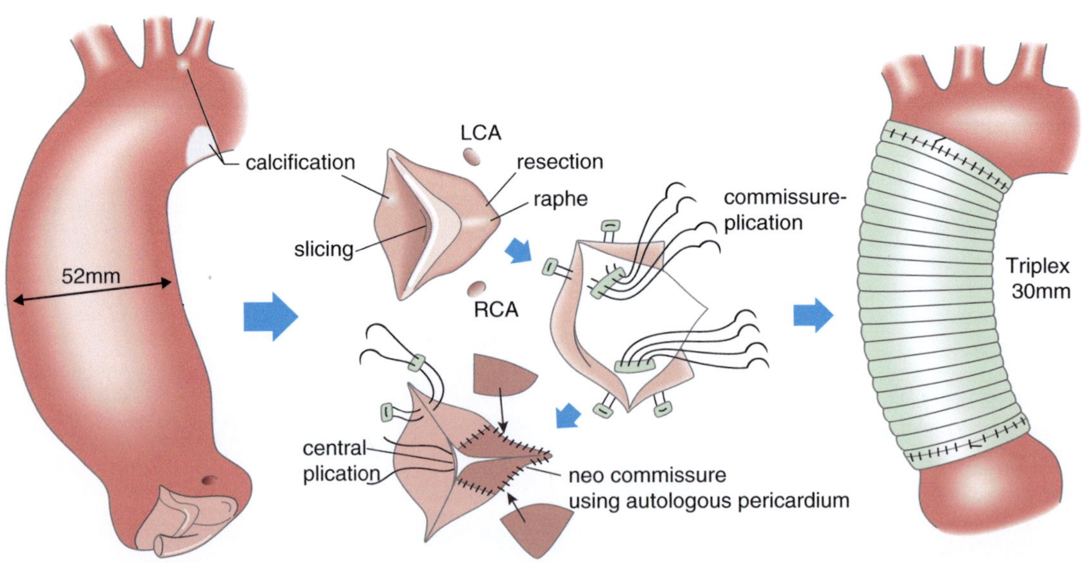

Fig. 29.1 The surgical schema for case 1

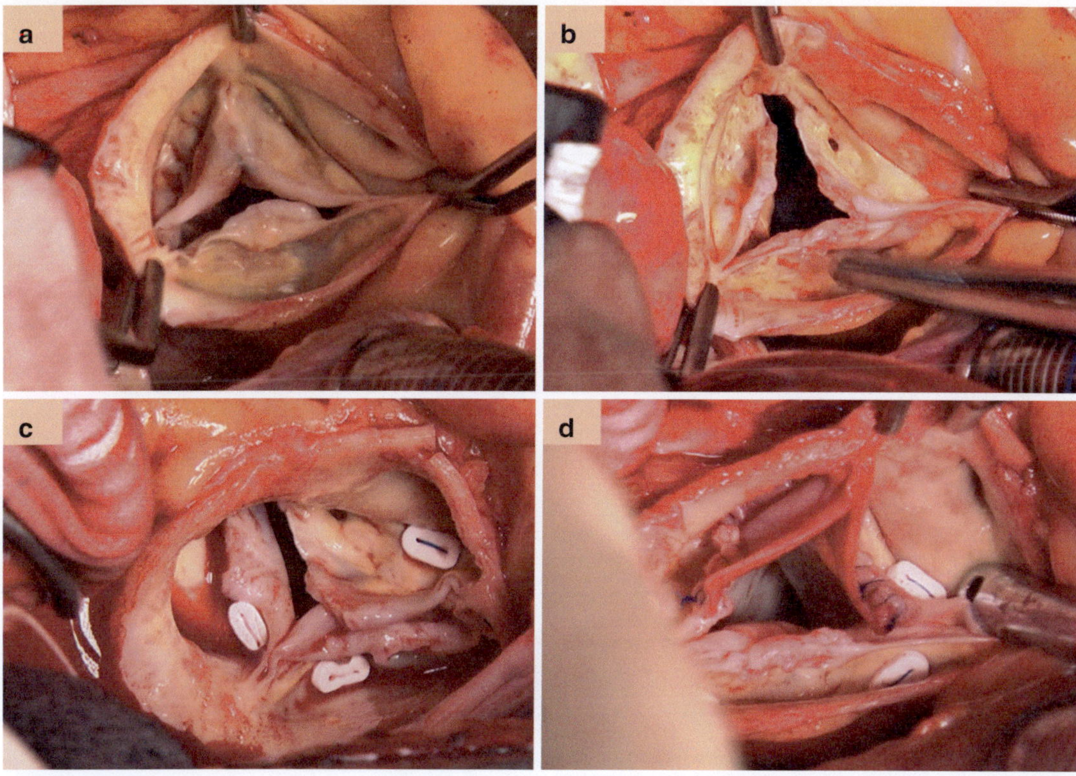

Fig. 29.2 Surgical findings in case 1. (**a**) Fusion of the RCC and LCC was observed and the raphe was calcified. (**b**) Resection of the calcified raphe (**c**) Additional subcommissural annuloplasty performed between the RCC and NCC and between the LCC and NCC. (**d**) The autologous pericardium, treated with glutaraldehyde, was used to replace the resected portions and new commissures were created

Patient 2	66-year-old woman, body height: 160 cm, body weight: 52 kg, BSA: 1.53 m^2
Medical history	Nothing notable
History of present illness	A chest CT scan performed during a health check-up in 2008 showed dilatation of the ascending aorta, and she was referred to and examined at our hospital. The diameter of her ascending aorta was 52 mm, and an echocardiogram showed a bicuspid aortic valve and mild AS. She therefore fulfilled the indications for surgery.
Preoperative echocardiogram	AR (−), mild AS, Vmax: 2.6 m/s, maximum AVG: 28 mmHg, AVJ: 28 mm, SV: 34 mm, STJ: 32 mm, LVDd/LVDs: 44/29 mm, LVEF: 63%, bicuspid aortic valve with fusion of the RCC and LCC and sclerosis of the raphe.
Preoperative CT scan	No significant coronary artery stenosis. The maximum diameter of the ascending aorta was 52 mm.

29.7 Surgical Technique

Replacement of the ascending aorta and partial aortic arch, aortic valvuloplasty (decalcification).

29.8 Surgical Method

We performed a median sternotomy, cannulated the ascending aorta, placed one drainage cannula in the right atrium and established cardiopulmonary bypass. We cross-clamped the aorta and then examined the aortic valve. Sclerosis of the raphe between the RCC and LCC was noted. We also determined that the cause of the AS was restricted opening of the fused leaflets associated with the sclerosis of the raphe, and we resected the calcification at this site using Pean forceps and surgical tweezers. We replaced the ascending aorta and

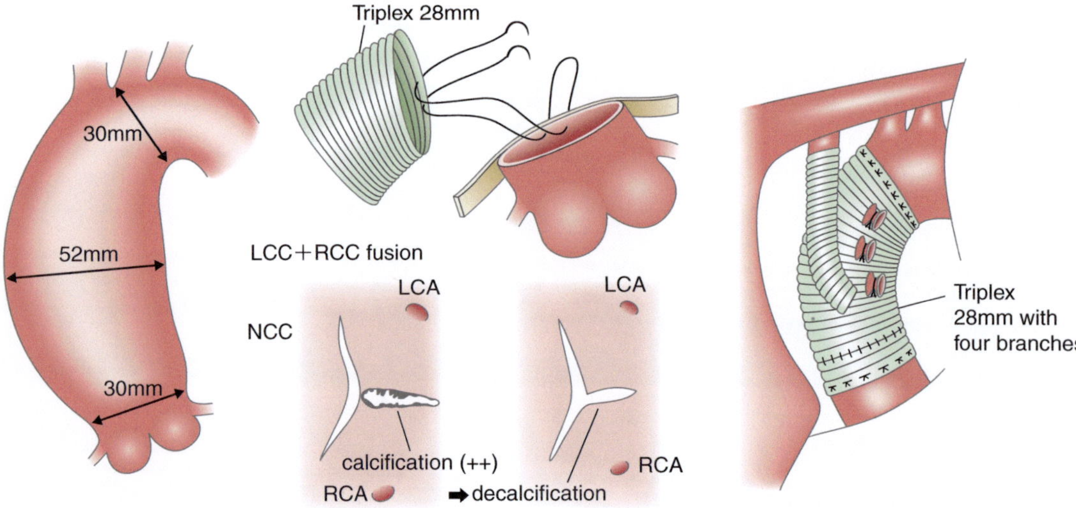

Fig. 29.3 The surgical schema for case 2

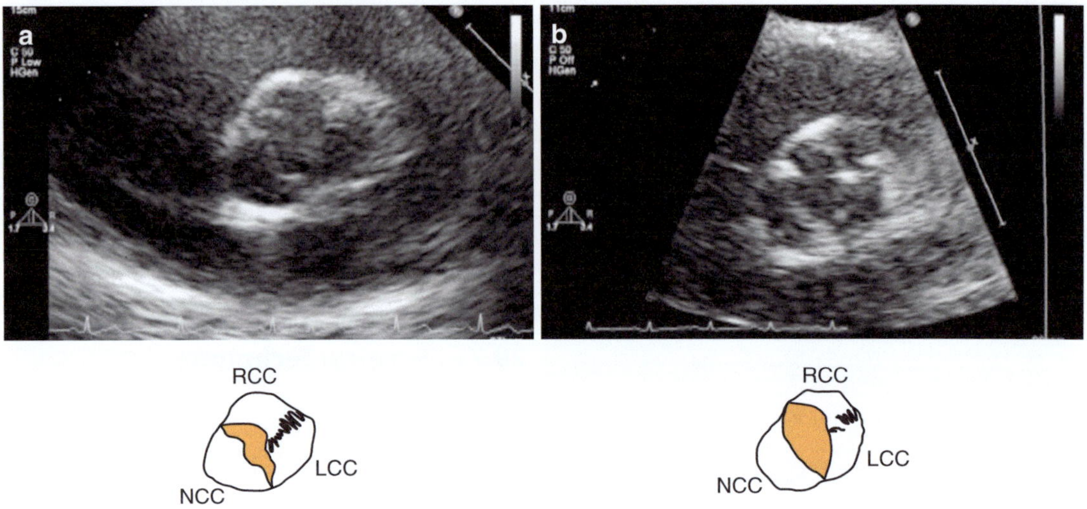

Fig. 29.4 Case 2. (**a**) Preoperative transthoracic echocardiogram. The raphe between the RCC and LCC was calcified, resulting in leaflet fusion and restricted opening. (**b**) Postoperative transthoracic echocardiogram. Reduced calcification of the raphe and reduction of the restricted opening of the fused leaflets

partial aortic arch and concluded the procedure (Figs. 29.3 and 29.4).

29.9 Personal Tips

Calcified lesions are normally present on the side facing the aorta, and the localized calcification can adequately be removed using Pean or Rongeur forceps. If a cavitron ultrasonic surgical aspirator (CUSA) is used, then it must be used with an understanding of the issues that are mentioned in the Key points below.

29.10 Postoperative Course

The patient was extubated on the day of surgery, discharged from the ICU on the POD 1 and then discharged from the hospital in an ambulatory state on the POD 9.

29.11 Postoperative Echocardiogram

AR:(–), Vmax: 1.7 m/s.
AVG: 13 mm Hg

29.12 Key Points

Two-thirds of bicuspid aortic valves that require aortic valve surgery are stenosed, and in most cases, it is difficult to perform a valvuloplasty. Requisite for valvuloplasty are that the calcified lesion is localized, and if there is no or very slight regurgitation, then this is a good candidate for decalcification. However, the long-term outcomes cannot be said to be favorable, and if the stenosis is advanced and the decalcification extends over a wide area, then we believe it is safer to investigate replacement. Because there are reports of remote sclerotic and calcific change due to inflammation when using a CUSA [1, 2], caution should be taken to minimize its usage even if needed. Meanwhile, it is possible to create a favorable coaptation zone by reconstruction methods using the autologous pericardium, and this is effective for cases that are associated with regurgitation [3, 4]. When compared to the tricuspid replacement method described by Ozaki (see Chap. 26), there are fewer portions that use autologous pericardium, which has unclear long-term outcomes, and even if these portions will be calcified in the future, it is possible to preserve the valve opening area using the residual native portions. If there are few calcified portions that are localized to the raphe and the fused leaflets is prolapsed, then it is one of the options to linealize the coaptation zone by resecting and reefing these sites and correcting the prolapse.

References

1. Cosgrove D, Ratliff N, Schaff H, Edwards W. Aortic valve decalcification: a new result. Ann Thorac Surg. 1990;49:689–90.
2. Craver J. Aortic valve debridement by ultrasonic surgical aspirator: a word of caution. Ann Thorac Surg. 1990;49:746–53.
3. Nezhad ZM, Kerchove L, Hechadi J, Tamer S, Boodhwani M, Poncelet A, et al. Aortic valve repair with patch in non-rheumatic disease: indication, techniques and durability. Eur J Cardiothorac Surg. 2014;46:997–1005.
4. Tolan MJ, Daubeney PE, Slavik Z, Keeton BR, Salmon AP, Monro JL. Aortic valve repair of congenital stenosis with bovine pericardium. Ann Thorac Surg. 1997;63:465–9.

30 How Do I Manage a Case with Borderline Dilatation of the Sinus of Valsalva?

Yoshiro Matsui

Patient	18-year-old man, body height: 169 cm, body weight: 67 kg, body surface area: 1.77 m^2
Medical history	Nothing notable
History of present illness	A murmur was detected when the patient was 13 years old, and he continued to be followed up. He played soccer and had experienced chest pain only once but could practice without difficulty. He underwent a detailed examination prior to joining a professional team, and surgical indications were detected.
Preoperative echocardiogram	Aortoventricular junction (AVJ): 35 mm, sinus of Valsalva (SV) diameter: 40 mm, sinotubular junction (STJ): 23 mm, left ventricular diastolic diameter (LVDd): 72 mm, left ventricular ejection fraction (LVEF): 50% (biplane modified method), bicuspid aortic valve (AV) (anteroposterior type), severe aortic regurgitation (AR), mild mitral regurgitation (MR), mild tricuspid regurgitation (TR), no aortic stenosis (AS), Vmax: 1.6 m/s
Preoperative computed tomography (CT) scan (Fig. 30.1)	Diameters: AVJ: 35 mm, SV: 35.7 mm, STJ: 23.5 mm, ascending aorta: 21 mm

30.1 Surgical Technique

Reimplantation procedure and aortic valvuloplasty.

30.2 Surgical Method

We performed a median sternotomy, cannulated the ascending aorta, placed a drainage cannula in the right atrium, and started cardiopulmonary bypass. The aortic root was dissected using a harmonic scalpel. The aorta was then cross-clamped, and cardiac arrest was achieved with both retrograde and anterograde cardioplegia. The aorta was transected immediately superior to the STJ. The AV was an anteroposterior bicuspid valve formed by fusion of the right coronary cusp (RCC) and left coronary cusp (LCC). The RCC had redundant tissue. There was no fenestration. The leaflet margins were hypertrophic, and the cusp height was 21 mm for the LCC, 21 mm for the RCC, and 24 mm for the noncoronary cusp (NCC). The commissural height was between 28 and 29 mm. First, we incised the hypertrophic raphe portion and sliced the raphe

Y. Matsui (✉)
Department of Cardiovascular and Thoracic Surgery, Hokkaido University Graduate School of Medicine, Sapporo, Hokkaido, Japan
e-mail: ymatsui@med.hokudai.ac.jp

T. Kunihara, S. Takanashi (eds.), *Aortic Valve Preservation*,
https://doi.org/10.1007/978-981-13-2068-2_30

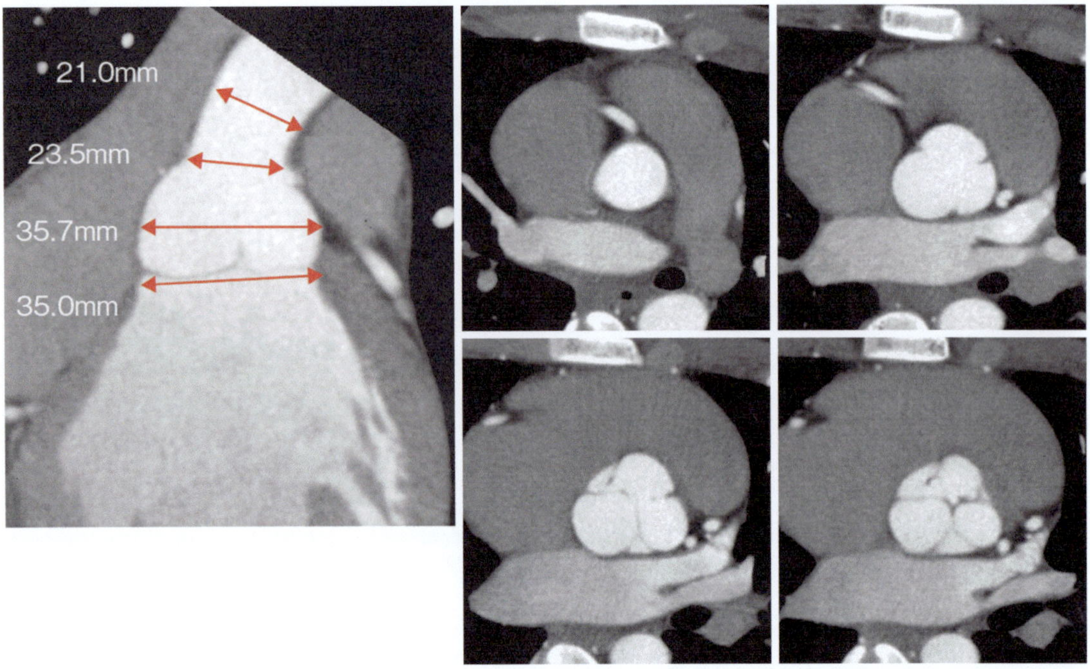

Fig. 30.1 Evaluation of the aortic root structure using preoperative CT. The valve was bicuspid with annular dilatation, and the sinuses of Valsalva measured less than 40 mm. The effective height was low

and free margin of the fused cusp. Next, we created the coronary buttons. The wall of the sinus of Valsalva was then resected and sewn to a 28-mm graft with sinuses as a first row with pledgeted mattress sutures that were placed from within the left ventricle (LV); three were placed in the commissures, three beneath the LCC, five beneath the NCC, and four beneath the RCC. After trimming, the aortic wall was sewn to the graft from the internal approach. The incised part of the raphe was readapted using nine sutures to adjust both leaflet free margins to equal length. Next, we attached the coronary buttons. Finally, we performed the distal anastomosis. The operation was concluded without transfusion. The patient was under cardiopulmonary bypass for 228 min and aortic cross-clamping for 193 min.

30.3 Postoperative Clinical Course

The patient was extubated 4 h after surgery and discharged from the intensive care unit on postoperative day 2. Four and a half years have elapsed since the surgery, and the patient enjoys playing sports without oral medication.

30.4 Postoperative Echocardiogram

In postoperative year 4, the patient had mild AR, mild MR, mild TR, an LVDd of 49 mm, an LVEF of 55% (biplane modification), no AS, and a V_{max} of 2.0 m/s through the AV (Fig. 30.2).

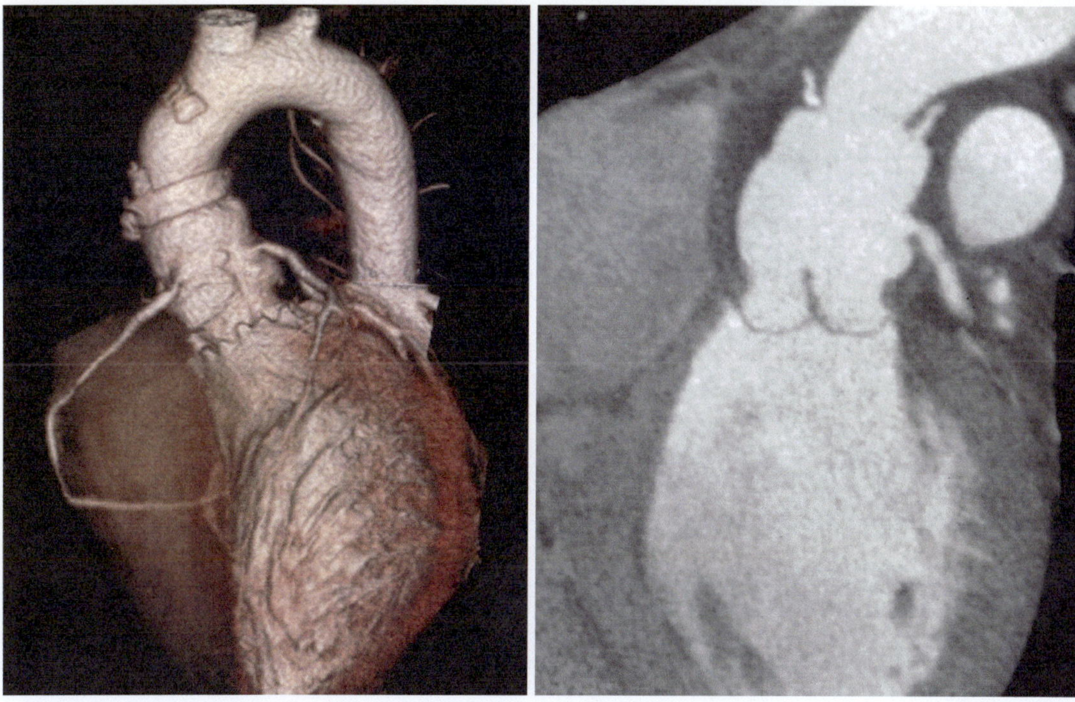

Fig. 30.2 Evaluation of the aortic root using CT on postoperative day 8. We confirmed favorable aortic root reconstruction using 3D CT. The effective height was high

30.5 Key Points

The 2006 American College of Cardiology (ACC)/American Heart Association (AHA) guidelines state that aortic root replacement (ARR) is a class I recommendation for an ascending aortic diameter (AAD) or aortic root diameter (ARD) ≥ 45 mm in patients with an underlying disease, such as a bicuspid AV or Marfan syndrome, and concomitant AS or AR [1]. However, according to a review exclusively of bicuspid AVs in 2009, ARR is indicated for patients with AAD or ARD ≥50 mm, patients at high risk based on family history or other factors, patients with small adult body size and AAD or ARD ≥45 mm, or patients with AAD or ARD ≥40 mm with a concomitant indication for elective AV surgery [2].

The 2012 European Society of Cardiology (ESC)/European Association for Cardio-Thoracic Surgery (EACTS) guidelines note that evidence is lacking for an AAD or ARD of 45 mm; therefore, they consider ARR to be a class I recommendation when the AAD is ≥50 mm, even in patients with Marfan syndrome. In addition, ARR is considered to be a class IIa recommendation when the AAD is ≥45 mm in patients with Marfan syndrome and risk factors (such as a family history of aortic dissection and/or aortic size increase >2 mm/year), or >50mm in patients with a bicuspid valve and similar risk factors, or >55 mm in other patients. However, in all cases, the level of evidence is grade C [3]. Still, these guidelines also mention that surgery can be indicated when the diameter reaches 45 mm in patients undergoing surgery on the AV depending on the patients' characteristics (bicuspid AV and others). Furthermore, lower thresholds of aortic diameters can be considered for low-risk patients in highly experienced centers.

The 2014 ACC/AHA guidelines also state that surgery is a class I recommendation for patients with a bicuspid valve with a diameter ≥50 mm, although they revised the recommendation that ascending aortic replacement or ARR is a class I recommendation with an evidence level of B in patients with an AAD or ARD exceeding 55 mm. However, ascending aortic replacement or ARR is a class IIa recommendation with an evidence level of C in patients at high risk with a family history of dissection or aortic size increase >5 mm/year when the diameter is ≥50 mm. Ascending aortic replacement is a class IIa (evidence level C) recommendation in patients with AAD ≥ 45 mm who require surgery on the AV, even though ARR may not absolutely be necessary [4].

Our patient was a young football player who wished to join a professional team. He fulfilled the indications for surgery due to a markedly dilated LVDd and a reduced LVEF. However, because he would frequently be involved in bodily contact with other players during games, the use of warfarin would be contraindicated, so we strongly recommended valve-sparing surgery. His sinus of Valsalva diameter was <40 mm, which fell below the 2006 guideline recommendation of 40 mm as a surgical indication. However, his STJ measured 23 mm, which clearly indicated the presence of annuloaortic ectasia. His AVJ was markedly enlarged to 35 mm, so we selected the reimplantation procedure because we considered reliable annular fixation to be mandatory. A bicuspid valve with a commissure angle of 180° can provide the maximum valve opening and is less likely to be associated with postoperative stenosis. Thus, ARR should be performed aggressively for better bicuspid valve morphology, although it can be challenging in patients without remarkable annular or SV enlargement. We selected the reimplantation procedure for our patient from this perspective. We also perform the remodeling procedure with external ring annuloplasty using the same cross-sectional vascular prosthesis. However, whether the outcomes are superior or inferior to those after the reimplantation procedure remains to be seen.

References

1. Bonow RO, Carabello BA, Chatterjee K, de Leon AC Jr, Faxon DP, Freed MD, et al. ACC/AHA 2006 guidelines for the management of patients with valvular heart disease: a report of the American College of Cardiology/American Heart Association Task Force on Practice Guidelines developed in collaboration with the Society of Cardiovascular Anesthesiologists endorsed by the Society for Cardiovascular Angiography and Interventions and the Society of Thoracic Surgeons. J Am Coll Cardiol. 2006;48:e1–148.
2. Tadros TM, Klein MD, Shapira OM. Ascending aortic dilatation associated with bicuspid aortic valve: pathophysiology, molecular biology, and clinical implications. Circulation. 2009;119:880–90.
3. Vahanian A, Alfieri O, Andreotti F, Antunes MJ, Barón-Esquivias G, Baumgartner H, et al. Guidelines on the management of valvular heart disease (version 2012): the Joint Task Force on the Management of Valvular Heart Disease of the European Society of Cardiology (ESC) and the European Association for Cardio-Thoracic Surgery (EACTS). Eur J Cardiothorac Surg. 2012;42:S1–44.
4. Nishimura RA, Otto CM, Bonow RO, Carabello BA, Erwin JP 3rd, Guyton RA, et al. 2014 AHA/ACC guideline for the management of patients with valvular heart disease: a report of the American College of Cardiology/American Heart Association Task Force on Practice Guidelines. J Thorac Cardiovasc Surg. 2014;148:e1–e132.

31 How Do I Manage Perforation and Fenestration?

Masanori Nakamura

31.1 Introduction

Valve-sparing root replacement is indicated when the underlying mechanism of aortic regurgitation (AR) is enlargement of the aortic root. Furthermore, central plication according to measurement of the effective height (eH) is considered to be a standard form of treatment for leaflet prolapse. However, the aortic valve, unlike the mitral valve, has a relatively small tissue volume, and it is difficult to perform direct suturing of leaflet defects, such as fenestration, perforation, and retraction, and thus, a pericardial patch is mandatory for repair. These are still considered to be challenging conditions because the technique for patchplasty has not still been standardized. However, recently, Schäfers et al. and El Khoury et al. reported favorable long-term outcomes, and this has been recognized as one of the forms of aortic valvuloplasty [1, 2].

Patient	60-year-old woman, body height: 150 cm, body weight: 48 kg, body surface area: 1.41 m^2
Medical history	Hypertension, cerebral infarction (no residual neurological deficit)
History of present illness	AR and an ascending aortic aneurysm were accidentally detected when the patient suffered a cerebral infarction, and she was referred to us for surgery.
Preoperative computed tomography scan	The ascending aortic aneurysm was dilated to 57 mm, the sinotubular junction (STJ) was somewhat dilated at 35 mm, although the diameter of the sinus of Valsalva was 36 mm, and the aortoventricular junction (AVJ) measured 20 × 26 mm, indicating no aortic root dilatation.
Preoperative echocardiogram	Grade III AR (vena contracta: 13 mm), grade II mitral regurgitation (MR), grade II tricuspid regurgitation, left ventricular dimension during diastole (LVDd): 56 mm, during systole (LVDs): 35 mm, left ventricular end-diastolic volume: 99 mL, end-systolic volume: 61 ml, indicating left ventricular dilatation. However, the left ventricular ejection fraction was favorable at 67%.
Preoperative transesophageal echocardiogram (TEE)	There was no obvious prolapse of the noncoronary cusp (NCC) or the right coronary cusp (RCC). There was severe regurgitation via the left coronary cusp (LCC), including at both commissures, and we believe that the AR was caused by retraction of the LCC (Figs. 31.1 and 31.2).

M. Nakamura
Department of Cardiovascular Surgery and Cardiology, Sapporo City General Hospital, Sapporo, Hokkaido, Japan
e-mail: masanori.nakamura@doc.city.sapporo.jp

T. Kunihara, S. Takanashi (eds.), *Aortic Valve Preservation*,
https://doi.org/10.1007/978-981-13-2068-2_31

31.2 Intraoperative Findings

The geometric height of the LCC was 18 mm, and there was no retraction, but we observed complete rupture of the chorda, which previously should have been attached to the commissure above the fenestration (Fig. 31.3).

31.3 Surgical Technique

1. We performed a partial aortic arch repair under hypothermic circulatory arrest. Then, systemic circulation was resumed by clamping the vascular graft.

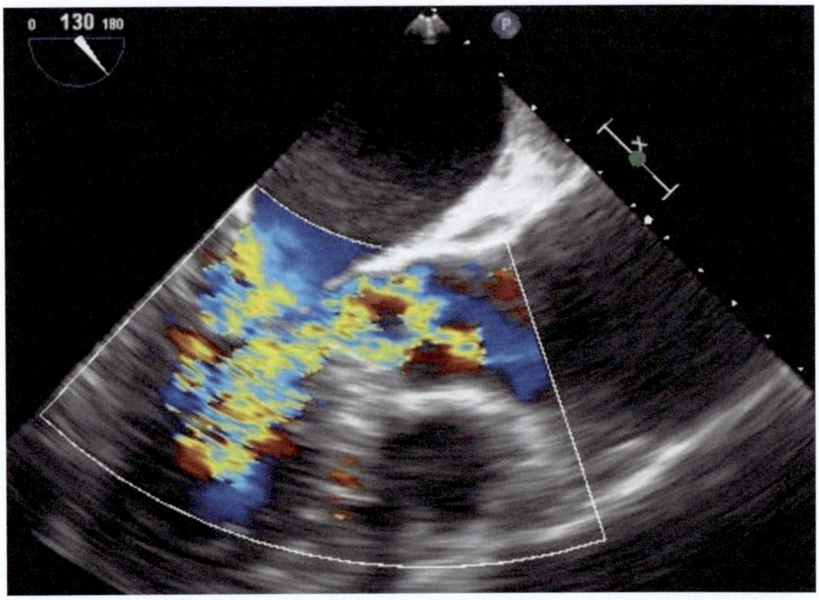

Fig. 31.1 Color-doppler image in the long-axis view from the preoperative transesophageal echocardiogram. Severe AR with eccentric jet was observed

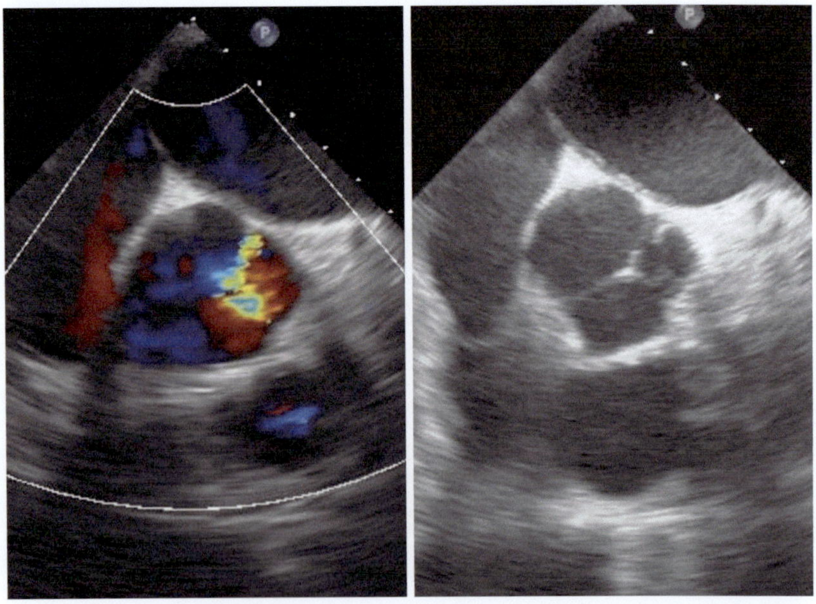

Fig. 31.2 Short-axis view from the preoperative transesophageal echocardiogram. AR jet was observed from both sides of the LCC suggesting retraction of the LCC

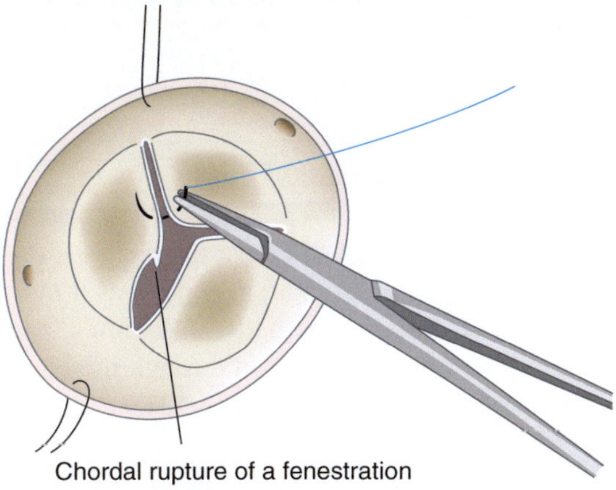

Fig. 31.3 The geometric height of the LCC was sufficient and the cause of AR was chordal rupture of the LCC. A pilot suture was placed between the node of Arantius of the RCC and LCC to maintain a consistent leaflet length between the RCC-LCC commissure and the node of Arantius of both leaflets

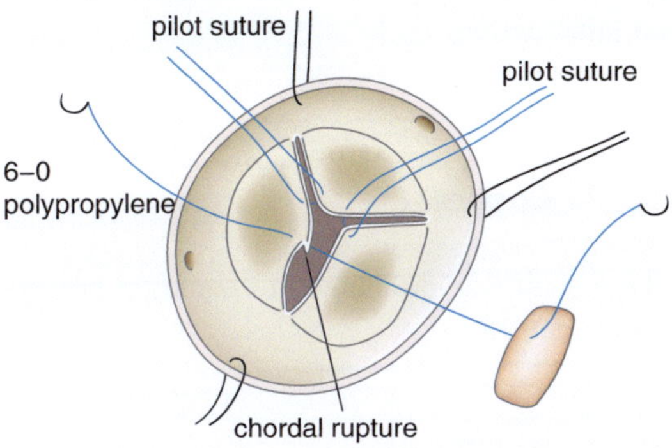

Fig. 31.4 Another pilot suture was placed between the node of Arantius of the RCC and NCC to determine the free margin length of the LCC defect by referring to the length of the NCC on the opposite side

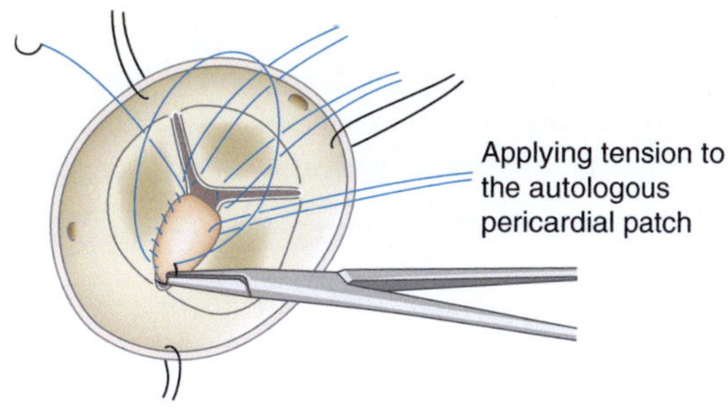

Fig. 31.5 The commissure was sutured up to the same height of the opposite commissure of the NCC and tied securely at the outside of the aorta

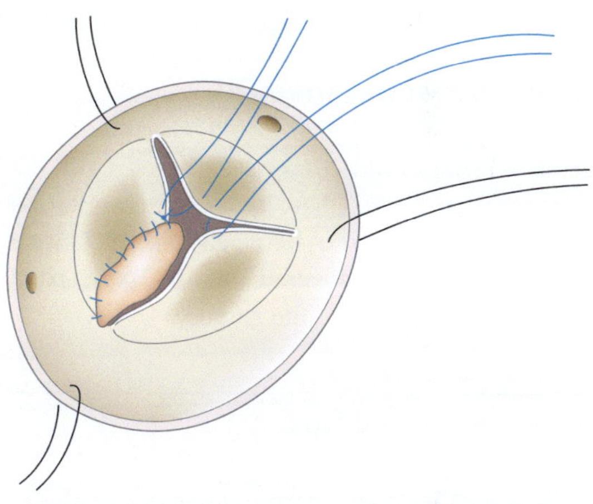

Fig. 31.6 The central portion was sutured to the pilot suture to maintain the same free margin length with the opposite cusp, resulting in a reproducible patch repair

2. Patch repair of the leaflet.

   From the intraoperative findings, we determined that this patient was an optimal candidate for patch repair, and we placed pilot sutures between the RCC and LCC, and between the RCC and NCC, to maintain a consistent leaflet length between the RCC-LCC commissure and the node of Arantius of both leaflets. We determined the free margin length of the LCC defect by referring to the length of the NCC on the opposite side and used a 10–20% larger patch (Fig. 31.4) [1]. The autologous pericardium was treated with 0.625% glutaraldehyde and attached to the defect of the LCC using continuous 6-0 polypropylene sutures. The commissure was sutured up to the same height of the opposite commissure of the NCC, and the sutures were securely tied with another suture at the outside of the aorta (Fig. 31.5). The central portion was sutured not to the base of the ruptured chorda but to the pilot suture and secured (Fig. 31.6). Finally, the free margin of the patch was cut and adjusted to the same height of the opposite leaflet.

3. Annuloplasty

   After dissecting the aortic root to the annulus, we used CV-0 expanded polytetrafluoroethylene sutures to perform external circular suture annuloplasty (21 mm) to prevent re-dilatation of the AVJ.
4. Reduction of the STJ and adjustment of the eH

   The STJ was anastomosed to a short, 26-mm vascular graft to remodel the aortic root geometry. Thereafter, we performed central plication of the prolapsing RCC and NCC at an eH of 8 mm using a 6-0 polypropylene suture. After fine tuning, the two vascular grafts were connected together and the aorta was unclamped.

31.4 Intraoperative TEE

Although only mild AR was observed from the center of the valve, there was no regurgitation from the commissure between the LCC and NCC, which was covered by the pericardial patch, so we concluded the surgery.

31.5 Personal Tips

1. When patients suffer from disorders similar to that of the present case, in which there are localized defects of the leaflets, we believe that they are good candidates for patch repair, as are patients with AR caused by infective endocarditis or fenestration, although it is very difficult to determine the optimal size of the patch. For this reason, pilot sutures are placed to maintain a consistent distance from each commissure and make the area of the defect more visible. This makes it easier to understand the size and morphology of the patch required. We obtained favorable results in the present case by placing a patch that extended beyond the ruptured chordae to the node of Arantius.
2. It is extremely important to secure fixation of the commissure, which is subject to stress [3]. No regurgitation occurs via the commissure when the patch is sutured right up to the same height of the opposite commissure and fixed to the aorta externally.

31.6 Postoperative TEE

Coaptation was obtained above the annulus, the eH was 12 mm, the coaptation depth was 8 mm, AR occurred through the node of Arantius, and no regurgitation was observed through the commissure repaired by the patch (Fig. 31.7).

31.7 Discharge Echocardiogram

The AR was mild (vena contracta: 3.2 mm) and located centrally, with a peak pressure gradient of 13 mmHg. The LVDd was reduced from the preoperative value of 56 mm to a postoperative value of 48 mm, and the grade II MR disappeared without intervention.

31.8 Postoperative Clinical Course

The patient was discharged to home on postoperative day 15.

31.9 Key Points

It was difficult to differentiate this condition from retraction preoperatively. However, the difficulty of patch repair for the two etiologies differs. Accordingly, it is important to keep valvuloplasty in mind in cases with chordal rupture of a fenestration when hypoplasia of a single leaflet is encountered preoperatively. This is caused by myxoid degeneration that results in cardiac failure due to a rapid increase in AR, and the RCC is also commonly implicated in reports [4].

Patch repair has been reported to be a risk factor for AR recurrence over the long term after aortic valvuloplasty [5]. However, patch repair is one of the durable valvuloplasty techniques to be mastered when treating a pathological etiology that requires the use of a patch. Aortic valvuloplasty with partial

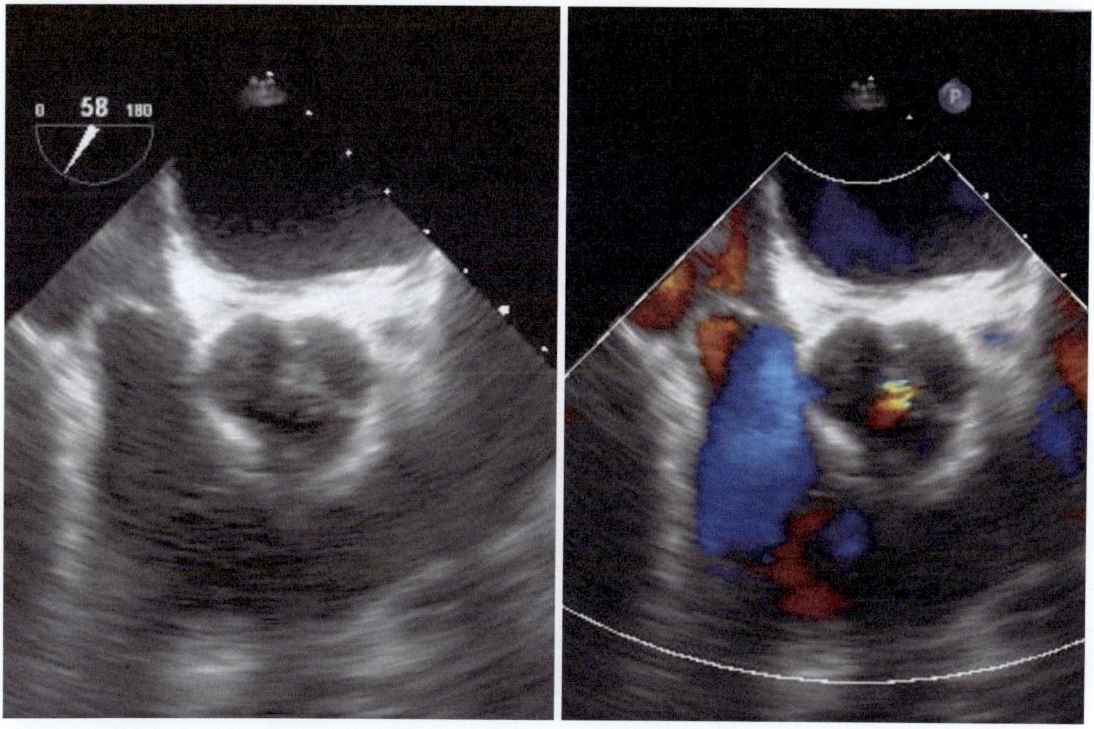

Fig. 31.7 Short-axis view from the postoperative transesophageal echocardiogram. A mild central AR jet was observed, but no regurgitation was observed through the LCC-NCC commissure repaired with the patch

use of a patch is a favorable surgical technique when treating chordal rupture of a fenestration. The connection between the autologous valve and the pericardium affects long-term outcomes, so naturally, these cases require long-term follow-up.

References

1. Schäfers HJ, Langer F, Glombitza P, Kunihara T, Fries R, Aicher D. Aortic valve reconstruction in myxomatous degeneration of aortic valves: are fenestrations a risk factor for repair failure? J Thorac Cardiovasc Surg. 2010;139:660–4.
2. Mosala Nezhad Z, de Kerchove L, Hechadi J, Tamer S, Boodhwani M, Poncelet A, et al. Aortic valve repair with patch in non-rheumatic disease: indication, techniques and durability. Eur J Cardiothorac Surg. 2014;46:997–1005.
3. Marom G, Halevi R, Haj-Ali R, Rosenfeld M, Schäfers HJ, Raanani E. Numerical model of the aortic root and valve: optimization of graft size and sinotubular junction to annulus ratio. J Thorac Cardiovasc Surg. 2013;146:1227–31.
4. Akiyama K, Hirota J, Taniyasu N, Maisawa K, Kobayashi Y, Tsuda M. Pathogenetic significance of myxomatous degeneration in fenestration-related massive aortic regurgitation. Circ J. 2004;68:439–43.
5. Kunihara T, Aicher D, Rodionycheva S, Groesdonk HV, Langer F, Sata F, et al. Preoperative aortic root geometry and postoperative cusp configuration primarily determine long-term outcome after valve-preserving aortic root repair. J Thorac Cardiovasc Surg. 2012;143:1389–95.

32 How to Manage Moderate Aortic Regurgitation in the Context of Combined Valvular Disease

Hideaki Takai

32.1 Introduction

Surgeons sometimes face difficulty when questioning how far to extend the surgical indications for valvuloplasty and valve replacement while taking the pathophysiology and surgical invasiveness into account when they consider surgical treatment for combined valvular disease (CVD). This would reflect the evidence that the mechanisms and pathophysiology of CVD are highly variable. Determination of the surgical indication is strongly affected by the cusp etiology, but the determination must be made with a comprehensive understanding of all examination results.

This chapter presents a patient with moderate aortic regurgitation (AR) in the context of CVD and discusses how we should evaluate and manage this condition as an example.

Patient	71-year-old man, body height: 164 cm, body weight: 64 kg, body surface area (BSA): 1.70 m^2
Medical history	Acute arterial occlusion of the lower extremity (10 years prior)
History of present illness	Atrial fibrillation (AF) was detected 12 years prior, and the patient received conservative treatment at another hospital. Onset of cardiac failure occurred 3 months prior and was managed by increasing the dose of diuretic agents, but we determined that surgery was indicated due to repeated episodes of cardiac failure.
Chest X-ray	Cardiothoracic ratio: 78%
Electrocardiogram	Long-standing, persistent AF, 56 beats per minute
Preoperative transthoracic echocardiogram (TTE) (Fig. 32.1)	Left ventricular end-diastolic diameter: 70 mm, end-systolic diameter: 42 mm, left ventricular ejection fraction: 69%, left atrial diameter: 99 mm, right ventricular systolic pressure: 57 mmHg, aorto-ventricular junction (AVJ): 21 mm, sinus of Valsalva (SV): 35 mm, grade 4 mitral regurgitation, grade 3 tricuspid regurgitation, grade 2 to 3 aortic regurgitation. A single straight regurgitant jet from the center of the aortic valve was present.
Preoperative transesophageal echocardiogram (TEE)	Aortic valve: tricuspid, no prolapse; AVJ: 21 mm
Preoperative Swan-Ganz catheter	Pulmonary capillary wedge pressure: 23 mmHg, pulmonary artery pressure: 50/26 mmHg (mean: 34 mmHg)
Preoperative computed tomography (CT) scan (Fig. 32.2)	AVJ: 37.8 × 22.5 mm, dilated with a mean value: 29.7 mm

H. Takai (✉)
Department of Cardiovascular Surgery, The Cardiovascular Institute, Tokyo, Japan
e-mail: cvstakai@yahoo.co.jp

T. Kunihara, S. Takanashi (eds.), *Aortic Valve Preservation*, https://doi.org/10.1007/978-981-13-2068-2_32

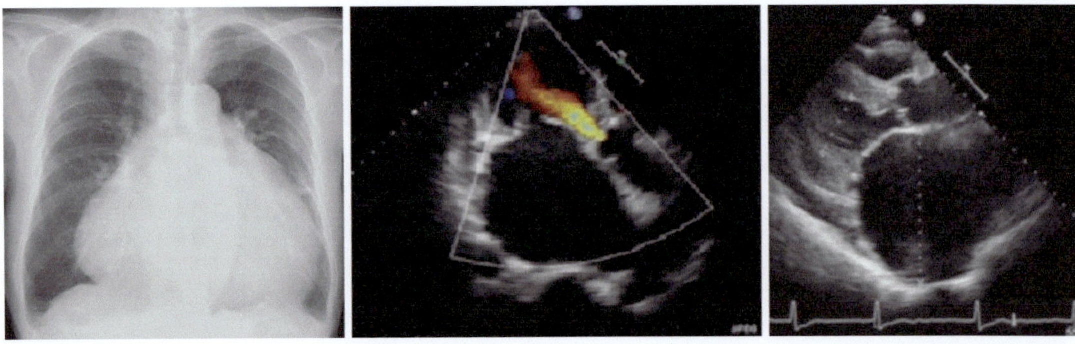

Fig. 32.1 The chest X-ray images (left) and preoperative transthoracic echocardiogram (middle and right)

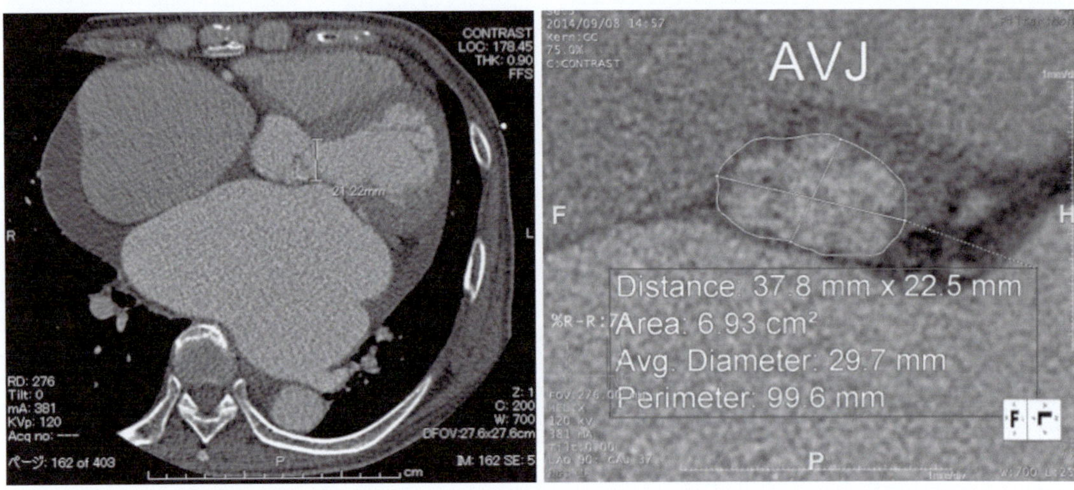

Fig. 32.2 Preoperative measurement of the aortic annulus using CT. This shows the max. and min. diameter (37.8 × 22.5 mm) and mean diameter (29.7 mm) at the level of the aortic annulus

32.2 Evaluation and Treatment Strategy

There are concerns regarding whether to perform bioprosthetic valve replacement or valvuloplasty to treat moderate AR. If these concerns are great, there are probably surgeons who would perform aortic valve replacement without hesitation. However, valvuloplasty deserves to be tried in patients without remarkable cusp degeneration and with reasonable macroscopic configuration, as in the presented case. If aortic valve replacement is performed first, this may halve the benefits of valvuloplasty for the other valves.

32.3 Surgical Findings

The geometric heights were all 20 mm, the effective heights were all 8 mm, and the AVJ was 26 mm.

32.4 Surgical Technique

- Mitral valvuloplasty (Seguine annuloplasty ring, 30 mm)
- Papillary muscle relocation
- Tricuspid annuloplasty (MC^3 annuloplasty ring, 32 mm)

- Aortic valvuloplasty (external suture annuloplasty, ø 22 mm)
- Left atrial plication, resection of the left atrial appendage, pacemaker lead implantation in the right ventricle
- Duration of cardiopulmonary bypass: 178 min, duration of aortic cross-clamping: 117 min

32.5 Postoperative Echocardiogram

The AVJ measured 20 mm postoperatively, and the aortic regurgitation had disappeared.

32.6 Postoperative Clinical Course

The patient was extubated 7 h after being admitted to the intensive care unit and was transferred to a general ward on postoperative day (POD) 3. The patient was discharged on POD 25 after rehabilitation was completed.

32.7 Key Points

Evaluation of the Aortic Root Geometry

According to the classification proposed by El Khoury et al. [1], the mechanism of AR in this case was mainly Type Ic (Fig. 32.3). If this were a case with mitral regurgitation caused by mitral annular dilatation, it would be classified as Carpentier Type 1. However, echocardiography (both TTE and TEE) revealed an annulus diameter of 21 mm, which cannot be said to represent dilatation. So, how did we diagnose annular dilatation?

Morphology of the AVJ

The aortic annulus is not round but rather a somewhat collapsed elliptical shape. Calleja et al. calculated the diameter of the aortic annulus using a variety of angles [2]. This is naturally possible by echocardiography as well, although multidetector CT measurements have provided extremely valuable information in recent years. Thin-slice

AI Class	Type I normal cusp motion with FAA dilatation or cusp perforation				Type II cusp prolapse	Type III cusp restriction
	I a	I b	I c	I d		
mechanism	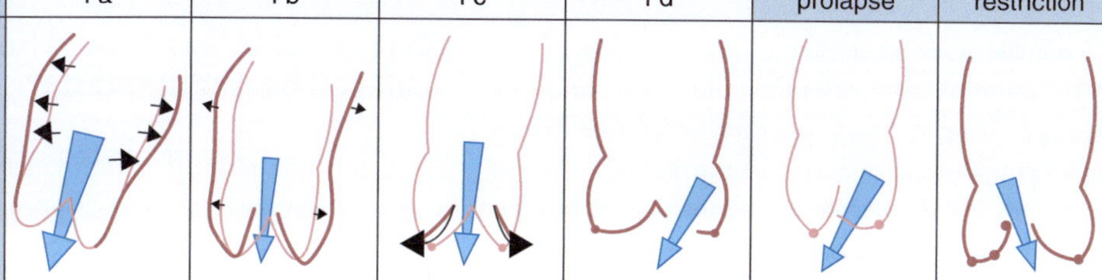					
repair techniques (primary)	STJ remodeling ascending aortic graft	aortic valve sparing : reimplantation or remodeling with SCA	SCA	patch repair autologous or bovine pericardium	prolapse repair plication triangular resection free margin resuspension patch	leaflet repair shaving decalcifcatio patch
(secondary)	SCA		STJ annuloplasty	SCA	SCA	SCA

Fig. 32.3 Schema for the mechanism of aortic regurgitation (reproduced with permission from Ref. [1])

Table 32.1 Mean aortic annulus diameters for various BSA ranges

	Male				Female			
	AVD (mm)		PVD (mm)		AVD (mm)		PVD (mm)	
BSA range (m²)	*n*	mean ± SD	*n*	mean ± SD	*n*	mean ± SD	*n*	mean ± SD
0.21–0.30	19	8.8 ± 1.0	39	14.0 ± 2.3	20	9.1 ± 0.8	30	10.0 ± 1.1
0.31–0.40	34	10.0 ± 1.6	38	11.7 ± 2.0	30	9.9 ± 0.8	36	11.2 ± 1.2
0.41–0.50	57	11.2 ± 0.9	58	13.3 ± 1.6	32	11.4 ± 1.4	31	13.2 ± 2.2
0.51–0.60	64	12.3 ± 1.2	68	14.5 ± 1.3	50	11.9 ± 1.2	54	13.9 ± 1.6
0.61–0.70	70	13.5 ± 1.3	73	16.0 ± 1.8	35	12.5 ± 1.3	36	15.0 ± 1.8
0.71–0.80	57	14.1 ± 1.1	64	16.6 ± 1.5	31	13.9 ± 1.5	36	16.4 ± 1.8
0.81–0.90	37	14.6 ± 1.5	39	17.6 ± 2.0	30	14.3 ± 1.3	30	17.5 ± 1.9
0.91–1.00	48	15.6 ± 1.3	61	18.7 ± 1.9	32	15.4 ± 1.4	35	18.1 ± 1.1
1.01–1.10	42	16.3 ± 1.5	51	19.5 ± 1.8	30	15.6 ± 1.4	36	10.0 ± 2.0
1.11–1.20	42	17.2 ± 1.9	45	20.4 ± 1.9	21	16.8 ± 1.8	22	19.6 ± 1.6
1.21–1.30	25	17.1 ± 1.6	39	20.6 ± 1.8	23	17.8 ± 2.1	27	20.7 ± 1.9
1.31–1.40	38	18.7 ± 1.7	55	21.6 ± 2.1	47	18.5 ± 2.2	71	21.6 ± 2.3
1.41–1.50	39	19.1 ± 2.3	44	22.3 ± 2.5	122	19.6 ± 2.0	150	22.4 ± 2.1
1.51–1.60	52	20.7 ± 2.4	69	23.5 ± 2.3	175	19.9 ± 1.9	218	22.8 ± 2.1
1.61–1.70	125	20.8 ± 2.1	135	23.7 ± 2.4	267	20.5 ± 1.8	317	23.5 ± 2.0
1.71–1.80	223	21.5 ± 2.0	230	24.5 ± 2.4	218	21.0 ± 1.6	285	24.1 ± 2.0
1.81–1.90	350	22.3 ± 2.1	417	25.2 ± 2.2	148	21.3 ± 1.6	167	24.1 ± 1.9
1.91–2.00	466	22.6 ± 1.7	518	25.7 ± 2.1	109	21.5 ± 1.4	122	24.6 ± 2.0
2.01–2.10	453	23.0 ± 1.8	525	26.2 ± 2.1	77	21.6 ± 1.4	75	24.8 ± 2.0
2.11–2.20	266	23.6 ± 1.9	309	26.8 ± 2.0	46	21.9 ± 1.5	68	25.0 ± 1.8
2.21–2.30	172	23.8 ± 1.8	210	26.8 ± 2.0	31	21.8 ± 1.5	39	25.5 ± 1.9
2.31–2.40	115	24.1 ± 1.9	134	27.3 ± 1.9	25	22.0 ± 1.5	34	25.0 ± 3.1
2.41–2.50	85	24.4 ± 1.9	133	27.5 ± 1.7	11	22.5 ± 1.6	14	26.0 ± 2.3
2.51–2.60	43	24.8 ± 1.8	45	27.8 ± 1.8				
2.61–2.70	33	25.2 ± 2.3	47	28.1 ± 1.9				

AVD Aortic valve anulus diameter, *PVD* pulmonary valve anulus diameter, *BSA* body surface area, *SD* standard deviation

Reproduced with permission from Ref. [5]

Sample size of 10 diameter measurements or less are not reported

CT can be used to depict a cross-section of the aortic annulus and calculate the mean annulus diameter from the annulus circumference or the leaflet coaptation zone. It is important to note that the annulus diameter measured by TEE is not the definitive value, and depending on the case, the accurate depiction and evaluation of the cross-section of the aortic annulus is important for determining the treatment plan. In the present case, the values measured using CT were 37.8 × 22.5 mm, with a mean value of 29.7 mm.

Surgical Annuloplasty Techniques

Two representative techniques are suture annuloplasty [3] and ring annuloplasty [4]. Please refer to the chapter on the types and outcomes of annuloplasty (Chap. 18) for further details.

What annulus Size Should be Achieved by Annuloplasty?

There are methods of annuloplasty that use the BSA as a standard (as an indication) [5] as can be seen in Table 32.1. In the present case, the aortic annulus diameter had a mean value of 29.7 mm, but the mean value based on the BSA was approximately 21 mm.

32.8 Conclusion

We believe that evaluation of the AVJ, SV, and STJ geometry using not only preoperative echocardiography but also CT is an important factor in the success of aortic valvuloplasty.

The greatest advantages of suture annuloplasty are that it is simple and not time-consuming.

However, we are awaiting the results of studies that are investigating whether the long-term outcomes are superior or inferior to those of other annuloplasty types.

References

1. Boodhwani M, de Kerchove L, Glineur D, Poncelet A, Rubay J, Astarci P, et al. Repair-oriented classification of aortic insufficiency: impact on surgical techniques and clinical outcomes. J Thorac Cardiovasc Surg. 2009;137:286–94.
2. Calleja A, Thavendiranathan P, Ionasec RI, Houle H, Liu S, Voigt I, et al. Automated quantitative 3-dimensional modeling of the aortic valve and root by 3-dimensional transesophageal echocardiography in normals, aortic regurgitation, and aortic stenosis: comparison to computed tomography in normals and clinical implications. Circ Cardiovasc Imaging. 2013;6:99–108.
3. Aicher D, Schneider U, Schmied W, Kunihara T, Tochii M, Schäfers HJ. Early results with annular support in reconstruction of the bicuspid aortic valve. J Thorac Cardiovasc Surg. 2013;145:S30–4.
4. Lansac E, Di Centa I, Bonnet N, Leprince P, Jault F, Rama A, et al. Aortic prosthetic ring annuloplasty: a useful adjunct to a standardized aortic valve-sparing procedure? Eur J Cardiothorac Surg. 2006;29:537–44.
5. Capps SB, Elkins RC, Fronk DM. Body surface area as a predictor of aortic and pulmonary valve diameter. J Thorac Cardiovasc Surg. 2000;119:975–82.

When Is Partial Remodeling Possible?

33

Tatsuhiko Komiya

33.1 Introduction

David et al. devised partial remodeling, which entails replacement of any dilatated sinuses of Valsalva in addition to replacement of the ascending aorta. The procedure is performed when there is no dilatation of the aorto-ventricular junction, and the dilatation mainly affects the sino-tubular junction (STJ). Among the sinuses of Valsalva, the non-coronary sinus (NCS) and right coronary sinus (RCS) tend to enlarge readily, whereas the left coronary sinus (LCS) tends not to enlarge and can be preserved in many cases (Fig. 33.1). During the procedure, we use prosthetic vascular grafts that are cut to match the lingulate shape of the area to be replaced. This decreases the length of the suture line, which is expected to decrease both the duration of surgery and intraoperative hemorrhage [1]. If type A acute aortic dissection (AAD) occurs, and an intimal tear extends into the sinuses of Valsalva and causes rupture, then it becomes essential to perform aortic root replacement (ARR). The Bentall procedure is usually performed, although valve-sparing aortic root replacement (VSARR) may also be considered. However, surgeons who have little experience with VSARR, which is associated with numerous challenges, may be able to shorten the duration of surgery by performing partial remodeling.

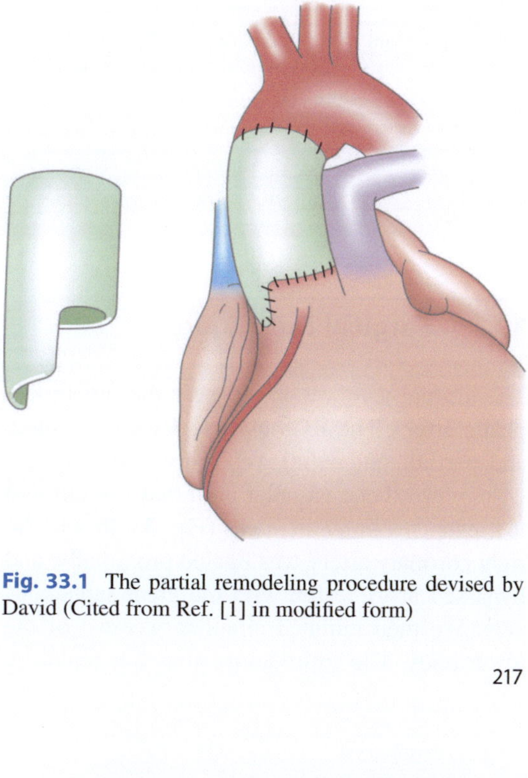

Fig. 33.1 The partial remodeling procedure devised by David (Cited from Ref. [1] in modified form)

T. Komiya (✉)
Department of Cardiovascular Surgery, Kurashiki Central Hospital, Okayama, Japan
e-mail: komiya@kchnet.or.jp

T. Kunihara, S. Takanashi (eds.), *Aortic Valve Preservation*,
https://doi.org/10.1007/978-981-13-2068-2_33

Patient 1	The patient was a 48-year-old woman. Body height 160 cm, body weight 58 kg, body surface area 1.60 m^2
Previous medical history	She suffered a lens dislocation at the age of 23 years.
Family history	Nothing of note.
History of present illness	The patient developed chest pain 2 months ago and subsequently developed exertional dyspnea. Her symptoms gradually deteriorated. Despite being diagnosed as having both aortic dissection (AD) and aortic regurgitation (AR), because it was not determined as acute onset, the patient was administered oral treatment for heart failure for 2 weeks.
Preoperative computed tomography (CT) scan	The CT scan showed a type A AD with a patent false lumen. Maximum ascending aorta diameter: 51 mm. Aortic arch: 36 mm. Descending aorta: 28 mm. The right coronary artery, the brachiocephalic artery, and the four visceral branches originated from the false lumen. The dissection extended into the sinuses of Valsalva (NCS and RCS) (Fig. 33.2). The RCS-NCS commissure was detached due to the dissection. The effective heights of the right-, left-, and non-coronary cusp were 3.7 mm, 9 mm, and 5.1 mm, respectively.
Preoperative echocardiogram	Severe AR, left ventricular diastolic diameter (LVDd): 52 mm, left ventricular systolic diameter (LVDs): 39 mm, left ventricular ejection fraction (LVEF): 49%, no asynergy. Basal annulus: 24 mm, sinus of Valsalva: 45 mm, STJ: 44 mm.

33.2 Surgical Technique

The intimal tear was found near the brachiocephalic artery. The RCS and NCS were resected, and partial remodeling was performed using a 24-mm prosthetic vascular graft that was tailored to create two lingulate areas (Fig. 33.2b, c). The right coronary artery was ligated proximally, and bypassed at #1 lesion with the great saphenous vein. We then initiated circulatory arrest of the lower body. The entire aortic arch was replaced. The aorta was cross-clamped for a total of 167 min, and cardiopulmonary bypass lasted for 235 min. Surgery lasted 6 h and 42 min.

Postoperative Clinical Course

The clinical course was uneventful, and the patient was discharged ambulatory on postoperative day 12.

Postoperative Evaluation

The AR disappeared postoperatively. LVDd: 44 mm, LVDs: 38 mm. A CT scan showed that a persistent dissection from the descending aorta onwards, although the sinus of Valsalva morphology had normalized (Fig. 33.2d).

33.3 Key Points

AR associated with aortic dissection can usually be eliminated simply by performing commissural fixation. However, when the dissection extends extensively to the aortic annulus, the adhesive strength of biological glue in the dissected lumen is usually inadequate, and VSARR needs to be considered. The above-mentioned patient required a total aortic arch replacement due to an extensive dissection, so we performed partial remodeling to preserve the LCS to shorten the duration of myocardial ischemia.

Patient 2	The patient was a 75-year-old man. Body height 166 cm, body weight 70 kg, body surface area 1.79 m^2
Medical history	Hypertension.
Family history	Nothing of note.
History of present illness	The patient suffered from back pain 1 year and 5 months ago, and detailed investigations revealed a thoracic aortic aneurysm.

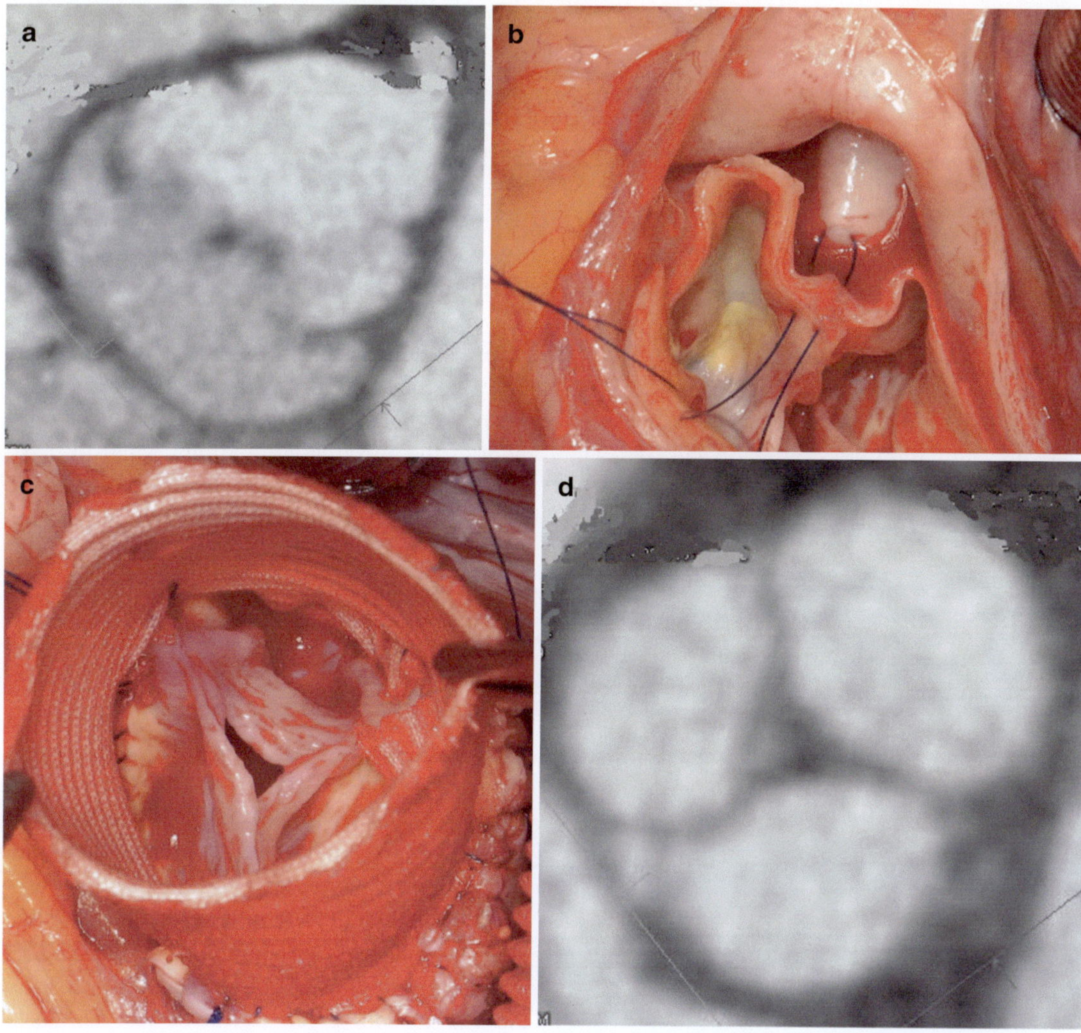

Fig. 33.2 Patient 1. (**a**) The preoperative CT scan showed dissection of the RCS and NCS. The commissure between them was detached. (**b**) Intraoperative photograph. Dissected commissure. (**c**) Intraoperative photograph. Partial remodeling of the RCS and NCS. (**d**) The postoperative CT scan showed that the sinus of Valsalva was repaired

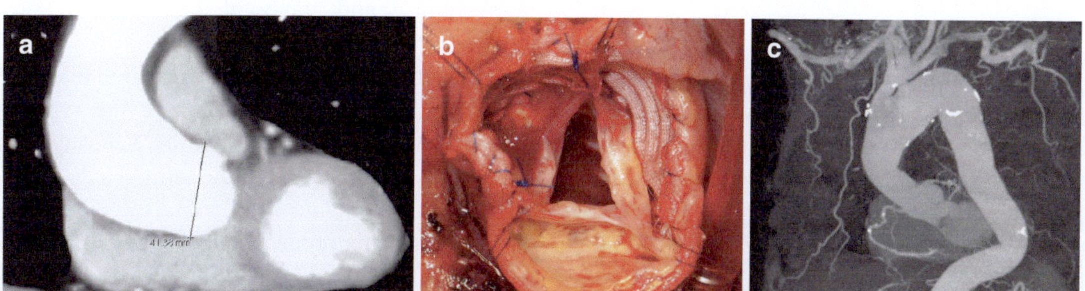

Fig. 33.3 Patient 2. (**a**) The preoperative CT scan showed enlargement of the ascending aorta and sinuses of Valsalva. (**b**) Intraoperative photograph showing partial remodeling of the RCS and NCS. (**c**) A postoperative CT scan shows the prosthetic vascular graft that has replaced the ascending aorta. The dilated sinuses of Valsalva are also repaired

Preoperative CT	Maximum ascending aorta diameter: 54 mm. Aortic arch: 38 mm. Descending aorta: 33 mm (Fig. 33.3a).
Preoperative echocardiogram	Mild AR, LVDd: 40 mm, LVDs: 23 mm, LVEF: 68%, basal annulus: 22 mm, sinus of Valsalva: 47 mm, STJ: 42 mm.

33.4 Surgical Technique

The aortic cusps presented a favorable shape. There were also mild atherosclerotic changes that were present within the sinuses of Valsalva. The enlargement of the LCS was determined to be mild. The walls of the NCS and RCS of Valsalva were preserved, and a semi-circular patch formed from a 26-mm prosthetic vascular graft was sutured within the sinuses to the deepest part of the aortic annulus using interrupted mattress sutures, while continuous sutures were used in other areas. The right coronary ostium button was created and anastomosed to the prosthetic vascular graft (Fig. 33.3b). The aorta was cross-clamped for a total of 110 min. The duration of cardiopulmonary bypass was 131 min. Surgery lasted 4 h and 53 min.

Postoperative Clinical Course

The clinical course was uneventful, and the patient was discharged on postoperative day 9 in an ambulatory condition.

Postoperative Evaluation

There was mild, residual, central AR at the time of discharge, although the sinus of Valsalva diameter had decreased to 36 mm (Fig. 33.3c). Three years have elapsed since surgery, but the AR has not deteriorated.

33.5 Discussion

Urbanski et al. performed partial remodeling in 71% of 236 ARRs, which included 30 patients suffering an AAD [2, 3]. Postoperative aortic valve replacement was performed on ten patients, and the freedom from AR (≥grade 3) at 8 years was 95%. When discussing this report, David stated that although partial remodeling is effective in the elderly, the reimplantation procedure should be performed on young patients suffering from conditions such as Marfan syndrome or bicuspid aortic valves, since enlargement of the aortic annulus might occur in these patients. Charitos et al. compared 108 patients who underwent total remodeling to 29 patients who underwent partial remodeling and reported significantly greater enlargement of the sinus of Valsalva and STJ diameter in the partial remodeling group, although the AR grade remained similar [4].

The Bentall procedure is usually performed when the dissection involves the aortic root and an adventitial tear extends into frank rupture, although VSARR may also be considered. Partial remodeling may shorten the duration of surgery in this state. Kazui et al. recommended performing partial remodeling with replacement of the NCS only because re-dissection of the NCS is commonly observed during repeat surgery after the use of biological adhesives [5]. Urbanski et al. reported that the native aortic valve was preserved in 56% of patients (n = 46) who underwent surgery to treat a type A AD involving the aortic root. The majority underwent partial remodeling, and favorable outcomes were reported [6].

The authors have previously reported that this procedure is expected to decrease the risk of bleeding from the aortic root by suturing the prosthetic vascular graft to the intimal side without resecting the sinuses of Valsalva (Fig. 33.4) [7]. To date, this procedure has been performed

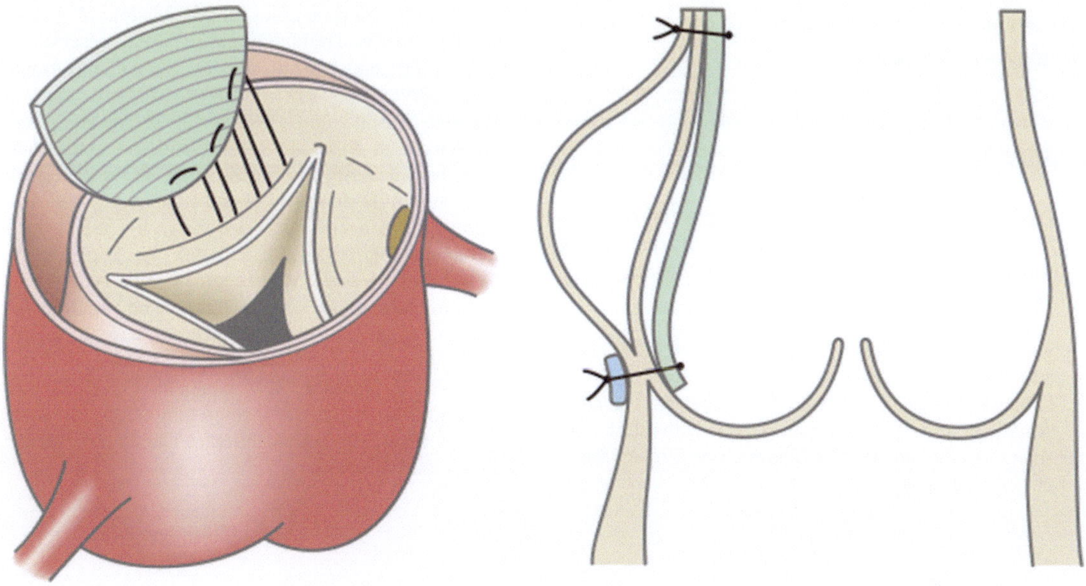

Fig. 33.4 Preservation of the autologous sinuses of Valsalva during partial remodeling to treat AAD. A prosthetic vascular graft is used to reinforce the intimal surface. Cited from Ref. [7] in modified form

on 20 patients. It was performed to manage the NCS in 17 patients, the RCS in 5 patients, and the LCC sinus in 1 patient. There were two operative mortalities, and AR was controlled in all patients at the time of discharge. The long-term outcomes in terms of repeat surgery to the aortic root showed that one patient underwent the Bentall procedure three-and-a-half years postoperatively due to infective endocarditis. Two patients were also found to develop moderate AR (after 4 and 7 years, respectively) when we evaluated the long-term outcomes.

33.6 Closing Remarks

Consideration needs to be given to patient age, etiology, and the extent of enlargement when deciding whether to replace all sinuses of Valsalva. It is difficult to define precisely, so we wonder whether it would be better to consider performing total remodeling or reimplantation instead. During AAD, there is a bleeding tendency and the patients are commonly treated by inexperienced surgeons. Partial remodeling offers the benefits of increased valve preservation and a shorter operation time. We should master the aortic root anatomy in routine practice.

33.7 Key Points

The Bentall procedure, which uses biological valves, was indicated in elderly patients with ascending aortic aneurysms associated with enlarged sinuses of Valsalva. The valve characteristics were not pathological, thus we decided valve-preservation was possible. The partial remodeling technique was used to shorten the duration of surgery and decrease the risk of bleeding. The control of AR was insufficient. However, there were no changes after 3 years had elapsed postoperatively, therefore valve sparing strategy was successful.

References

1. David TE, Feindel CM, Bos J. Repair of the aortic valve in patients with aortic insufficiency and aortic root aneurysm. J Thorac Cardiovasc Surg. 1995;109:345–51.
2. Urbanski PP. Valve-sparing aortic root repair with patch technique. Ann Thorac Surg. 2005;80: 839–43.
3. Urbanski PP, Zhan X, Hijazi H, Zacher M, Diegeler A. Valve-sparing aortic root repair without downsizing of the annulus. J Thorac Cardiovasc Surg. 2012;143:294–302.
4. Charitos EI, Stierle U, Sievers HH, Misfeld M. Valve-sparing aortic root remodeling with partial preservation of the intact native aortic sinuses. Eur J Cardiothorac Surg. 2009;36:589–91.
5. Kazui T, Washiyama N, Bashar AH, Terada H, Suzuki K, Yamashita K, et al. Role of biologic glue repair of proximal aortic dissection in the development of early and midterm redissection of the aortic root. Ann Thorac Surg. 2001;72:509–14.
6. Urbanski PP, Hijazi H, Dinstak W, Diegeler A. Valve-sparing aortic root repair in acute type A dissection: how many sinuses have to be repaired for curative surgery? Eur J Cardiothorac Surg. 2013;44: 439–43.
7. Komiya T, Tamura N, Sakaguchi G, Kobayashi T. Modified partial aortic root remodeling in acute type A aortic dissection. Interact Cardiovasc Thorac Surg. 2009;8:306–9.

Aortic Valvuloplasty to Treat Aortic Regurgitation Accompanied by a Ruptured Sinus of Valsalva Aneurysm

34

Takeshi Miyairi

Patient	48-year-old man, body height: 170 cm, body weight: 77 kg, body surface area: 1.88 m^2
Medical history	The patient was noted to have a ventricular septal defect (VSD) in childhood. From the age of 30 years, he suffered from hyperlipidemia and hepatic steatosis, and these were both untreated.
History of present illness	From 10 days prior to consultation, the patient developed a fever and cough. He visited his local practitioner, who prescribed antibiotics, but he did not improve. From 5 days prior to consultation, the patient developed dyspnea and general malaise, so he was admitted by his local practitioner. Blood cultures were negative. Blood tests showed hepatic dysfunction, so an abdominal ultrasound was performed, which suggested acute cholecystitis. The patient then underwent endoscopic retrograde biliary drainage, but his hepatic function did not improve. He was transferred by ambulance to our hospital, where we observed marked symptoms of cardiac failure. We performed detailed examinations and diagnosed the patient as having a type I VSD, a ruptured sinus of Valsalva (SV) aneurysm, and aortic insufficiency.
Preoperative echocardiogram	Type I VSD, grade II aortic regurgitation, prolapse of the right coronary cusp (RCC) There was a short shunt jet observed from the right SV into the right ventricular lumen. The left ventricular end-diastole and systole diameter (LVDd/Ds) were 56/34 mm, the aortic diameter (AoD) was 29 mm, the left atrial diameter (LAD) was 47 mm, the left ventricular ejection fraction (LVEF) was 69%, the left ventricular fractional shortening (LVFS) was 39%, estimated pulmonary artery (PA) pressure was 75 mmHg, and the Qp/Qs ratio was 2.88. Left ventricular systolic function was maintained, but left ventricular diastolic function was moderately to severely impaired.
Preoperative cardiac catheterization results	Right atrium: 34/26/24 mmHg, PA: 66/31/52 mmHg, pulmonary capillary wedge pressure: 42/40/33 mmHg, aorta: 91/42/64 mmHg, LV: 92/11/33 mmHg, Qp/Qs ratio: 2.3

T. Miyairi (✉)
Department of Cardiovascular Surgery, St. Marianna University School of Medicine, Kawasaki, Japan
e-mail: miyairitakeshi@gmail.com

T. Kunihara, S. Takanashi (eds.), *Aortic Valve Preservation*, https://doi.org/10.1007/978-981-13-2068-2_34

34.1 Surgical Technique

Closure of the ruptured SV aneurysm, patch closure of the VSD, and aortic valvuloplasty.

34.2 Surgical Method

The patient was placed in the supine position, and general anesthesia was induced. Thereafter, the patient went into cardiac arrest due to ventricular tachycardia, so we immediately started cardiopulmonary resuscitation (CPR), performed as much skin sterilization as possible during CPR, and draped the patient. Next, we performed a median sternotomy, and when a moderate volume of pericardial fluid was drained, spontaneous maintenance of his heart rate returned.

The ascending aorta was cannulated, two drains were placed from the right atrium into the superior vena cava (SVC) and inferior vena cava (IVC), and cardiopulmonary bypass was initiated.

We first taped the SVC and IVC, then inserted a retrograde cardioplegic route via the right atrium, inserted a vent cannula from the right superior pulmonary vein into the left ventricle, and inserted an antegrade cardioplegia cannula via the aortic root, which was left in situ.

The aorta was cross-clamped, a longitudinal incision was created in the main PA, and we confirmed the presence of a Type I VSD measuring 12 × 16 mm immediately below the pulmonary valve. When we examined the right ventricle through the pulmonary valve, we found the SV aneurysm extending through the middle of the VSD from the aortic valve, which was projecting into the right ventricle. We also observed rupture of the distal end and lateral wall of the aneurysm. The right SV aneurysm had a rough surface, the tissue was extremely fragile, and we strongly suspected the presence of infection, so we resected the entire area. We also sent part of these fragile tissues for culture. Virtually the entire right SV was resected, excluding the origin of the right coronary artery, and only the RCC and the annulus remained. The resected portion was repaired using autologous pericardium treated with 0.6% glutaraldehyde solution and secured at four points using 5-0 polypropylene sutures, whereas the rest of the patch was secured with continuous sutures. The areas with fragile tissue were supplementarily secured using mattress sutures with autologous pericardial pledgets (Fig. 34.1).

Next, we used an autologous pericardial patch in a similar manner to close the VSD, using interrupted sutures of 5-0 polypropylene (Fig. 34.2).

We observed prolapse of the RCC, so we added a single cusp plication suture and ensured that the length matched that of the other leaflets. We then performed a commissural annuloplasty on the left coronary cusp and non-coronary cusp commissures using pledgeted mattress sutures of 5-0 polypropylene.

We confirmed no residual VSD leaks by inflating the lung, and then we closed the PA using a single continuous suture. The aortotomy was closed using double-layered sutures.

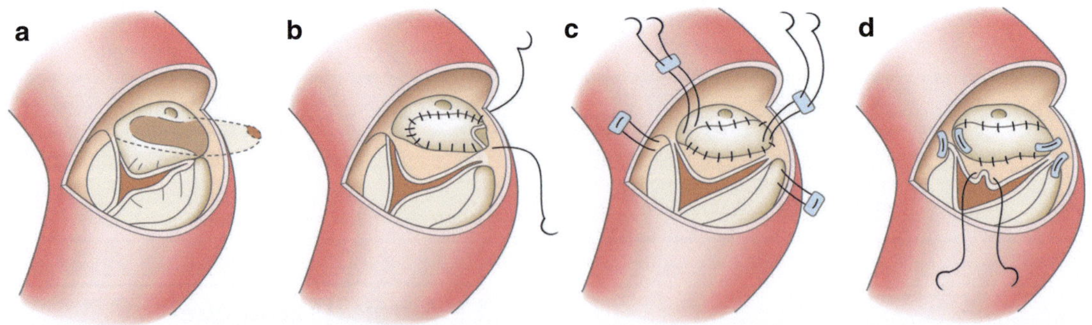

Fig. 34.1 Transverse aortotomy of the ascending aorta. (**a**) The ruptured sinus of Valsalva aneurysm at the right coronary sinus. (**b**) Closure of the defect using an autologous pericardial patch. (**c**) Subcommissural annuloplasty. (**d**) Central cusp plication

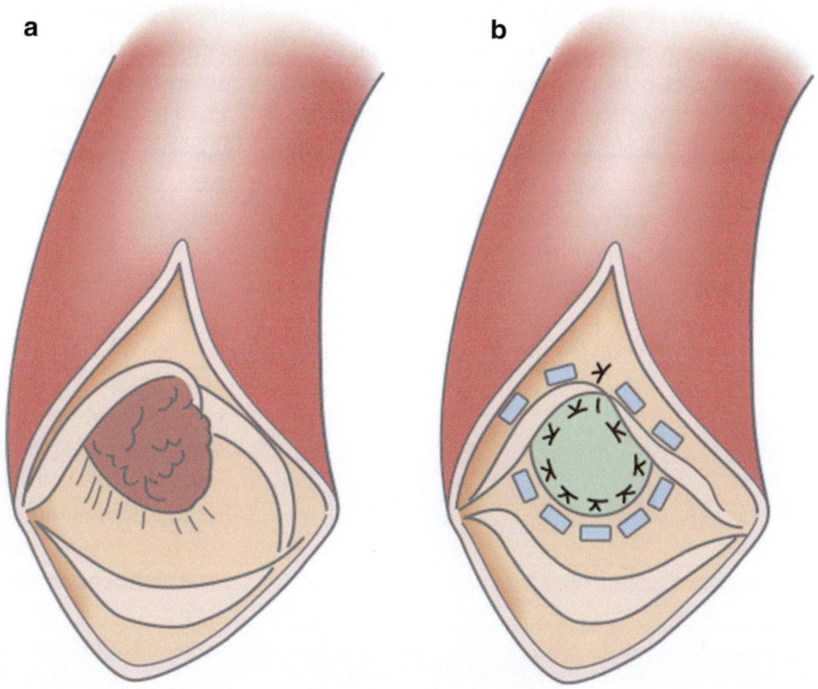

Fig. 34.2 Longitudinal incision in the main pulmonary artery. (**a**) The right SV aneurysm extended through the middle of the VSD and projected into the right ventricle. (**b**) Closure of the VSD using an autologous pericardial patch

34.3 Personal Tips

Suspected infectious tissues should thoroughly be resected. The resected parts of the SV should be reconstructed using an autologous pericardial patch treated with 0.6% glutaraldehyde to prevent tissue shrinkage. Particularly the areas where the tissues are fragile should be secured with mattress sutures pledgeted with autologous pericardium. As the SV must be resected up to the margin of the annulus, suturing should be performed with appropriate caution to ensure that the pericardial patch sutures do not compromise the leaflet.

34.4 Postoperative Clinical Course

Postoperative management was challenging due to the prolonged cardiac failure that started preoperatively, the hepatic dysfunction caused by hepatic congestion and the associated coagulation disorder, and acute renal failure. The patient was extubated on postoperative day (POD) 13, discharged from the intensive care unit on POD 20, and transferred to a rehabilitation hospital on POD 80.

34.5 Postoperative Echocardiogram

Neither a left-to-right shunt nor aortic regurgitation was present. LVDd/Ds: 47/29 mm, AoD: 26 mm, LAD: 35, LVEF: 70%, LVFS: 40%, estimated PA pressure: 33 mmHg.

34.6 Key Points

The authors addressed the following points during aortic valvuloplasty.

1. Approach: A transverse incision is made approximately 1 cm superior to the sinotubular junction of the ascending aorta. The incision is rather long, measuring greater than two-thirds of the circumference, to enable exposure of the commissures without distortion.

2. Exposure of the visual field: 2-0 polyester sutures are placed at the three commissures and retracted in a straight line externally to prevent distortion of the leaflets, and then the sutures are secured by the suture holder used for valve replacement (Fig. 34.3).
3. Central plication: While applying adequate traction to the commissure between two leaflets unaffected by prolapse, a 5-0 polypropylene suture is attached to an area close to the nodes of Arantius of both leaflets to make the length from the commissures equivalent and is then tied loosely. Two other 5-0 polypropylene sutures are placed immediately next to each of the previous sutures on both leaflets. While applying adequate traction to the two commissures of the prolapsing leaflet, the sutures are affixed to the prolapsed leaflet to determine the extent of plication to ensure that the distances from the commissures are equivalent (Fig. 34.4).
4. Finally, the effective height is measured, and if it is ≤9 mm, then additional plication of each leaflet is performed.
5. Commissural annuloplasty: reduction of the commissures is performed by placing 2-0 polyester mattress sutures with Teflon felt pledgets to the commissures to step over them. The suture is directed externally, away from the SV next to the commissure, and the surgeon ensures that it is not directed inferiorly to the commissure. In addition, by suturing at an adequate distance away from the aortic annulus, the felt will not come into contact with the leaflets and will not interfere with their motion. Accordingly, we tend to use smaller felt pledgets.
6. Resection: Coaptation is impeded by areas where the leaflet free margins are calcified or hypertrophic and sclerotic, so a small portion is resected and sutured, and additional plication of the other leaflets is performed to create a good fit.

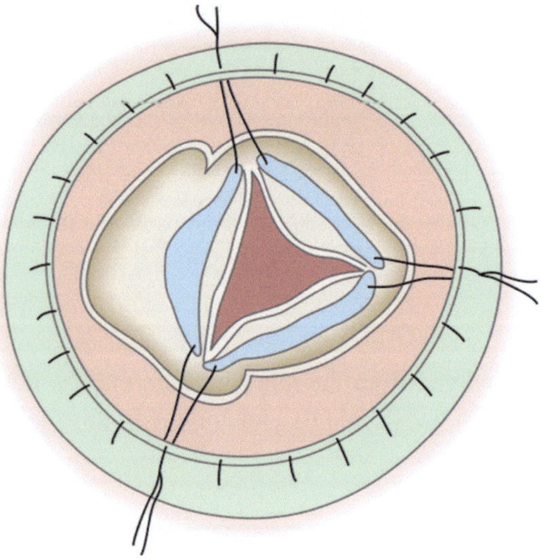

Fig. 34.3 Resuspension of the commissures

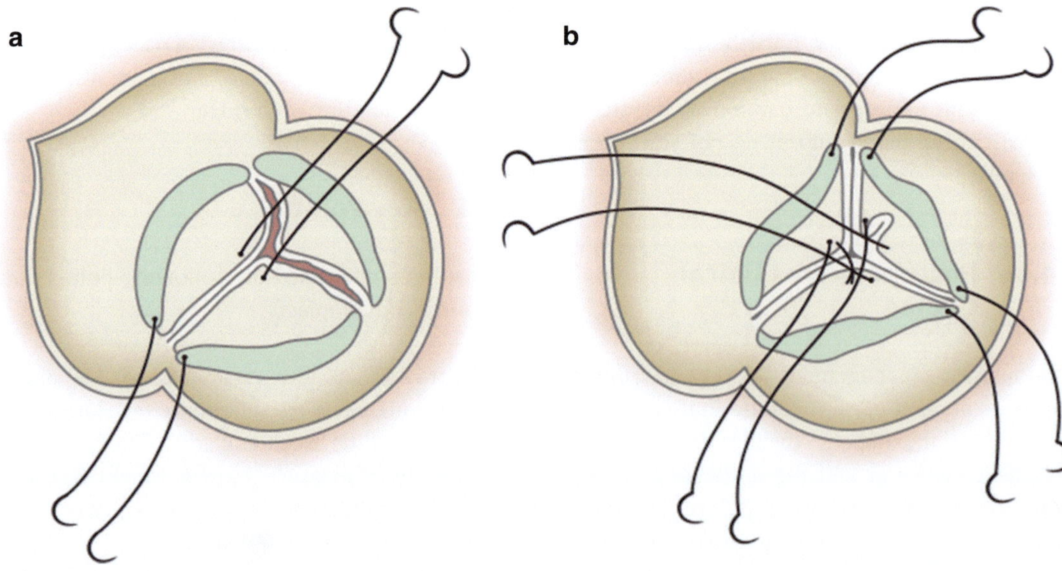

Fig. 34.4 Central plication. (**a**) Pilot sutures to adjust the free margin length of each cusp. (**b**) Central cusp plication

Valvuloplasty to Treat Aortic Regurgitation Associated with a Ventricular Septal Defect

35

Takayoshi Ueno and Yoshiki Sawa

35.1 Introduction

The ventricular septal defects (VSDs) known to cause aortic regurgitation (AR) are doubly committed VSDs, perimembranous VSDs, and muscular outlet VSDs [1]. Surgery is naturally often indicated in patients with a high shunt volume that causes cardiac failure or pulmonary hypertension, although it is possible to prevent the progression of AR by closing the VSD before AR worsens due to aortic valve (AV) prolapse [2]. If the AR is graded as trivial or more, then we believe that this is an acceptable indication for surgery [3]. Consider early closure if there are concerns for a patient with a doubly committed VSD, which can be closed through an incision made only in the pulmonary artery. However, if the concomitant AR is graded as moderate or greater, then consider surgical management of the AV.

Patient	71-year-old woman, height: 155 cm, body weight: 51 kg, body surface area: 1.48 m^2 30 years after ventricular septal defect closure and aortic valve plasty.

History of present illness	A heart murmur was detected at birth. The patient suffered from difficulty in breathing and noticed palpitations from 1 year prior to presentation. Echocardiography revealed AR associated with a VSD. She was referred to our hospital and underwent surgery.
Echocardiography findings	VSD: muscular outlet type. Right coronary cusp (RCC) herniation was observed, and we found moderate AR and elongation of the RCC with thickening of the free margin.
Surgery	VSD closure, aortic valvuloplasty
Intraoperative findings	The AV was tricuspid, and the RCC sinus was larger than the others. The RCC itself possessed excess tissue due to elongation and was hypertrophic. We observed a partial cleft-like gap on the RCC and performed direct closure. The commissure between the RCC and left coronary cusp was secured to the aortic wall by folding up the cusps, and the other commissures were secured in a somewhat suspended state while the coaptation with the noncoronary cusp (NCC) was reinforced. An intraoperative transesophageal echocardiogram showed trivial AR only.

T. Ueno (✉) · Y. Sawa
Department of Cardiovascular Surgery, Graduate School of Medicine, Osaka University, Suita, Japan
e-mail: uenotm@surg1.med.osaka-u.ac.jp

T. Kunihara, S. Takanashi (eds.), *Aortic Valve Preservation*, https://doi.org/10.1007/978-981-13-2068-2_35

Postoperative course	AR was mild during the first 5 postoperative years, although it subsequently worsened. The patient underwent AV replacement 7 years after the operation. When the AV was replaced, we found that the NCC was also elongated, in addition to the RCC that had previously undergone valvuloplasty. There was also a partial slit in the RCC, so we decided that a repeat valvuloplasty would be difficult.

35.2 AR Etiology

AR may be caused by either a lack of support for the cusp adjacent to the VSD or the Venturi effect. During systole, the shunt flow through the VSD causes the adjacent cusp to become deformed and drawn in the direction of the right ventricle. If the cusp is heavily drawn toward the right ventricle, then the prolapse worsens, resulting in AR. Accordingly, there are few cases of VSDs causing AR that meet the indications for surgery in early infancy. Conversely, the cases that do meet the indications for surgery will commonly occur from the ages of 5 to 10 years onward. In cases with a surgical indication to treat the AV with moderate or greater AR, if either their AV cusps are commonly associated with deformation, enlargement, and elongation or annular enlargement is seen, then the success of valvuloplasty is less likely. Accordingly, although these operations usually become challenging, valvuloplasty is often performed as an initial intervention while taking growth into consideration when the surgical intervention is performed in childhood.

35.3 Valvuloplasty Surgery

The valvuloplasty technique is important to reshape the cusps that are causing the AR. Historically, the first reports of aortic valvuloplasty for VSD-AR started to appear in 1960 [4], although in the initial stages, the main objective was to shorten the elongated cusps. A stay suture was placed to match the nodules of Arantius for this purpose, and maintenance of cusp coaptation was thought to be important. However, patients frequently had to undergo reoperation due to AR recurrence when this technique was used, and it has further been improved. A resuspension stitch is used to suspend the cusps from the aortic wall, and the accuracy of the valvuloplasty is improved by reinforcing the commissure [5]. There were reports on valvuloplasty from various perspectives in the 1990s, and in 1997, Yacoub et al. reported on aortic valvuloplasty from the perspective of correcting the anatomical features of VSD-AR [6]. Specifically, a mattress suture is placed along the VSD margin and passed through the aortic annulus, and then the enlarged sinus of Valsalva is folded and plicated. This corrects the position of the aortic annulus, reinforces the annulus, plicates the sinus, and corrects the cusp prolapse. These maneuvers in turn facilitate an aortic valvuloplasty that reconstructs an almost anatomically normal AV configuration (Fig. 35.1a). However, we still believe that this method has a potential risk associated with VSD recurrence. One reason is that direct VSD closure causes excessive tension. Another is that when dealing with the complete doubly committed type (which is commonly seen in Asian patients) without muscular tissue between the AV and pulmonary valve (PV), a suture needs to be passed through the fibrous tissue between the AV and PV, and thus the support is weak.

For this reason, we use the following strategies when we treat VSD-AR: (1) We first measure the original size of the VSD, including the tissue of the prolapsing Valsalva sinus rather than the actual size of the defect. We then use a patch that is the same size as, or slightly smaller than, the VSD and close the VSD through the right ventricle. This achieves some reduction of the enlarged aortic annulus and can also return the prolapsing sinus to the left ventricle (Fig. 35.1b). (2) We make an aortotomy and coapt the nodules of Arantius together in the center to estimate the length of the elongated cusps. Thereafter, the elongated cusps are folded and plicated close to

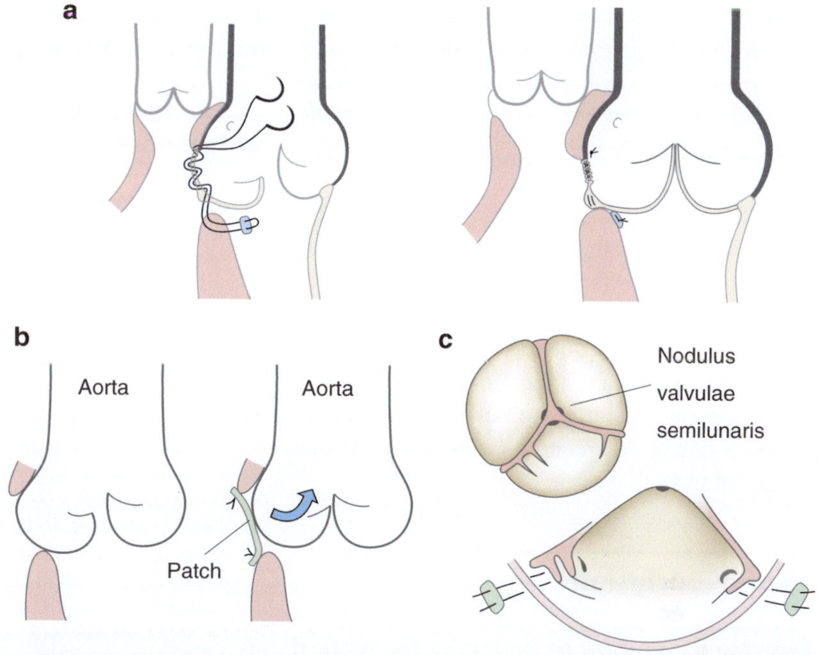

Fig. 35.1 Surgical technique for aortic valvuloplasty. (**a**) Schema for the surgical technique described by Yacoub et al. (cited from Ref. [6]). (**b**) A patch is sutured from the right ventricle, and the prolapsing sinus is returned into the left ventricle while simultaneously performing reduction of the adjacent annulus. (**c**) Elongated cusps are suspended from the aortic wall to fold them back

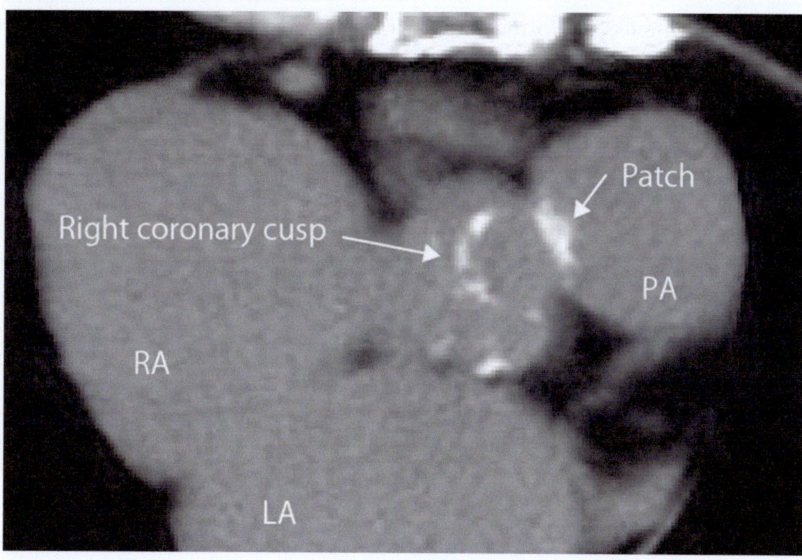

Fig. 35.2 A computed tomographic image of a horizontal cross-section of the AV 30 years after surgery to treat a VSD-AR. Calcification of the RCC, which was treated by valvuloplasty, can be seen. *PA* Pulmonary artery, *RA* right atrium, *LA* left atrium

the commissure using a polypropylene mattress suture to ensure an adequate length of the coaptation zone. This suture is drawn out of the aortic wall to somewhat suspend the cusp and then ligated (so-called "Trusler stitch") [5] (Fig. 35.1c). This is considered to be the primary technique for aortic valvuloplasty and VSD closure to treat VSD-AR.

35.4 Long-Term Outcomes

Based on the above, a certain degree of surgical invasiveness that affects the cusps and sinuses is unavoidable when performing valvuloplasty to treat VSD-AR. In addition, the procedure is commonly performed on young patients, and a long period of postoperative follow-up is required. In some cases, the surgical manipulations to the cusps may cause cusp sclerosis or deformation of the sinuses at a later point in life, so periodic follow-up is extremely important. Figure 35.2 shows a computed tomographic image from a patient 30 years after surgery performed to treat VSD-AR that was based on the above-mentioned surgical technique. A horizontal cross-section of the operated AV shows calcification of the plicated RCC. Echocardiography showed mild to moderate AR due to poor mobility of the RCC. There is still no indication for reoperation in this patient, although we believe that there is always a risk of AR recurrence in future, as this patient shows.

35.5 Conclusion

This chapter provides an outline of the surgical technique used to perform valvuloplasty to treat VSD-AR. Patients will often require long-term follow-up. In addition, when valve tissues are subjected to surgical manipulations, this poses the risk of future reoperation due to factors such as valvular sclerosis or deformation, so long-term postoperative follow-up is essential.

References

1. Jacobs JP, Burke RP, Quintessenza JA, Mavroudis C. Congenital heart surgery nomenclature and database project: ventricular septal defect. Ann Thorac Surg. 2000;69(Suppl 4):S25–35.
2. Sim EK, Grignani RT, Wong ML, Quek SC, Wong JC, Yip WC, et al. Outcome of surgical closure of doubly committed subarterial ventricular septal defect. Ann Thorac Surg. 1999;67:736–8.
3. Elgamal MA, Hakimi M, Lyons JM, Walters HL 3rd. Risk factors for failure of aortic valvuloplasty in aortic insufficiency with ventricular septal defect. Ann Thorac Surg. 1999;68:1350–5.
4. Starr A, Menashe V, Dotter C. Surgical correction of aortic insufficiency associated with ventricular septal defect. Surg Gynecol Obstet. 1960;111:71–6.
5. Trusler GA, Moes CA, Kid BS. Repair of ventricular septal defect with aortic insufficiency. J Thorac Cardiovasc Surg. 1973;66:394–403.
6. Yacoub MH, Khan H, Stavri G, Shinebourne E, Radley-Smith R. Anatomic correction of the syndrome of prolapsing right coronary aortic cusp, dilatation of the sinus of Valsalva, and ventricular septal defect. J Thorac Cardiovasc Surg. 1997;113:253–60.

Valvuloplasty for Aortic Regurgitation Associated with Infective Endocarditis

36

Kazuyoshi Tanigawa and Kiyoyuki Eishi

Patient	60-year-old man, body height: 171 cm, body weight: 80 kg, body surface area: 1.92 m^2
Medical history	Gastric ulcer
History of present illness	The patient experienced marked pain due to a carious tooth but did not seek treatment. He subsequently developed lower back pain, a fever of 39 °C, and a cough. He was examined by his local practitioner and prescribed antipyretic analgesics, an antitussive agent, and oral antibiotics. He remained feverish, however, and subsequently suffered from increasing respiratory distress, so he underwent a detailed examination. Echocardiography revealed vegetations on the anterior leaflet of the mitral valve (MV), and the patient was referred to the Department of Cardiology at our hospital. Blood cultures led to the detection of *Streptococcus mitis*, and antibiotics were switched to 2 g of ampicillin 6 times per day and 70 mg of gentamicin 3 times per day intravenously. A lumbar magnetic resonance imaging (MRI) scan revealed pyogenic spondylitis, although we decided to continue conservative therapy with antibiotics after consultation with the Department of Orthopedics. However, the inflammatory response did not normalize and the fever persisted, so we scheduled cardiac surgery after we had drained the epidural abscess.
Preoperative echocardiogram	Aortic diameter: 40 mm, aortic valve (AV) opening: 19 mm, left atrial diameter: 47 mm, interventricular septum: 16 mm, posterior wall of the left ventricle: 15 mm, left ventricular end-diastolic diameter: 50 mm, left ventricular end-systolic diameter: 26 mm, left ventricular fractional shortening: 48%, left ventricular ejection fraction: 79%, moderate aortic regurgitation (AR), moderate mitral regurgitation (MR). There was a 15-mm vegetation attached to the anterior leaflet of the mitral valve (A3), facing the left ventricular outflow tract. Systolic anterior motion (SAM) was observed. The AV was tricuspid—we noted calcification of the bodies of Arantius but did not see any obvious vegetations (Fig. 36.1).

36.1 Surgical Technique

Aortic valvuloplasty, mitral valve replacement (MVR).

K. Tanigawa
Division of Cardiovascular Surgery, Nagasaki University, Graduate School of Biomedical Sciences, Nagasaki, Japan

K. Eishi (✉)
Division of Cardiovascular Surgery, Nagasaki University, Graduate School of Biomedical Sciences, Nagasaki, Japan
e-mail: keishi@nagasaki-u.ac.jp

T. Kunihara, S. Takanashi (eds.), *Aortic Valve Preservation*, https://doi.org/10.1007/978-981-13-2068-2_36

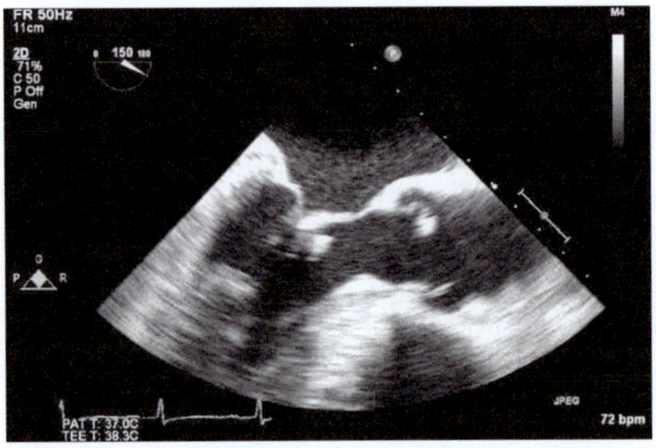

Fig. 36.1 Preoperative transesophageal echocardiogram. Vegetations on the AV and anterior leaflet of the MV

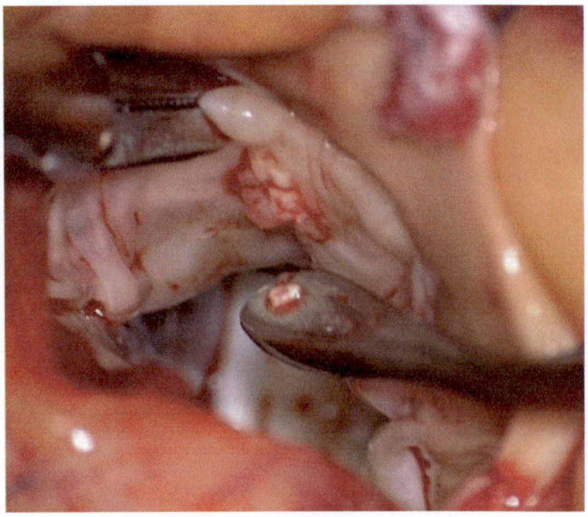

Fig. 36.2 Intraoperative findings. Vegetations noted on the left coronary cusp facing the outflow tract. A curette was used to remove the vegetations

36.2 Surgical Method

We cannulated the ascending aorta, placed drains in the inferior and superior vena cava, and initiated cardiopulmonary bypass. After cross-clamping the ascending aorta, an incision was made into the right side of the left atrium. The patient had hypertrophic cardiomyopathy accompanied by systolic anterior motion (SAM), although the visual field was somewhat unfavorable. We performed debridement of the infectious foci on the MV using a curette, scalpel, and electric scalpel. This resulted in a defect in the clear zone from the lateral A2 area to A3, which we closed using an autologous pericardial patch. We performed fixation between the lateral A3 area and the posterior commissure and then performed an annuloplasty using a 28-mm Memo 3D annuloplasty ring (Sorin Biomedica Cardio S.R.L., Saluggia, Italy). Next, we opened the ascending aorta and noted vegetations on all three AV leaflets. There was no evident valve destruction, so we performed debridement and electrocautery and concluded the surgery. After the patient was weaned from cardiopulmonary bypass, we observed MR due to SAM by transesophageal echocardiography, so we re-initiated cardiac arrest and unfastened the prosthetic valve ring. This did not improve the MR, however. We then performed MV replacement with a 27-mm St. Jude Medical prosthetic valve (St. Jude Medical, St. Paul, MN, USA). There were no issues with the AV (Fig. 36.2).

36.3 Personal Tips

Although the surgical techniques for aortic valvuloplasty are fascinating, if we consider preservation of the AV morphology to be important, then clearance of the infected tissues could be inadequate. When performing valvuloplasty in patients with infective endocarditis, we believe the procedure should be limited to either debridement of the infected tissues alone, or repair of cusp perforations with a pericardial patch, or repair by means of a relatively simple technique (leaflet plication, commissural plication).

36.4 Postoperative Course

The patient was extubated on postoperative day (POD) 1, and there were no notable complications. On POD 2, the patient was transferred to a general ward for further management. We did not suspect any infectious cerebral aneurysms when we examined postoperative confirmatory cranial MRI images. Antibiotics were administered for 6 weeks postoperatively, and the patient continued cardiac rehabilitation. Thereafter, the inflammatory response normalized, and we observed no AR, no functional insufficiency of the prosthetic MV, and no persistent vegetations, so we discharged the patient home.

36.5 Key Points

The purposes of surgical treatment during infective endocarditis may be to control cardiac failure due to valve dysfunction associated with the infection, to perform curettage of the infectious foci causing septicemia, to prevent embolization of the vegetations, and to prevent and repair structural damage to tissues such as the annulus. Although it may initially appear possible to manage cardiac failure, emergency surgery may occasionally be required for patients who experience either worsening cardiac failure caused by sustained cardiac volume overload or myocardial ischemia due to diastolic hypotension, particularly when acute AR occurs due to AV destruction.

Compared to valve replacement, valvuloplasty is expected to reduce the need for anticoagulant therapy, decrease prosthetic valve infection, and decrease postoperative mortality and complications. The effectiveness of mitral valvuloplasty for mitral infective endocarditis has already been widely acknowledged from this perspective [1, 2]. There are very few reports in the literature that deal with the efficacy of aortic valvuloplasty, whereas there are many reports that support the efficacy of AV replacement (AVR) [3]. However, there can be challenges in cases associated with severe conditions such as infection or deterioration of the annulus, even if thorough curettage and patch reconstruction, or even valve replacement, are performed.

Mayer et al. [4] compared the surgical techniques for AV procedures to treat infective endocarditis. They studied an aortic valvuloplasty group (33 patients) and an AVR group (67 patients) and then reported on their respective in-hospital mortality (9 and 18%, $p = 0.37$), 5-year survival rates (88 and 65%, $p = 0.047$), reoperation rates (35 and 10%, $p = 0.021$) and freedom from AR $\geq$ grade II at 5 years (66 and 87%, $p = 0.066$). The reoperation rates were higher and freedom from AR rates were lower in the aortic valvuloplasty group. However, we cannot ignore the fact that both the postoperative mortality and 5-year survival were better in the valvuloplasty group than in the AVR group, despite the inclusion of severe cases, such as those associated with aortic root abscesses.

36.6 Conclusion

We performed AV surgery on 31 patients (AVR in 29 and valvuloplasty in 2 patients) suffering from infective endocarditis affecting the AV at our hospital between April 1999 and December 2014. The indications for aortic valvuloplasty for infective endocarditis were limited, and the two valvuloplasty patients did not show severe preoperative regurgitation. Aortic valvuloplasty to treat infective endocarditis is commonly complicated by challenges related to infection of the AV or annulus. However, we believe that there are increasing cases that will meet the indications for this form of treatment thanks to advances in aortic valvuloplasty, and we will need to address further improvements and perform investigations going forward.

References

1. Zegdi R, Debièche M, Latrémouille C, Lebied D, Chardigny C, Grinda JM, et al. Long-term results of mitral valve repair in active endocarditis. Circulation. 2005;111:2532–6.
2. Miura T, Hamawaki M, Hazama S, Hashizume K, Ariyoshi T, Sumi M, et al. Outcome of surgical management for active mitral native valve infective endocarditis: a collective review of 57 patients. Gen Thorac Cardiovasc Surg. 2014;62:488–98.
3. David TE, Gavra G, Feindel CM, Regesta T, Armstrong S, Maganti MD. Surgical treatment of active infective endocarditis: a continued challenge. J Thorac Cardiovasc Surg. 2007;133:144–9.
4. Mayer K, Aicher D, Feldner S, Kunihara T, Schäfers HJ. Repair versus replacement of the aortic valve in active infective endocarditis. Eur J Cardiothorac Surg. 2012;42:122–7.

Valvuloplasty to Treat Traumatic Aortic Regurgitation

37

Hitoshi Okabayashi

37.1 Introduction

Blunt chest trauma commonly occurs during road traffic accidents in up to 20% of cases although traumatic aortic regurgitation (AR) is said to be rare. Reports indicate that cardiac injury is observed in 15–20% of autopsy cases, whereas valve injury is observed in 5% [1]. Valve injury may affect the aortic, mitral, or tricuspid valve. The most commonly observed lesions of the aortic valve (AV) in these cases are leaflet injury and disruption of the leaflets from the annulus, which most commonly affect the noncoronary cusp (NCC) [2–7]. The mechanism of AV injury involves the application of compressive force to the sternum from an anterior direction during early diastole; the aorta is compressed between the sternum and the vertebrae while the AV is closed, which leads to excessive pressure being exerted on the AV, thus causing injury [8]. There is speculation that the NCC might be more commonly injured because the leaflets with coronary ostia are able to avoid this pressure by diverting blood flow into the coronary arteries [9].

Patient 1	A 21-year-old man was involved in a road traffic accident on his motorcycle and suffered a right femoral fracture, mandibular fracture, and rib fractures. He was transported to the emergency center via ambulance. During his hospital stay, he was found to be suffering from a concomitant antithrombin III deficiency, and a cranial computed tomography (CT) scan revealed findings indicating a cerebral infarction. We initiated warfarin administration and transferred him to a local hospital for rehabilitation. Moderate AR was detected during transthoracic echocardiogram (TTE), and he was diagnosed as having traumatic AR. He was transferred to our hospital 6 months after the road traffic accident.
TTE	We noted prolapse due to a tear in the right coronary cusp (RCC) and AR of moderate to severe grade. The left ventricular ejection fraction (LVEF) was 67%, the left ventricular end-diastolic diameter (LVEDd) was 59 mm, and B-type natriuretic peptide (BNP) measured 120 pg/mL. RCC prolapse was similarly observed during transesophageal echocardiography (TEE).

H. Okabayashi (✉)
Department of Cardiovascular Surgery,
Mitsubishi Kyoto Hospital, Kyoto, Japan
e-mail: okabayashihitoshi@gmail.com

T. Kunihara, S. Takanashi (eds.), *Aortic Valve Preservation*,
https://doi.org/10.1007/978-981-13-2068-2_37

Cardiac catheterization	The pressure in the ascending aorta was 109/43 (76) mmHg, LV pressure was 112/13 mmHg, pulmonary artery pressure was 18/6/12 mmHg, the LVEF was 62%, and the LV end-diastolic volume index (LVEDVI) and end-systolic volume index (LVESVI) measurements were 205 and 77 mL/m^2, respectively.
Thoracic computed tomography (CT) scan	Suspected RCC tear. The aortic annulus diameter was 27 mm.

37.2 Examination and Diagnosis

The diagnosis of traumatic AR is achieved by noting (1) a history of blunt chest trauma, (2) no history of cardiac disease, (3) the sudden appearance of AR symptoms, and (4), severe AR during aortography or echocardiography [4].

37.3 Timing of Surgery

When road traffic accidents occur, patients commonly suffer multiple traumatic injuries other than AR, and even when it is diagnosed, it is usually challenging to choose the appropriate timing of surgery. Reports indicate that echocardiographic findings are useful when choosing the timing of surgery, and early surgery is required if the patient has an LVEDd >55 mm, LV fractional shortening <0.3, an LVEF <50% and/or pulmonary hypertension [9].

37.4 Key Point

In terms of surgical treatment for traumatic AR, there have been reports of attempts to perform aortic valvuloplasty initially. However, increasing numbers of reports indicate that these patients require reoperation due to persistent regurgitation and recurrence, so AV replacement is considered the valid choice. Recently, reports on aortic valvuloplasty have also been published, but at present, the decision to perform valvuloplasty or valve replacement is made based on the severity of the leaflet injury [10]. Valvuloplasty may be performed using an autologous pericardial patch in the event of leaflet perforation, whereas disruption of the annulus can be repaired by re-suturing, and commissural prolapse can be managed by performing refixation. We have also reported a case in which we successfully performed aortic valvuloplasty to treat AR caused by a traumatic AV injury [11].

37.5 Surgery

Through a median sternotomy, the ascending aorta was cannulated, a single drain was placed in the right atrium, and cardiopulmonary bypass was initiated. We cross-clamped the ascending aorta and then made a transverse aortotomy. Cardioplegic solution was selectively infused to achieve cardiac arrest. When we examined the AV, we noted a 14 × 12-mm perforation at the center of the RCC (Fig. 37.1). The autologous pericardium was first treated with glutaraldehyde and then sutured to the leaflet to perform a patch valvuloplasty (Fig. 37.2). In addition, CV-7 was used to suspend the free margin of the RCC. After we confirmed with TEE that the AR had disappeared, we weaned the patient from extracorporeal circulation. The patient was discharged uneventfully. Mild AR was present postoperatively.

Patient 2	A 54-year-old man who fell from a tree sustained multiple fractures and was admitted to a local hospital. A pelvic fracture, right humeral fracture, and pulmonary contusions were noted and were complicated by left peroneal nerve paralysis. He received treatment from the Department of Orthopedics and developed cardiac failure 1 month after the accident.
TTE	An RCC tear and severe AR were observed. The LVEF was 60%, LVDd/s were 68/46 mm, respectively, and the aortic annulus diameter was 24 mm.
Cardiac catheterization	The ascending aortic pressure was 135/55 (88) mmHg, the LV pressure was 135/8 mmHg, and the pulmonary artery pressure was 20/2/7 mmHg. The LVEF was 64%, and the LVEDVI and LVESVI were 140 and 50 mL/m^2, respectively. Grade IV AR was also observed.

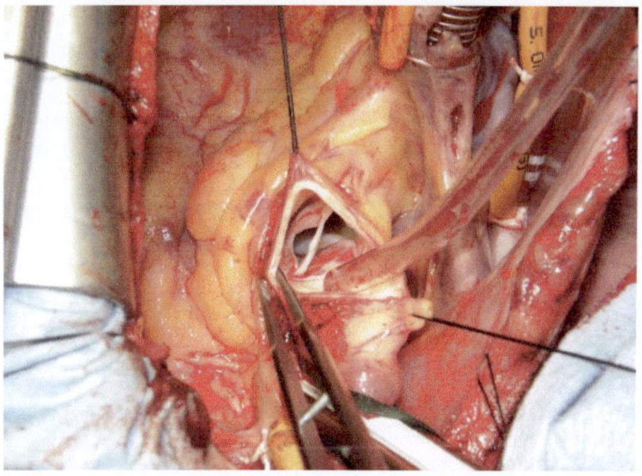

Fig. 37.1 Intraoperative findings of patient 1: A perforation of the RCC was observed, but the commissure was intact

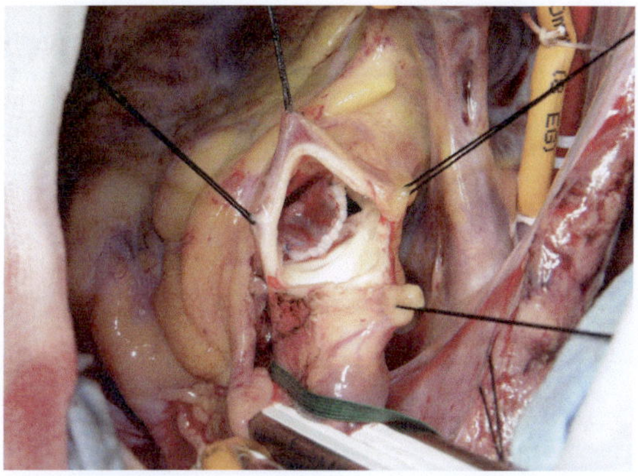

Fig. 37.2 Intraoperative findings of patient 1: The perforated area of the RCC was closed using glutaraldehyde-treated autologous pericardium and 8-0 polypropylene sutures

37.6 Surgery

Through a median sternotomy, the ascending aorta was cannulated, a single drain was placed in the right atrium, and extracorporeal circulation was initiated. We cross-clamped the ascending aorta and then made a transverse aortotomy. Cardioplegic solution was selectively infused to achieve cardiac arrest. When we examined the AV, we noted that the half of the RCC that was closest to the NCC had torn away from the commissure, although the portion closest to the LCC was still intact (Fig. 37.3). We trimmed a glutaraldehyde-treated autologous pericardial patch to a size of 45 × 22 mm. We first

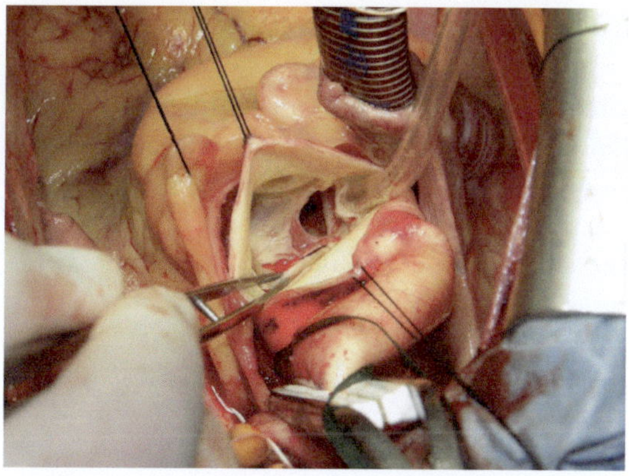

Fig. 37.3 Intraoperative findings of patient 2: There was disruption of the commissure between the RCC and NCC and prolapse of one-half of the RCC

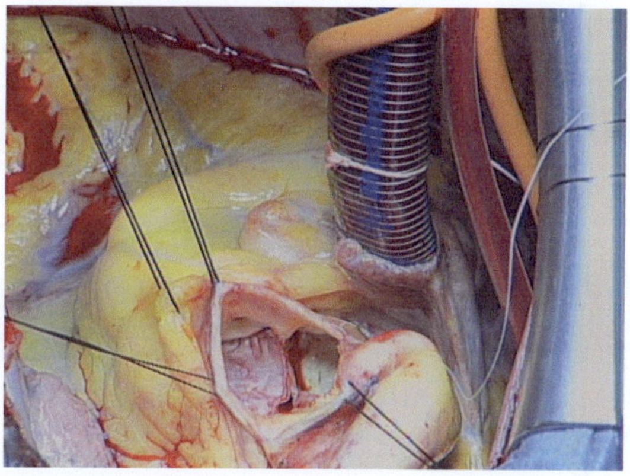

Fig. 37.4 Operative procedure of patient 2: The glutaraldehyde-treated autologous pericardium was sutured to the RCC using 6-0 polypropylene sutures. We performed a commissuroplasty using autologous pericardium-pledgeted 5-0 polypropylene sutures

passed a 5-0 polypropylene suture through the two commissures and the center of the annulus and then performed a patch valvuloplasty using 6-0 polypropylene sutures to fix the autologous pericardium to the RCC. Additional commissuroplasty was performed using pericardium-pledgeted 5-0 polypropylene sutures at the two commissures (Fig. 37.4). There was slight prolapse of the NCC, so CV-7 was passed through the free margin of the NCC to perform additional suspension. The patient was easily weaned off extracorporeal circulation. TEE showed trivial AR, and TTE after 6 months also showed mild AR.

37.7 Conclusion

The timing of surgery for traumatic AR should be decided after taking the echocardiographic findings into consideration. However, in most cases, the surgery is delayed after careful observation of the injury. Aortic valvuloplasty is possible if the injury is confined to the cusps.

References

1. Prfere R, Chilcott M. Blunt trauma to the heart and great vessels. N Engl J Med. 1997;336:626–32.
2. Traumatic valvular injury. CARPENTIER'S reconstructive valve surgery –from valve analysis to valve reconstruction. Philadelphia: Sunders Elsevier; 2010. p. 311–4.
3. Esmaeilzadeh M, Alimi H, Maleki M, Hosseini S. Aortic valve injury following blunt chest trauma. Res Cardiovasc Med. 2014;3:e17319.
4. Egoh Y, Okoshi T, Anbe J, Akasaka T. Surgical treatment of traumatic rupture of the normal aortic valve. Eur J Cardiothorac Surg. 1997;11:1180–2.
5. Kan CD, Yang YJ. Traumatic aortic and mitral valve injury following blunt chest injury with a variable clinical course. Heart. 2005;91:568–70.
6. Vocke D, Moarof I, Matt P, Anabitarte P. Aortic valve rupture due to a motorcycle accident. Cardiovasc Med. 2011;14:192–4.
7. Obadia JF, Tatou E, David M. Aortic valve regurgitation caused by blunt chest injury. Br Heart J. 1995;74:545–7.
8. Matteucci ML, Rescigno G, Altamura G, Manfrin M, D'Alfonso A, Piccoli G, et al. Delayed traumatic aortic cusp detachment mimicking aortic dissection. Ann Thorac Surg. 2006;82:1093–5.
9. Camarasa P, Berkane N, Joly L, Theissen MA, Carles M, Samat-Long C, et al. Safe and delayed repair in acute aortic traumatic insufficiency based on echocardiographic criteria. J Trauma. 2004;57:385–8.
10. Girardi L, Isom OW. Repair of traumatic aortic valve disruption and descending aortic transection. Ann Thorac Surg. 2000;69:1251–3.
11. Kin H, Minatoya K, Mukaida M, Okabayashi H. Successful valve repair in traumatic aortic valve regurgitation. Interact Cardiovasc Thorac Surg. 2011;12:869–71.

How to Manage Aortic Regurgitation from an Allograft

38

Hideaki Kado

38.1 Introduction

The benefits of Ross operation include the elimination of postoperative anticoagulant therapy, and the favorable postoperative valve function. The procedure has widely been performed as autologous pulmonary valve (PV) transplantation to treat aortic valve (AV) disease predominantly in young patients. Example of good indications for the procedure include women who wish to fall pregnant or athletes who want to avoid anticoagulants, young patients for whom a suitable prosthetic valve size cannot be found, and patients with infective endocarditis.

Meanwhile, drawbacks include the complex surgical technique associated with elevated risk of early postoperative complications, late pulmonary autograft failure (AGF), and the durability of the substitute PV [1]. There are still ongoing debates regarding the selection of surgical techniques to treat root dilatation or regurgitation of the transplanted autologous PV.

Patient	15-year-old boy, body weight: 50 kg, suffering from AR as a complication after the Ross-Konno procedure
Medical history	Three months after birth, the patient underwent single-stage curative surgery to treat a coarctation of the aorta (CoA) and a ventricular septal defect (VSD) (complicated by 22q11.2 deficiency syndrome). At the age of 7 years, the patient underwent the Ross-Konno procedure to treat aortic stenosis (AS) due to bicuspid valve and an expanded polytetrafluoroethylene (ePTFE) composite vascular graft (Yamagishi valve) with an 18-mm valve was used to repair the right ventricular outflow tract (RVOT). AR gradually progressed postoperatively, and we observed advanced stenosis affecting the ePTFE valved-conduit and tricuspid regurgitation (TR).
Preoperative examinations	Preoperative transesophageal echocardiography showed a left ventricular end-diastolic diameter (LVDd) of 59 mm, a left ventricular ejection fraction (LVEF) of 74%, and enhanced intensity at the center of the leaflets with moderate central regurgitation (Fig. 38.1). There was no obvious leaflet prolapse. Preoperative catheter angiography and computed tomography (CT) images showed an ascending aortic diameter of 34 mm, a sinus of Valsalva (SV) diameter of 40 mm, and a left ventricular outflow tract (LVOT) diameter of 28 mm (Figs. 38.2 and 38.3). The maximum RVOT pressure gradient was 100 mmHg, and there was moderate tricuspid regurgitation.

H. Kado (✉)
Department of Cardiovascular Surgery,
Cardiovascular Centre, Fukuoka Children's Hospital,
Fukuoka, Japan
e-mail: kadohideaki@gmail.com

T. Kunihara, S. Takanashi (eds.), *Aortic Valve Preservation*,
https://doi.org/10.1007/978-981-13-2068-2_38

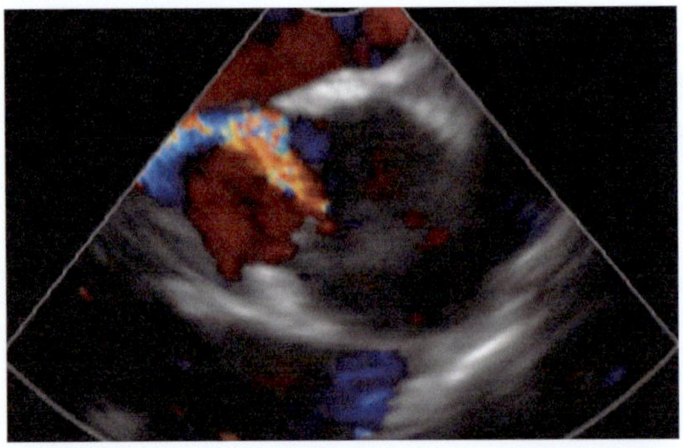

Fig. 38.1 Preoperative transesophageal echocardiogram. Moderate regurgitation from the center of the leaflets and dilatation of the SV were observed

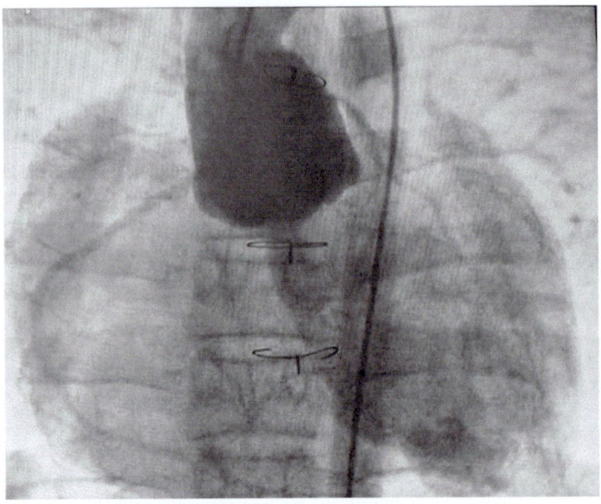

Fig. 38.2 Preoperative aortogram. Ascending aortic diameter: 34 mm, SV diameter: 40 mm, LVOT: 28 mm

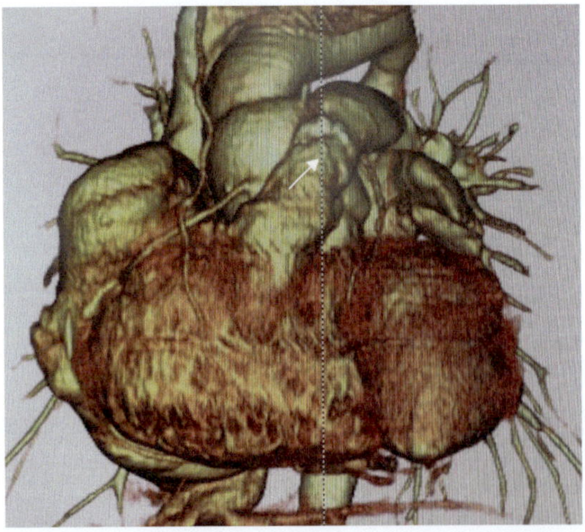

Fig. 38.3 Preoperative 3D CT image. Stenotic ePTFE composite 18 mm-valved-conduit at RVOT (white arrow)

38.2 Surgical Plan

Either aortic valvuloplasty or valve-sparing root replacement (VSRR) was the first choice of treatment for AR, and the plan was to avoid aortic valve replacement (AVR) to the greatest possible extent. We also intended to increase the size of the composite ePTFE graft used to reconstruct the RVOT and simultaneously perform tricuspid valvuloplasty.

38.3 Surgery

We cross-clamped the aorta, then transected the anastomosis distal to the autologous PV. The valve morphology was that of a balanced tricuspid valve, and we noted relatively severe hypertrophy and shortening at the center of the leaflets at the non-coronary cusp (NCC) and left coronary cusp (LCC) position (Fig. 38.4). A water test confirmed markedly unfavorable leaflet coaptation due to the hypertrophy and shortening at the center of the leaflets. We determined that it would be difficult to perform a VSRR, and believed that leaflet supplementation or extension were indicated. Use of autologous pericardium was impossible, as there was a high degree of tissue atrophy and hypertrophy, so instead, we decided to use a 0.1-mm thick ePTFE membrane. The free margin length was 30 mm for all three leaflets. We did not resect the leaflets but attach a 10 × 42 mm ePTFE strip to the three leaflet free margins using continuous 6-0 polypropylene sutures (Fig. 38.5). The new commissures were created by sewing the tips of two ePTFE strips to the aortic wall superior to the commissures, and each suture was reinforced and secured at the aortic wall externally (Fig. 38.6). The strip height was set at 8 mm at the center of the leaflets and 6 mm at the commissures, and favorable coaptation of the three leaflets was confirmed. After removing the aortic cross-clamp, we performed an RVOT reconstruction using a 22-mm composite ePTFE velved-conduit and tricuspid valvuloplasty. Postoperative transesophageal echocardiography showed a flow velosity of 1.2 m/s across the AV and trivial AR through the posterior commissure

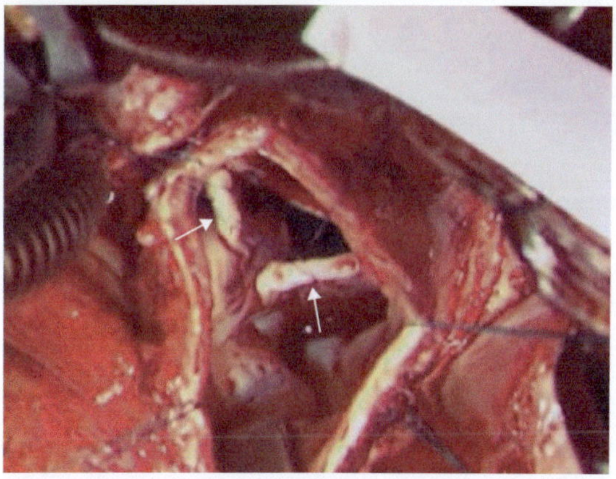

Fig. 38.4 Intraoperative findings for the transplanted autologous PV. Hypertrophy and shortening (white arrow) observed at the center of the leaflets at the NCC and LCC position

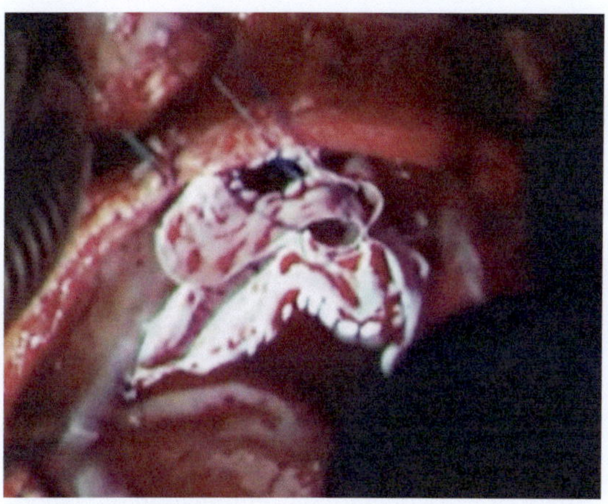

Fig. 38.5 Leaflet extension using an ePTFE membrane (0.1 mm)

(Fig. 38.7). The postoperative course was uneventful. Transthoracic echocardiography 1 year after surgery showed an aortic flow velosity of 1.3 m/s and mild AR through the posterior commissure.

38.4 Key Points

AGF is observed in the early postoperative period after Ross operation in 2–5% of patients, and may be caused by technical error or infection. Freedom from AGF due to late root disease is 70–86% at 10 years and 56–78% at 15 years

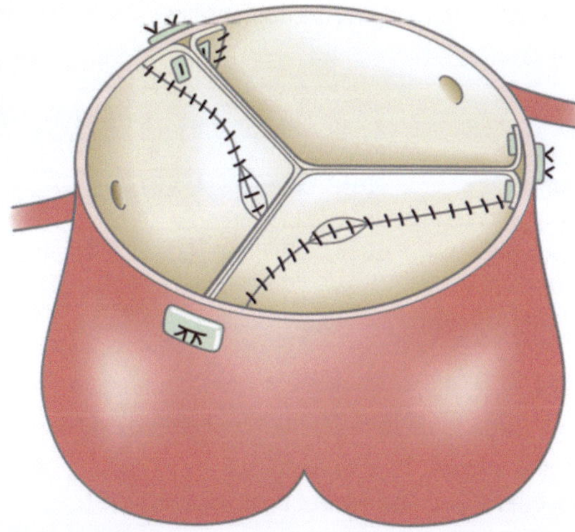

Fig. 38.6 Schema for leaflet extension

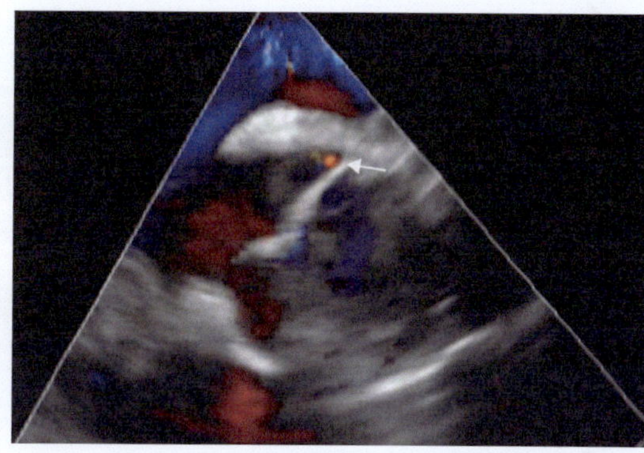

Fig. 38.7 Postoperative transesophageal echocardiogram. The transvalvular flow velocity at aortic position was 1.2 m/s, and trivial AR was observed through the posterior commissure

postoperatively, so the incidence of AGF increases over time. Risk factors include complicating AR prior to Ross operation, a bicuspid AV, and the surgical technique used to perform Ross operation [1, 2]. The incidence of AGF is low in patients who undergo additional reinforcement of the root using strips during Ross operation or who undergo subcoronary method rather than root replacement [3].

The aortic root dilates over time and patients with an SV diameter of ≥40 mm at 10 years postoperatively increases over 40. This tendency is particularly marked in pediatric patients. In addition, when AGF occurs after Ross operation, 25–50% of patients have normal or almost nor-

Table 38.1 Recently reported surgical cases of AGF treatment

First authors	Year	Number of reoperations	Valve-sparing: Root replacement	Valve-sparing: Valvuloplasty	Non-valve-sparing: Valve replacement/root replacement
Elkins [1]	2008	38	0	11	27
Stulak [2]	2010	42	0	0	42
De Kerchove [4]	2010	28	12 (Yacoub: 1, David: 11)	14	2
Luciani [5]	2012	27	11 (Yacoub: 10, David: 1)	6	10
Liebrich [6]	2014	46	18	3	25
Nelson [7]	2015	46	16	1	29

mal aortic leaflets. Valve lesions include prolapse at the center of the leaflets, hypertrophy and degeneration, and leaflet perforation [4, 5].

The indications for reoperation to treat AGF are the same as the standard surgical criteria to treat aortic root dilatation or AR. Most reports state that surgery is indicated when the SV diameter is ≥45–50 mm irrespective of the presence of AR, or when severe AR is accompanied by the symptoms related to left ventricular (LV) dilatation or dysfunction.

The surgical technique for reoperation is usually conventional, simple prosthetic valve replacement or root replacement, although the number of reports of valvuloplasty and VSRR have increased in recent years (Table 38.1) [4–7]. Reports have mentioned valve plication, leaflet plication, leaflet suspension, and leaflet supplementation as valvuloplasty techniques. Opinions are divided regarding the selection of the remodeling or reimplantation procedure when performing VSRR [4, 5].

In the present case, the authors found that it was impossible to use autologous pericardium, so instead we used a 0.1-mm thick ePTFE membrane as a supplementary material.

Generally, the supplementary material widely used during leaflet extension or supplementation surgery is autologous pericardium treated with glutaraldehyde. However, Nosál et al. [8] used the same 0.1-mm ePTFE membrane as a supplementary material for leaflet extension in 13 patients, and reported favorable results after a mean follow-up period of 14.8 months (maximum: 30 months). In addition, 0.1-mm ePTFE membrane is reported to yield favorable long-term outcomes when used to supplement the low-pressure pulmonary substitute valve, and we believe it may even be a useful supplementary material when performing surgery on the aortic leaflets. However, there are no reported cases of long-term use for AV repair, and insufficient strength is indicated, so strict follow-up is required going forward.

38.5 Conclusion

We believe that the selection of the surgical technique to treat AGF is affected not only by the patient age and severity of the root lesions, but also by the background, i.e. which surgical technique was used to perform the initial Ross operation, as well as how the patient or surgeon feels about the reoperation. In addition, it should also be kept in mind that late RVOT reoperation after Ross operation is unavoidable throughout their lives. A major benefit of Ross operation is elimination of postoperative anticoagulant therapy by using the autologous pulmonary valve to replace the aortic valve. Aortic valvuloplasty or VSRR would primarily be chosen as the redo procedure to respect this benefit of previous Ross operation. However, anatomically, the autologous PV is different from the AV, and we do not know whether this valve is durable over the long-term when VSRR is performed. Accordingly, prosthetic valve replacement or root replacement using a composite graft should be performed to achieve accurate repair of aortic root lesions and avoid multiple reoperations, although concerns with regard to bileaflet prosthetic valve still remain.

Anyhow, there will always be issues when selecting a surgical technique for AGF and we believe discussions will need to continue going forward.

References

1. Elkins RC, Thompson DM, Lane MM, Elkins CC, Peyton MD. Ross operation: 16-year experience. J Thorac Cardiovasc Surg. 2008;136:623–30.
2. Stulak JM, Burkhart HM, Sundt TM 3rd, Connolly HM, Suri RM, Schaff HV, et al. Spectrum and outcome of reoperations after the Ross procedure. Circulation. 2010;122:1153–8.
3. David TE, David C, Woo A, Manlhiot C. The Ross procedure: outcomes at 20 years. J Thorac Cardiovasc Surg. 2014;147:85–93.
4. de Kerchove L, Boodhwani M, Etienne PY, Pasquet A, Poncelet A, Ovaert C, et al. Preservation of the pulmonary autograft after failure of the Ross procedure. Eur J Cardiothorac Surg. 2010;38:326–32.
5. Luciani GB, Lucchese G, De Rita F, Puppini G, Faggian G, Mazzuccoet A. Reparative surgery of the pulmonary autograft: experience with Ross reoperations. Eur J Cardiothorac Surg. 2012;41:1309–15.
6. Liebrich M, Weimar T, Tzanavaros I, Roser D, Doll KN, Hemmeret WB. The David procedure for salvage of a failing autograft after the Ross operation. Ann Thorac Surg. 2014;98:2046–52.
7. Nelson JS, Pasquali SK, Pratt CN, Yu S, Donohue JE, Loccoh E, et al. Ross procedure across the pediatric age spectrum. Ann Thorac Surg. 2015;99:2086–95.
8. Nosál M, Poruban R, Valentík P, Šagát M, Nagi AS, Kántorová A. Initial experience with polytetrafluoroethylene leaflet extensions for aortic valve repair. Eur J Cardiothorac Surg. 2012;41:1255–7.

Part IV

Aortic Valve Repair: Specialists in the World

39 Leaders in Valvuloplasty Around the World

Takashi Kunihara and Shuichiro Takanashi

39.1 Tirone E. David

Professor Tirone E. David (Fig. 39.1) is a giant star among cardiac surgeons, and it is no exaggeration to say that every surgeon knows his name. For a cardiac surgeon, I think there can be nothing more honorable than having one's own name represent the name of a surgical procedure. As everyone knows, the "David procedure", valve-sparing aortic root reconstruction, is a surgery in which the three Valsalva sinuses are excised and the crown-shaped aortic annulus is enclosed within a vascular graft, and it can be said that this represents Prof. David's aggressive approach to new cardiovascular surgery and his superior surgical technique that enables it. In the early stage of development, a straight graft without the Valsalva sinus was used (David-I) [1] with the cusp free margin length as its diameter. However, in the latest technique, it has been changed to use a larger graft creating a Valsalva sinus (David-V). Previously, the David procedure could only be performed by Prof. David, but I appreciate his great contribution to the standardization and popularization of this procedure by analyzing anatomical theory and proving excellent long-term results.

Prof. David was born in Brazil in 1944 and graduated from the Universidade Federal do Paraná in 1968. He received his cardiac surgery training in the United States as a surgical resident at Downstate Medical Center, State University of New York, then became a cardiac surgical resident at the Cleveland Clinic, and finally became a staff surgeon at Toronto General Hospital (TGH) in 1978. He was the head of Toronto Western Hospital from 1980 to 1989 and TGH from 1989 to 2011, and he still remains active as a cardiac surgeon at TGH today.

I was a clinical fellow at TGH for 2 years, from 1987 to 1989. My permission to train at TGH was granted by the former head, Professor Baird, but I had the honor to see Prof. David become the head of the department during my stay there. The other candidate was Prof. Rick D. Weisel. I remember that the decision was made not in the open council of a Japanese selection committee but in a very closed council.

Prof. David's success after transferring to TGH was remarkable, and the number of operations he performed also increased dramatically. However, I remember him being on TV and in a newspaper for a campaign entitled "Cardiac surgeon cannot sleep well thinking about waiting patients" because there was a long waiting period for surgery, and some of his patients had unfortunately

T. Kunihara (✉)
Department of Cardiac Surgery, The Jikei University School of Medicine, Tokyo, Japan
e-mail: kunihara@jikei.ac.jp

S. Takanashi
Cardiovascular Surgery, Sakakibara Heart Institute, Fuchu, Tokyo, Japan

T. Kunihara, S. Takanashi (eds.), *Aortic Valve Preservation*, https://doi.org/10.1007/978-981-13-2068-2_39

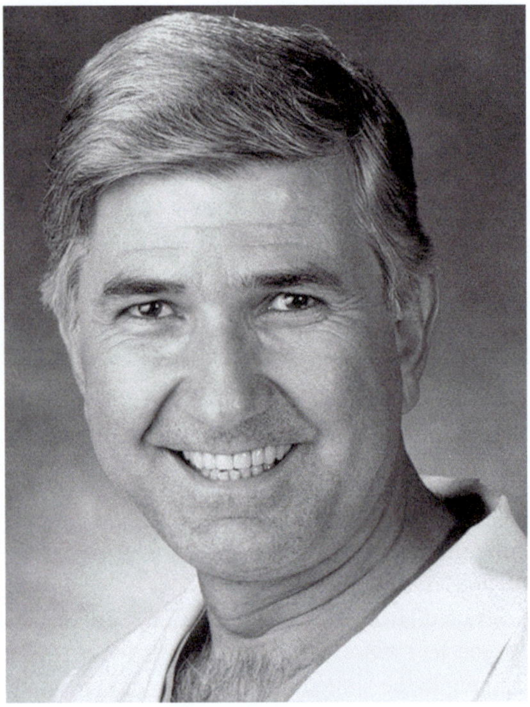

Fig. 39.1 Professor Tirone E. David

died while waiting for surgery. Prof. David lives in another world for me, but I always feel proud that I am one of his trainees. When I became a chief professor of Nagoya University, I immediately received a message from him: "Congratulations Aki. This is wonderful news. All the best in the future." He is always a mentor who supports and takes his followers into consideration.

In an interview with Prof. Cosgrove at the AATS meeting, I remember Prof. David mentioning that "A good surgeon must have an eagle's eye, lion's heart, a lady's hand and an elephant's bladder". This phrase, "A good surgeon must have an eagle's eye, lion's heart and a lady's hand" is a British proverb, and I feel Prof. David's humor when he added "an elephant's bladder" to this. Prof. David is blessed with the eagle's eyes and the lion's heart, but his right hand, which I have shaken, was big and was not a lady's hand. Moreover, I think that the elephant's bladder is unnecessary for Prof. David because he is an extremely superior surgeon. I'd like to start aiming to get an elephant's bladder.

(Akihiko Usui, Department of Cardiac Surgery, Nagoya University Graduate School of Medicine, Nagoya, Japan)

39.2 Magdi Habib Yacoub

I first met Professor Yacoub back in my resident era at Kobe General Hospital in 1985 (Fig. 39.2). The following year, I visited Harefield Hospital in the UK and witnessed a heart transplantation for the first time. During 1992–1994, I received direct training from him on heart transplantation and artificial hearts. Starting with heart, heart-lung, and lung transplantation including domino transplantation, I was greatly fascinated by his surgical technique full of creativity that I had never experienced before and his skill, which I did not have an opportunity to experience first-hand, in mitral valve repair on a beating heart, aortic valve/root replacement using a homograft, and various surgeries for congenital heart disease and arch repair with retrograde cerebral perfusion. Among the procedures that Professor Yacoub performed, the aortic root remodeling procedure was a boldly challenging technique that established preservation of the aortic valve, even in the era when mitral valve repair itself was also only sometimes performed. He made three slits in a prosthetic graft in both the position and the length as measured by estimation, and in the operation, a suture was placed from the center of the leaflet to the commissure. When coaptation of the aortic valves was not ideal, without hesitation, he placed a "central plication".

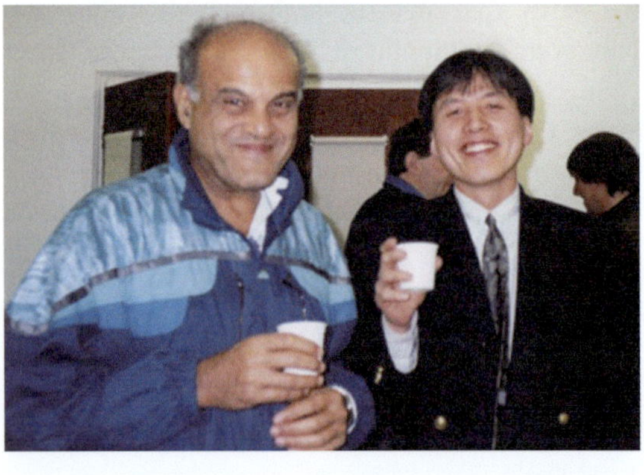

Fig. 39.2 March 13, 1994 One photo from the farewell party for the author. Professor Yacoub was 57 years old and I was 36 years old. Behind the author is Professor John Pepper who is now a consultant surgeon and Director of Clinical Research at the Royal Brompton and Harefield NHS Foundation Trust

Professor Yacoub was 79 years old when I met him again in 2014. The "Prof" was still vigorous and still operating in Egypt and working on research into biological valves. He is a truly the "world's best cardiac surgeon" for me, an example that can never be surpassed, due to his neverending desire to explore and study by reading Nature and The Lancet, his rare and superior surgical skills, and his attitude of continuing to work without sleep or breaks.

(Hitoshi Ogino: Cardiovascular Surgery, Tokyo Medical University, Tokyo, Japan)

39.3 Hans-Joachim Schäfers

Professor Hans-Joachim Schäfers (Fig. 39.3) was born in Lünen, Nordrhein-Westfalen, Germany in 1957 and graduated from Essen University in 1982. He received his surgical training mainly at Hannover Medical School and studied abroad as a respiratory surgery fellow at Toronto University (1987–1988). After obtaining board certification as a surgeon (1989), a vascular surgeon (1991), and a cardiothoracic surgeon (1991), he has served as chief professor of the Department of Thoracic and Cardiovascular Surgery at Saarland University Medical Center (Universitätsklinikum des Saarlandes: UKS) since 1995. He is also a visiting professor at Malaga University in Spain and Tel Aviv University in Israel. Now, he is the world's leading expert in aortic valvuloplasty and valve-sparing aortic root replacement using the aortic root remodeling procedure.

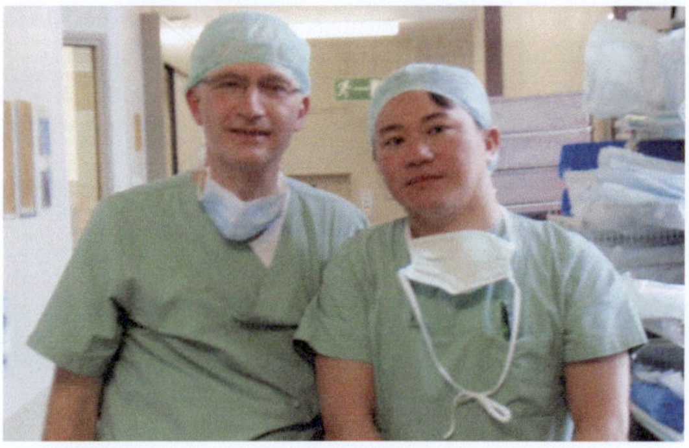

Fig. 39.3 Hans-Joachim Schäfers

In the area of aortic valvuloplasty, he proposed the concept of effective height (EH) in 2006, and in 2010 he introduced reference values by measuring the EH of healthy subjects. By measuring the dimensions of the aortic root, it can be said that he was revolutionary in inventing aortic valvuloplasty that is supported not only by subjectivity but also by mathematics. There are no readers who do not know Schäfers' caliper, which measures EH. He has already performed the remodeling procedure in over 700 patients, and he has extensive experience in the surgical treatment of ischemic mitral valve insufficiency with the "ring and string" technique and of chronic thromboembolic pulmonary hypertension.

Besides his daily clinical practice of adult cardiac surgery, he also performs pediatric cardiac surgery, respiratory surgery, peripheral vascular surgery, and various other surgical procedures. He is considered a pioneer of lung transplantation in Europe (receiving the 1993 Presidential Award of the International College of Chest Physicians), and at UKS, they still perform about 20 lung transplantations per year.

He has written more than 300 academic papers including those as a co-author and 5 textbooks, so his academic works are too numerous to mention, and he is also a reviewer and editor for many famous academic journals. He is very strict in conferences, during surgery, and rounds, and thus his staff are always concentrated on clinical practice. In his private life, he has a wife, four children, and a dog, and during vacations, he spends his time relaxing in Spain and Italy with his family as a good father.

(Mitsuru Asano: Department of Cardiovascular Surgery, Seirei Mikatahara Hospital, Hamamatsu, Japan)

39.4 Emmanuel Lansac

Dr. Emmanuel Lansac (Fig. 39.4) is a senior specialist in cardiac surgery at the Department of Cardiac Pathology of Institut Mutualiste Montsouris in Paris, France. His main area of interest is aortic valve repair surgery for dystrophic aortic roots (aneurysms and/or isolated aortic

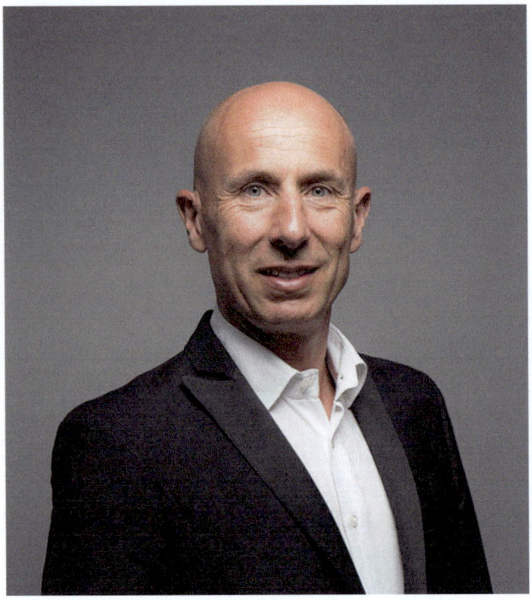

Fig. 39.4 Emmanuel Lansac

insufficiency). In 2000, he worked on research on the dynamics of the aortic root with Professors C. Duran and C. Acar at The International Heart Institute of Montana Foundation, Missoula, Montana, USA. Since then his research has focused on the development and evaluation of a physiological approach to aortic valve repair based on an expansible aortic ring annuloplasty device, a new medical device he patented in association with the Assistance Publique Hôpitaux de Paris. He is the main investigator of the French prospective multicentric CAVIAAR (Conservative Aortic Valve surgery for aortic Insufficiency and Aneurysm of the Aortic Root) trial comparing this aortic valve repair approach (130 patients) with the mechanical Bentall procedure (131 patients). He chairs the Aortic Valve Repair working group of Heart Valve Society, which aims to gather international physicians and scientists involved in the development of aortic valve repair with the goal to combine forces and share experiences to advance knowledge in this field. An international prospective multicenter registry of aortic valve repair, AVIATOR (Aortic Valve insufficiency and ascending aorta aneurysm InternATiOnal Registry), has been settled, as it will play a key role in clarifying and standardizing the place of repair in aortic valve surgery (http://shvd.org/Working-Groups/AV-repair/). Dr. Lansac is involved in teaching aortic valve repair during EACTS courses and symposia, such as the one he organizes yearly in Paris: Aortic Valve Repair: a step by step approach (www.caviaar.com). He is married and has a son. Both in his work and life, he continues to be deeply interested in social politics.

(Isabella Di Centa: Institut Mutualiste Montsouris, Paris)

39.5 Gebrine El Khoury

Professor Gebrine El Khoury (Fig. 39.5) is the head of the Cardiovascular and Thoracic Surgery Department of the Cliniques universitaires Saint-Luc and professor of the Cardiosurgery Department at the Université Catholique de Louvain in Brussels, Belgium. Born in Lebanon, he graduated from the Université Catholique de Louvain in 1984, where he did his surgical internship. Afterwards, he studied at Toronto General Hospital and in Paris under Professor A. Carpentier, and since 1996, he has been active as a professor of thoracic and cardiovascular surgery at his current institution. He has actively been working on aortic valve (AV) repair since 1996 and experienced 554 cases by 2011. After more than 15 years of experience, his patients

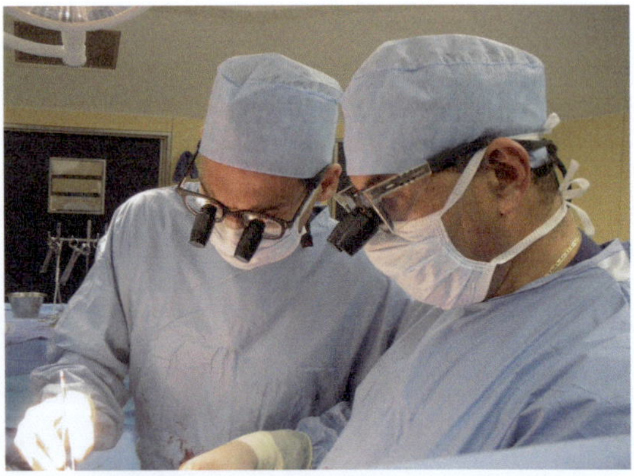

Fig. 39.5 Gebrine El Khoury

undergoing AV repair for the tricuspid valve have an average age of 58 years, and 66% have undergone aortic root repair for aortic lesions. His 10-year freedom from AV reoperation is 89%, and that from aortic regurgitation (AR) ≥ class II is 86%. His patients undergoing AV repair for a bicuspid valve have an average age of 44 years, and 65% have undergone aortic root repair for aortic lesions, with a 10-year survival rate of 94% and freedom from AV reoperation of 81%. Furthermore, with regard to long-term valve-related events, the rates of thromboembolism (<0.7%/patient-year), hemorrhage (<0.3%/patient-year), and infective endocarditis (<0.2%/patient-year) are quite low. In 2009, he classified the causes of AR into types 1 to 3, similar to Carpentier's classification for the mitral valve, and published a paper on establishing repair methods for each classification. In addition, he is working vigorously to make this technique reproducible by publishing articles on cusp repair (free margin plication, PTFE [polytetrafluoroethylene] resuspension, and patch repair) and releasing video presentations of actual surgeries, etc.

When I worked with Professor El Khoury from April to November 2011, AV repair was performed in 30 cases, of which about half were bicuspid valves. Normally, he performed the reimplantation method as the valve-sparing operation, but actually there were many complicated cases such as raphe shaving for type 3 calcification and tricuspidization of the bicuspid valve using a patch.

Professor El Khoury has a unique personality. He usually speaks French, has a great spirit of service, and shows us detailed videos of his surgeries with a Panasonic High-Vision camera. He has extensive experience with the Ross operation, and he once mentioned that he had already done some Ross operations before beginning to perform CABG surgery. At the Aortic Valve Repair Summit, which is held annually in Brussels every June 5 to 6, live surgery cases are presented over 2 days. This is a symposium definitely worth attending, and I would strongly recommend it.

(Hitoshi Minami: Department of Cardiovascular Surgery, Hyogo Prefectural Awaji Medical Center, Awaji, Japan)

39.6 D. Craig Miller

I had the privilege to be appointed as a Carl and Leah McConnell Cardiovascular Surgical Research Fellow for three-and-one-half years from March 1993.

Dr. Miller (Fig. 39.6), who is famous for proposing the Stanford classification for aortic dissection, has an established reputation in both thoracic aortic surgery and aortic root reconstruction and has welcomed patients from all over the United States of America. I would like to say that his technique is superb, although I actually never saw Dr. Miller operate, so this is merely my assumption. A fundamental aspect of his value is that he always makes the residents perform difficult and challenging operations successfully, and they later become experienced and active surgeons worldwide.

Dr. Miller worked with one of his personal pupils, Dr. Scott Mitchell, and a radiologist, Dr. Michael Dake, to implement thoracic endovascu-

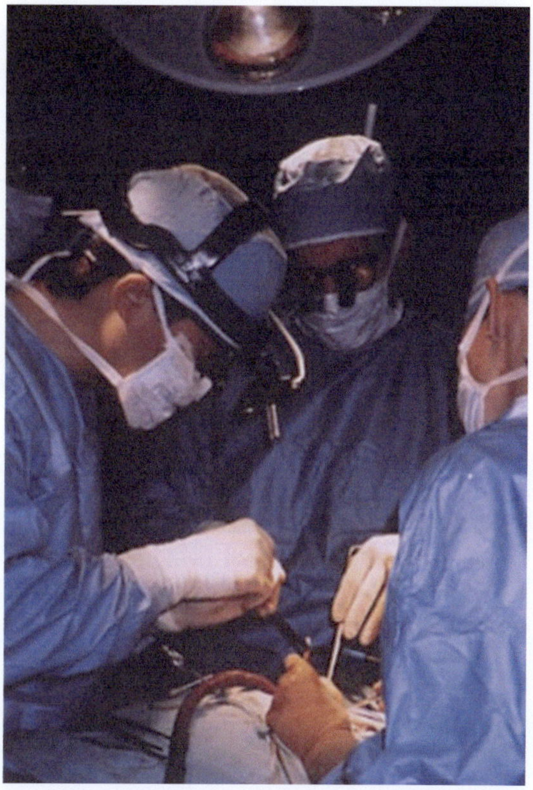

Fig. 39.6 D. Craig Miller

lar aortic repair (TEVAR), which led to the publication of this technique in The New England Journal of Medicine in the first half of the 1990s.

Dr. Miller is one of the American leaders in the field of cardiac physiology and mechanics and particularly in the analysis of torsional deformation of the left ventricle. Previously, studies in physiology that focused on cardiac mechanics were declining, National Institute of Health grants were hard to come by, and there were few suitable laboratories. I had no choice but to apply for my fellowship when I was developing the geometric research and surgical technique for ischemic mitral regurgitation. I developed animal models, published many papers, and thereafter, it was my personal honor to work on what had been the central topic at Dr. Miller's laboratory for a long time. Dr. Miller believes that it is always necessary for young academic surgeons to conduct laboratory investigations by themselves. His laboratory has produced a great number of professors who are active across the globe.

Dr. Miller is a leading academic surgeon, a surgical educator of the highest caliber, and a philosopher who is always lost deep in thought. It is my pleasure to introduce him to young readers.

(Masashi Komeda, Department of Cardiovascular Surgery, Jinsenkai Hospital and Iseikai Hospital, Osaka, Japan)

39.7 Hans-Hinrich Sievers

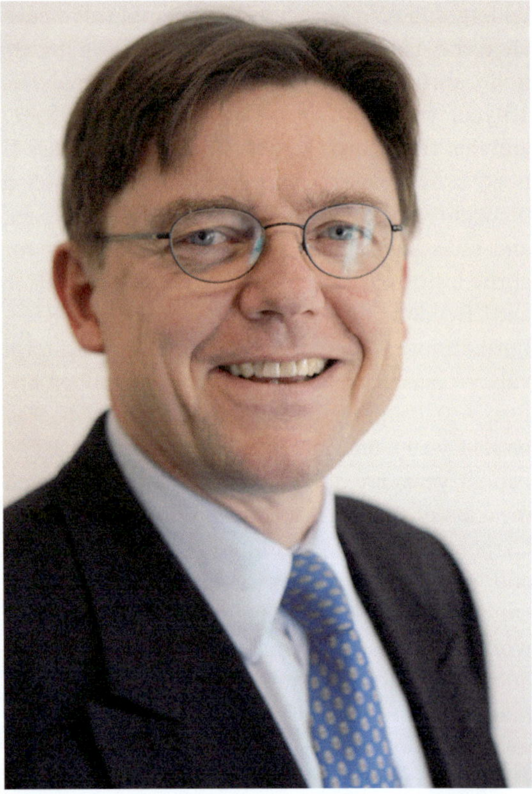

Fig. 39.7 Hans-Hinrich Sievers

Professor Hans-Hinrich Sievers (Fig. 39.7) is a senior specialist in cardiac surgery and head of the Department of Cardiac and Thoracic Vascular Surgery at the University Clinic Schleswig Holstein Campus in Lübeck, Germany, where since 1994, he has focused scientifically on the aortic valve and aortic root pathology, and the mechanism of aortic valve repair is of major interest. With respect to aortic root pathology and treatment, he has worked closely together with Professor Sir Magdi Yacoub and other pioneers in the surgical treatment of aortic root pathologies.

He has performed extended scientific workups with numerous publications to his name and has implemented of a classification system for the bicuspid aortic valve, the so-called "Sievers BAV Classification".

He chaired the development of a special sinus prosthesis for root reconstruction and an anuloplasty ring for stabilization of the aortic root. The ring can be implanted inside the aortic root to facilitate reconstruction.

He has also performed a tremendous amount of research on an autograft procedure, the Ross procedure, which he first performed in Germany in 1992 in collaboration with Dr. Donald Ross.

By founding the "Ross Registry", which contains more than 2000 patients with a follow-up of more than 18 years, Professor Sievers has had a major impact on standardization of the Ross procedure with very good long-term follow-up results.

He also chaired the aortic valve working group of the German Society of Cardiothoracic and Vascular Surgeons and is a member of various national and international cardiovascular societies.

He is married and has two sons. He is interested in nature-preserving strategies, hunting, and sculpture art.

(Thorsten Hanke, Asklepios Clinic Harburg, Hamburg, Germany)

39.8 Axel Haverich

Professor Axel Haverich (Fig. 39.8) graduated from Hannover Medical School (MHH) in 1978 and then received his surgical training from Professor Hans Borst. He studied abroad at Stanford University from mid 1983 till mid 1984. In 1993, he left for Kiel University to take up a post as the Director of the Division of Cardiac and Vascular Surgery. Professor Borst's idea was to appoint Professor Haverich as his successor at MHH, but due to internal university unwritten regulations, thus he applied for the post at Kiel University.

On May 1, 1996 Professor Haverich returned to MHH being appointed the Director of the Department Thoracic, Cardiac and Vascular Surgery. While he was still at Kiel University, he was awarded the Gottfried Wilhelm Leibniz Prize, the highest scientific award in Germany.

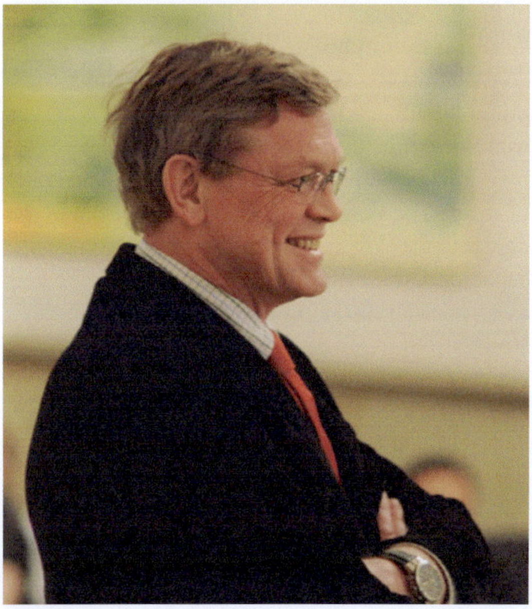

Fig. 39.8 Axel Haverich

This money was used to establish the Leibniz Forschungslaboratoiren für Biotechnologie und künstliche Organe (Leibniz Research Laboratory for Biotechnology and artificial Organs: LEBAO). Research on decellularized valves at the LEBAO yielded favorable results. Decellularized aortic and pulmonary valves are already starting to be used in clinical practice, and favorable short- and medium-term outcomes have been reported.

This form of surgery is elaborate and impressive. The reimplantation procedure was rapidly adopted and by the year 2000, the greatest number of cases were being treated with this procedure around the world. It is without exaggeration to say that the excellent clinical research promoted the dissemination of valve-preserving surgery.

Professor Haverich is well educated and has a humble character. He is also known as being quite knowledgeable about Japan, and many doctors from Japan have studied abroad at MHH. His pupils are not limited to those in Germany, however; he has also been a mentor to several professors around the world, including Japan. He is also very knowledgeable about wines and has struck up a close friendship with the Scorpions, a famous rock band from Hannover.

(Kenji Minatoya, Department of Cardiovascular Surgery, Graduate School of Medicine, Kyoto University, Kyoto, Japan; Hannelore Laue, Reg. Manager CORTISS c/o Prof. Dr. A. Haverich Klinik für HTTG-Chirurgie, Hannover, Germany).

39.9 Ruggero De Paulis

It is a great honor to introduce in this column Professor Ruggero De Paulis (Fig. 39.9), a dear friend whom I met while studying abroad. He is already known as the Italian surgeon who devised the Valsalva graft, but to the best of my knowledge, in terms of specialization, he is also an experienced cardiovascular surgeon who can perform off-pump coronary artery bypass surgery and mitral valvuloplasty.

I worked with him probably for 6 months during the 1990s. At that time, I was working as an

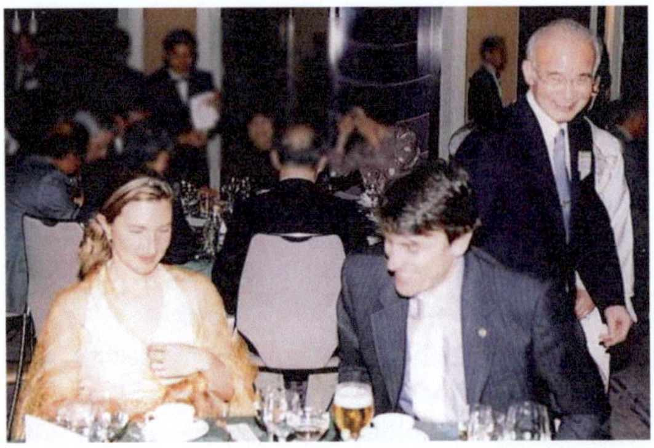

Fig. 39.9 Ruggero De Paulis

adult cardiovascular surgery resident while engaged in research related to prosthetic organ/heart transplantation at the Henri-Mondor Hospital and the Surgical Research Centre, both affiliated with the University of Paris. The head of the cardiovascular surgery department at the Henri-Mondor Hospital was the late Professor J. P. Cachera, and the head of the research laboratory was Professor D. Y. Loisance, who later became the head of the cardiovascular surgery department. Prof. Loisance is known as the first surgeon in the world to put the wearable Novacor left ventricular assist system to clinical use.

Prof. Ruggero came to the Henri-Mondor Hospital in the 1990s after being introduced by Dr. Phillippe Deleuze, who was working as a Chef de Clinique at the Henri-Mondor Hospital (a position equivalent to an assistant professor in Japan). Dr. Phillippe became friends with Prof. Ruggero when they worked on research together while Prof. Ruggero was studying abroad as a postdoctoral fellow in the field of artificial organs at the University of Utah in the USA (1986 to 1987) researching the Jarvik7 total artificial heart. Thereafter, Prof. Ruggero was asked by Professor G. C. Bloch, who was due to transfer from Henri-Mondor Hospital, to move with him to Lariboisière Hospital (also affiliated with the University of Paris) where he took up a position as a Chef de Clinique in France.

In 1992, he obtained a staff position at the University of Rome Tor Vergata and returned to Italy. Prof. Ruggero subsequently developed the Valsalva graft in the latter part of the 1990s. There is a famous anecdote involving his wife Stefania, who cut a vascular graft and sewed it back together to create prototype. What makes Prof. Ruggero amazing is that he was not only an inventor and exceptional surgeon but he also scientifically verified the benefits of the Valsalva graft from many perspectives. For example, he first studied rapid valve motion velocity in valve-sparing aortic root replacement, showed the significance of the sinus of Valsalva, and verified with finite element analysis that there was little tension placed on the coronary artery anastomosis to the Valsalva graft.

We came into contact again after he was employed as an associate professor at the University of Roma Tor Vergata in 2002. He was invited to the 33rd Annual Meeting of the Japanese Society for Cardiovascular Surgery in 2003, which was presided over by the late Emeritus Professor Keishu Yasuda at Hokkaido University. The photographs taken at the official society social gathering include a single shot of Stefania and Prof. Yasuda together. I remember impressively that Stefania was happily confirming the fact that her husband was a genius while we were dining together privately.

Prof. Ruggero's achievements were duly recognized, and in 2006, he was promoted to Director of the European Hospital in Rome and transferred there. He is currently an active EACTS (European Association for Cardio-Thoracic Surgery) committee member in the vascular domain. When he was speaking at EACTS in Milan in 2014, he mentioned that he might return to the University of Roma Tor Vergata (probably as the head of the department). We expect him to be active in this capacity in the future.

(Norihiko Shiiya, First Department of Surgery, Hamamatsu University School of Medicine, Hamamatsu, Japan)

39.10 Kohei Kawazoe

To describe Dr. Kohei Kawazoe (Fig. 39.10) in a few words, he is a "Samurai Valvuloplasty Surgeon". He was passionate about valvuloplasty more than 5 years before Dr. Carpentier pub-

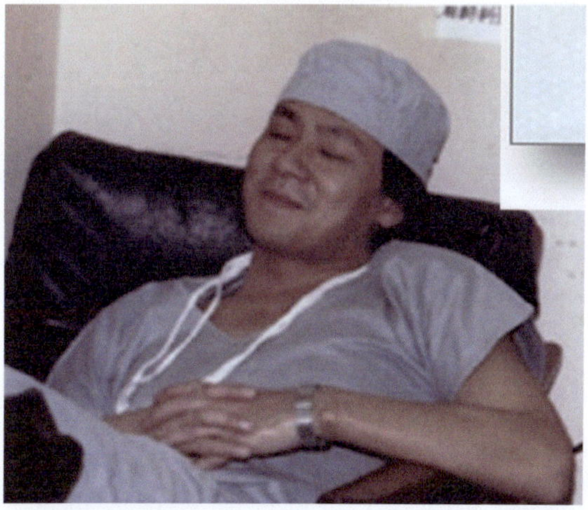

Fig. 39.10 Kohei Kawazoe

lished the "French Correction", which was considered the bible of valvuloplasty at the time. I cannot count all of the legendary stories regarding his valvular research, such as taking dogs with lead embedded in the annulus to the cath lab in the cardiology department to observe the movement of the mitral valve annulus. This photo shows him taking a nap 6 years after he graduated in 1977. From this time, he had an image of aortic valvuloplasty in his mind. At the age of 34, he was appointed as a valvular disease surgery specialist at the National Cardiovascular Centre. After that, he performed a number of valvuloplasties and became a professor at Iwate Medical University at the age of 46. At the Japan Cardiovascular Surgery Society in 2006, organized during the time that he assumed his role as professor at Iwate Medical University, he titled his presidential lecture "Valve disease is my lover". His passion for valvuloplasty was stronger than anyone's, and he fought a lonely battle back in the time when mitral valve replacement was the mainstream surgical method. The footprints he has left on valvuloplasty and the results he has obtained are remarkable. Many surgeons admire his attitude, and those he has inspired are now active professors nationwide. He had long been active in the TWO HUNDREDS CLUB of cardiac surgeons hosting live cardiovascular surgery seminars from 2002 to 2017 and continues to sponsor a valvular disease conference.

When participating in his golfing hobby, he can coax a sharp shot from his large body. However, he also has many cultural hobbies, such as reading books and appreciating images of the Buddha and he is very talented. In the future, he dreams of carving statues of the Buddha by himself, and when he returned to Osaka, I gave him a sculpting knife, but as he is still an active physician, it seems that he won't be using it for a long time to come.

(Kohei Abe, Cardiovascular Center, St. Luke's International Hospital, Tokyo, Japan)

39.11 Tsuyoshi Ito

A major achievement in aortic valvuloplasty developed by Dr. Tsuyoshi Ito (Fig. 39.11) was the introduction of intraoperative endoscopy, but there were several others. He proposed to divide aortic root morphology into two major categories and to modify the graft design according to this morphology, which improved valve-sparing root replacement with high originality. The aortic root morphology in patients who require valve-sparing surgery is not always pear-shaped as one would see in those with Marfan syndrome. Dr. Ito

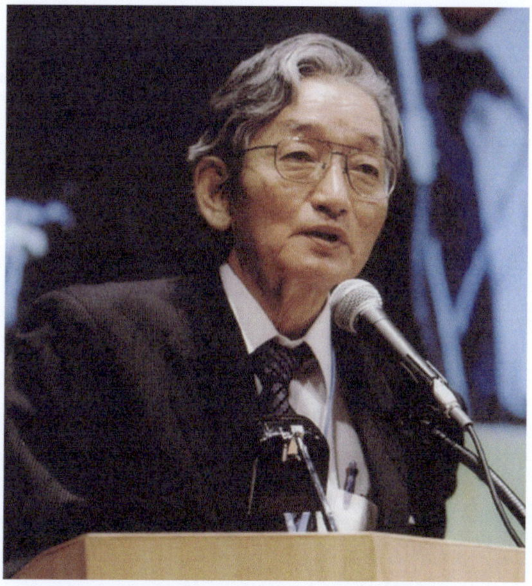

Fig. 39.11 Tsuyoshi Ito

defined the cases with the pear-shaped aortic root as "the root type" and those with more predominant dilatation of the ascending aorta than the aortic root as "the ascending type". He selected the vascular graft for the root type to be 4 mm larger in diameter than that for the ascending type, and customized the configuration of the three scallops depending on the height and length of the annulus. This restored the three-dimensional annulus structure without distortion. Dr. Ito prefers the remodeling procedure over the reimplantation procedure because he does not appreciate losing this morphology. Although his method seems to require a state-of-the-art surgical sense, it reproducibly results in elegant cusp coaptation.

I do not ever remember Dr. Ito raising his voice or becoming worked up during surgery. Instead, he always stayed cool when performing surgery and created a relaxing atmosphere for the surrounding staff by telling jokes. I remember him telling me that "this is because performing surgery is like conducting an orchestra". There was a large television in the doctor's lounge, and at night, the surgical staff surrounding Dr. Ito would enjoy Yomiuri Giants baseball games and follow the activities of overseas Japanese baseball players, although by the same token, we would also review the videos of that day's surgeries and discuss them with everyone. We also repeatedly watched a video of surgical procedures performed by Dr. Yacoub, which I obtained while visiting Harefield Hospital in England. Even today, when I face challenging cases, I always imagine how Dr. Ito would perform the surgery under pressure. I appreciate that I have such a strong mentor because I am always encouraged by him in this scenario.

(Satoshi Otsubo, Department of Cardiovascular Surgery, Tokyo Saiseikai Central Hospital, Tokyo, Japan)

39.12 Joseph Bavaria

Dr. Joseph Bavaria (Fig. 39.12), the immediate past president of the Society of Thoracic Surgeons (STS) [2], is an internationally renowned cardiovascular surgeon. He is currently the Brooke Roberts-William M. Measey Professor of Surgery and Vice-Chief, Division of Cardiovascular Surgery at the University of Pennsylvania (UPenn). Raised in Cincinnati, Ohio, Dr. Bavaria spent many of his adolescent years living abroad, moving across Europe with his family. He started high school at the American School in Paris, France, before returning to the United States to complete his high school education. Dr. Bavaria received a Bachelor of Science degree in Chemical Engineering from Tulane University in New Orleans, where he later earned his medical degree and participated in the Honors Chemical Engineering Exchange Program at the University of Edinburgh in Scotland. Obviously, that portion of his life spent abroad has helped him keep a global focus.

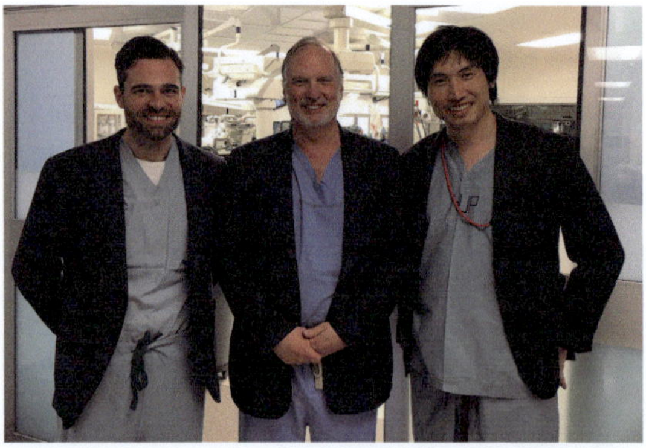

Fig. 39.12 Daniel Dohle, MD (left, aortic surgeon at the University of Mainz, Germany), Joseph Bavaria, MD (middle) and myself (right) in the operating room at UPenn

His primary clinical interests include thoracic aortic surgery and more broadly, cardio-aortic surgery. As the director of the Thoracic Aortic Surgery Program at UPenn, which is a leading institution with one of world's busiest aortic programs, he performs over 400 major cardiovascular procedures a year. The majority of these procedures are complex thoracic aortic surgeries and aortic valve repairs. Additionally, Dr. Bavaria recently hosted the 1st, 2nd and 3rd North American Aortic Valve Repair Symposiums. The deep-dive discussion with him prior to each aortic valve repair case is the best moment for his fellows to learn all about the key concepts of aortic valve repair. Dr. Bavaria routinely tries to expand the concepts used in the mitral valve repair arena to aortic valve pathology.

Of note, Dr. Bavaria takes immense pride in teaching trainees in the operating room. Despite the complexity of the procedures, he is always standing on the left-hand side of the table and letting his residents/fellows actually operate. To the best of my knowledge, Dr. Bavaria's ability to effectively control the operation, regardless of its complexity or the level of the operating trainee, and maintain excellent outcomes despite being on the left side of the table, is second to none in the world. In this great environment, his fellows become real cardio-aortic surgeons who are familiar with the "true" key concepts of aortic valve repair. Another notable thing I must relate about Dr. Bavaria is how enjoyable it is in the operating room. He always shows up wearing a nice blue jacket (Bavaria Jacket; photo). His first words are always "Is this my room? What do you got?" What I eventually realized over time was that he was testing me on how thoughtful and knowledgeable I was in every phase of the conduction of the operation. As he is extremely busy and often performs four major complex cases a day, it is not uncommon that we are operating until midnight. In such busy circumstances, he orders pizza for everyone working late in the operating room team (so-called "Pizza Night"). Sausage mushroom pizza is a MUST.

Finally, there are a number of words of wisdom from Dr. Bavaria that I would like to share.

Just do the right thing.

Stay with me!!

Sinus rhythm is the rhythm of success.

Go Go Go!!

Cardiac surgery is a contact sport.

Be a cerebral surgeon.

This is a Mainline Stitch!!

UUhhggg, another pizza night!

I am extremely proud to have spent a year with Dr. Bavaria as his thoracic aortic fellow and performed so many complex procedures including a number of David procedures and aortic valve repairs as the primary operator. I would not be in my current position as a cardio-aortic surgeon without his great support.

(Shinichi Fukuhara, M.D., Department of Cardiac Surgery, University of Michigan)

References

1. David TE, Feindel CM. An aortic valve-sparing operation for patients with aortic incompetence and aneurysm of the ascending aorta. J Thorac Cardiovasc Surg. 1992;103:617–21.
2. Bavaria JE, Fukuhara S, Desai ND. Thoracic aortic surgery enters the era of big data. Eur J Cardiothorac Surg. 2017;52:499–500.

Part V

Closing Remarks

40 Cardiologists' Expectations of Aortic Valvuloplasty

Hiroyuki Watanabe

40.1 Development of Aortic Valvuloplasty

In recent years, aortic stenosis and mitral regurgitation have stolen the limelight from other forms of valvular disease. However, treatment of aortic regurgitation (AR) has made solid advancements, of which the greatest have been the improved outcomes for aortic valvuloplasty, which has already become a practical option in a few institutions.

This increase in options has also influenced echocardiographic diagnosis. For example, the functional classification of leaflet motion as type I when normal, type II in the event of prolapse, and type III when restricted has been well received by internists [1]. This classification differs from the etiological classification that has traditionally been proposed by internists as it is based on structural and functional abnormalities. The introduction of valvuloplasty has begun to influence the diagnostic course of AR.

40.2 From Mechanical Valves to Bioprosthetic Valves

The standard treatment for AR is aortic valve replacement (AVR), and the two options for replacement are mechanical and bioprosthetic valves. These two options have become standard forms of treatment.

The benefit of mechanical valves is their long-term durability, and the structural valve deterioration (SVD) that affects bioprosthetic valves does not occur. However, these patients need to take warfarin lifelong. Warfarin is extremely efficacious in preventing thromboembolism, but it is accompanied by dietary, alcohol, and drug restrictions and necessitates anticoagulant monitoring. Hemorrhagic complications due to warfarin also present a major risk.

Mechanical valves such as the On-X valve are expected to reduce the required warfarin dose [2], although withdrawal of warfarin is not recommended.

The administration of direct oral anticoagulants (DOAC) has been studied for some time to resolve these disadvantages of warfarin. Eikelboom et al. focused on dabigatran, which has been shown to be a useful anticoagulant in atrial fibrillation patients, and attempted to confirm whether this drug was useful as an anticoagulant in patients with mechanical heart valves. However, the study was terminated after 252 patients were enrolled because the dabigatran

H. Watanabe (✉)
Department of Cardiology, Cardiac Center, Tokyo Bay Urayasu Ichiwaka Medical Center, Urayasu, Chiba, Japan
e-mail: hiroyukiw@jadecom.jp

T. Kunihara, S. Takanashi (eds.), *Aortic Valve Preservation*,
https://doi.org/10.1007/978-981-13-2068-2_40

group suffered more hemorrhagic complications, and thromboembolism was also more common than in those in the non-dabigatran group [3]. This shows that DOAC, which were expected to succeed warfarin as second-generation anticoagulants, appear to have no benefit in patients with prosthetic heart valves.

If anticoagulants are well-tolerated, then mechanical valves are the first-line treatment for young AR patients, although currently, there are a number of patients who cannot undergo anticoagulant treatment for various reasons. These include young women who wish to become pregnant, patients who do not have access to anticoagulant monitoring for social reasons or due to their location, and patients who are at risk of hemorrhage.

The number of cases that prioritize quality of life are increasing under these circumstances, with the result that bioprosthetic valves have been increasingly selected for AVR in recent years. A report from 2015 analyzed 76,000 patients with AVR and found that 53.3% had received a bioprosthetic valve. It should be noted that the rate of bioprosthetic valve use increased from 37.7% between 1998 and 2001 to 63.6% between 2007 and 2011. Furthermore, the greatest increase was observed in patients between the ages of 55 to 64 years [4]. Generally, bioprosthetic valves are considered to be treatment for elderly patients, although this report shows that major changes have occurred in the generations that are heading towards their elderly years.

40.3 Challenges with Bioprosthetic Valves

Bioprosthetic valves are gradually becoming the first choice for AVR, although the challenge of SVD is by no means resolved. According to a report by Chan et al., bioprosthetic valves that are implanted in young patients require reoperation at an earlier stage. Factors affecting the duration until reoperation are the age at the time of surgery and the type of bioprosthetic valve used. We also know that patients aged <40 years who are fitted with a stented aortic bioprosthetic valve require reoperation after a mean period of 7 years, whereas patients aged between 40 and 60 years require reoperation after a mean period of 13 years [5].

One factor that contributes to the deterioration of bioprosthetic valves is patient-prosthetic mismatch (PPM). PPM occurred in 12% of 387 patients who underwent AVR with a bioprosthetic valve. The freedom from reoperation in these patients at 10 years was 74.3%, although the reasons for reoperation were SVD in 96 patients, paravalvular leaks in 10 patients, and infective endocarditis in 5 patients. SVD frequently occurs in patients with PPM, and a multivariate analysis showed age at the time of surgery and PPM to be risk factors for SVD. This analysis also concluded that the reoperation rate was twice as high in patients with PPM than in those without PPM [6].

Johnston et al. also published the results of a prognostic survey of AVR in 12,569 patients using Carpentier-Edwards valves (PERIMOUNT; Edwards Lifesciences, Irvine, CA). Bioprosthetic valves were removed from 344 patients, with the causes being infective endocarditis in 41% and SVD in 44%. When we examined all subjects, we found actuarial estimates of explant for SVD of 1.9% and 15% at 10 and 20 years, respectively. However, these explant rates were 5.6% and 46% at 10 and 20 years, respectively, in patients aged <60 years. Factors related to SVD are younger age, the intake of lipid-lowering drugs, PPM, and a higher transvalvular pressure gradient. The effect of postoperative transvalvular pressure gradient on explantation for SVD was most pronounced in patients aged <60 years. We also noted that bioprosthetic valves exhibit much better durability in young patients than expected, although the intention to minimize the postoperative transvalvular pressure gradient by means of annular enlargement or use of valves with better effective orifice area should be encouraged [7].

There is also a study that compared the postoperative mortality and valve-related complications for biological and mechanical valves in patients aged <65 years. During a follow-up period of 18 years, the respective freedom from reoperation was 95% and 55% for mechanical and biological valves, whereas that from hemorrhagic complications was 78% and 98%. Significant differences were noted in both cases. These results also showed that there were no significant differences between two types of prosthetic valves in terms of mortality rates during long-term follow up [8].

There also remain challenges regarding postoperative anticoagulant therapy for prosthetic valves. The guidelines recommend 3 months of warfarin administration after valve replacement using a bioprosthetic valve. However, a study by Mérie et al. reported that withdrawal of warfarin within 6 months postoperatively is related to an increase in cardiovascular deaths [9]. Meanwhile, another report followed up patients without administering warfarin from 5 days after AVR using a bioprosthetic valve if the patients had no atrial fibrillation, if no other valves had been treated, if there was no history of cerebral hemorrhage, no mitral valve stenosis, and no history of warfarin use. The results indicated that the risk of thromboembolic events within 90 postoperative days was low at 2.2%, and no myocardial or cerebral infarctions occurred [10].

40.4 Expectations of Aortic Valvuloplasty

When performing surgical treatment for AR, at present, biological valves are selected for elderly patients and mechanical valves for young patients. Expectations for biological valves have been in increasing regardless of generation by overcoming the disadvantage of SVD. Higher expectations have been placed on valvuloplasty as the newest option for treatment because it is believed to have potential as a new form of treatment for valvular disease that does not require anticoagulant therapy but offers high durability.

The challenges of aortic valvuloplasty from the perspective of internists include the fact that it is difficult to determine for which patients the procedure is indicated. Factors influencing patient selection are the surgical technique, the surgeon, the institution, and the success rates. Compared to valve replacement, valvuloplasty appears to depend on a greater degree of surgical skill. Specifically, when compared to valve replacement, which will function only if the prosthetic valve is accurately seated in the aortic annulus, valvuloplasty requires the normalization of valve mobility, coaptation area, and the morphology of the sinuses of Valsalva to be effective.

For this form of surgery to be popularized, we believe that patient indications need to be established by standardizing the surgical techniques, and this includes a discussion about optimal timing.

40.5 Conclusion

The surgical treatment of AR to date has involved the selection of mechanical valves for young patients and bioprosthetic valves for older patients. However, in recent years, the number of young patients who request bioprosthetic valves that overcome the risks of mechanical valves has increased. The risks related to warfarin and valve deterioration are significant for patients. Going forward, we will need to determine forms of surgical treatment that decrease patient risk, regardless of age, and high expectations have been placed on aortic valvuloplasty. We believe that the first step in this process will be the standardization of surgical techniques.

References

1. Boodhwani M, de Kerchove L, Glineur D, Poncelet A, Rubay J, Astarci P, et al. Repair-oriented classification of aortic insufficiency: impact on surgical techniques and clinical outcomes. J Thorac Cardiovasc Surg. 2009;137:286–94.
2. Puskas J, Gerdisch M, Nichols D, Quinn R, Anderson C, Rhenman B, et al., PROACT Investigators. Reduced anticoagulation after mechanical aortic valve replacement: interim results from the prospective randomized on-X valve anticoagulation clinical trial randomized Food and Drug Administration investigational device exemption trial. J Thorac Cardiovasc Surg. 2014;147:1202–10.
3. Eikelboom JW, Connolly SJ, Brueckmann M, Granger CB, Kappetein AP, Mack MJ, et al., RE-ALIGN Investigators. Dabigatran versus warfarin in patients with mechanical heart valves. N Engl J Med. 2013;369:1206–14.

4. Isaacs AJ, Shuhaiber J, Salemi A, Isom OW, Sedrakyan A. National trends in utilization and in-hospital outcomes of mechanical versus bioprosthetic aortic valve replacements. J Thorac Cardiovasc Surg. 2015;149:1262–9.e3.
5. Chan V, Malas T, Lapierre H, Boodhwani M, Lam BK, Rubens FD, et al. Reoperation of left heart valve bioprostheses according to age at implantation. Circulation. 2011;124:S75–80.
6. Urso S, Calderón P, Sadaba R, Mahillo I, Tuñón J, Aldamiz G, et al. Patient-prosthesis mismatch in patients undergoing bioprosthetic aortic valve implantation increases risk of reoperation for structural valve deterioration. J Card Surg. 2014;29:439–44.
7. Johnston DR, Soltesz EG, Vakil N, Rajeswaran J, Roselli EE, Sabik JF 3rd, et al. Long-term durability of bioprosthetic aortic valves: implications from 12,569 implants. Ann Thorac Surg. 2015;99:1239–47.
8. McClure RS, McGurk S, Cevasco M, Maloney A, Gosev I, Wiegerinck EM, et al. Late outcomes comparison of nonelderly patients with stented bioprosthetic and mechanical valves in the aortic position: a propensity-matched analysis. J Thorac Cardiovasc Surg. 2014;148:1931–9.
9. Mérie C, Køber L, Skov Olsen P, Andersson C, Gislason G, Skov Jensen J, et al. Association of warfarin therapy duration after bioprosthetic aortic valve replacement with risk of mortality, thromboembolic complications, and bleeding. JAMA. 2012;308:2118–25.
10. Berger PB, Vedamurthy D, Casale A, Sun H, Benoit C, Ferrari A, et al. The risk of thromboembolic complications without anticoagulation after surgical aortic valve replacement with a bioprosthesis. J Am Coll Cardiol. 2015;65:A2041. https://doi.org/10.1016/S0735-1097(15)62041-1.

Correction to: Aortic Valve Preservation

Takashi Kunihara and Shuichiro Takanashi

Correction to:
T. Kunihara, S. Takanashi (eds.), *Aortic Valve Preservation*, https://doi.org/10.1007/978-981-13-2068-2

This book was inadvertently published with the following line missing in the copyright page "The Work was first published in 2015 by Bunkodo Co., Ltd. with the following title: DAIDOUMYAKUBEN KEISEIJUTSU NO SUBETE." This line is included in this book version.

The updated online version of the front matter can be found at https://doi.org/10.1007/978-981-13-2068-2

T. Kunihara, S. Takanashi (eds.), *Aortic Valve Preservation*,
https://doi.org/10.1007/978-981-13-2068-2_41

MIX
Papier aus verantwortungsvollen Quellen
Paper from responsible sources
FSC® C105338

If you have any concerns about our products,
you can contact us on
ProductSafety@springernature.com

In case Publisher is established outside the EU,
the EU authorized representative is:
Springer Nature Customer Service Center GmbH
Europaplatz 3, 69115 Heidelberg, Germany

Printed by Libri Plureos GmbH
in Hamburg, Germany